D1251996

The Thoracic Spine and Rib Cage: Musculoskeletal Evaluation and Treatment

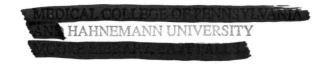
MEDICAL COLLEGE OF PENNSYLVANIA
AND HAHNEMANN UNIVERSITY

The Thoracic Spine and Rib Cage: Musculoskeletal Evaluation and Treatment

Timothy W. Flynn, P.T., M.S., O.C.S.

Instructor of Continuing Medical Education, College of Osteopathic Medicine, Michigan State University, East Lansing, Michigan; Doctoral Candidate, Center for Locomotion Studies, Pennsylvania State University, State College, Pennsylvania

Foreword by

Philip E. Greenman, D.O., F.A.A.O.

Professor of Osteopathic Manipulative Medicine and Professor of Physical Medicine and Rehabilitation, Michigan State University, East Lansing, Michigan

With 14 Contributing Authors

Butterworth–Heinemann

Boston   Oxford   Melbourne   Singapore   Toronto   Munich   New Delhi   Tokyo

Copyright © 1996 by Butterworth–Heinemann

 A member of the Reed Elsevier group

All rights reserved.

No part of this publication may be reproduced, stored in a retrieval system, or transmitted in any form or by any means, electronic, mechanical, photocopying, recording, or otherwise, without the prior written permission of the publisher.

Every effort has been made to ensure that the drug dosage schedules within this text are accurate and conform to standards accepted at time of publication. However, as treatment recommendations vary in the light of continuing research and clinical experience, the reader is advised to verify drug dosage schedules herein with information found on product information sheets. This is especially true in cases of new or infrequently used drugs.

Chapters 4, 5, 7, 9: The views or assertions contained herein are the private views of the individual author(s) and are not to be construed as official or as reflecting the views of the Department of the Army or the Department of Defense.

∞ Recognizing the importance of preserving what has been written, Butterworth–Heinemann prints its books on acid-free paper whenever possible.

WE
725
T4873
1996

Library of Congress Cataloging-in-Publication Data

The thoracic spine and rib cage : musculoskeletal evaluation and
treatment / Timothy W. Flynn ; forward by Philip E. Greenman ; with
14 contributing authors.
p. cm.
Includes bibliographical references and index.
ISBN 0-7506-9517-X (hardcover : alk. paper)
1. Thoracic vertebrae. 2. Chest pain. 3. Backbone. 4. Ribs.
5. Intercostal muscles. I. Flynn, Timothy W.
[DNLM: 1. Thoracic Vertebrae. 2. Ribs. 3. Diagnosis,
Differential. 4. Chest Pain. 5. Musculoskeletal System. 6. Back
Pain. WE 725 T4873 1996]
RD766.T47 1996
617.5'4--dc20
DNLM/DLC
for Library of Congress   95-45707
                                                                CIP

British Library Cataloguing-in-Publication Data
A catalogue record for this book is available from the British Library.

The publisher offers discounts on bulk orders of this book.
For information, please write:

Manager of Special Sales
Butterworth–Heinemann
313 Washington Street
Newton, MA 02158-1626

10 9 8 7 6 5 4 3 2 1

Printed in the United States of America

Contents

PART IV   CLINICAL PERSPECTIVES AND CONCERNS

Contributing Authors

Mark R. Bookhout, M.S., P.T.
Instructor of Continuing Medical Education, College of Osteopathic Medicine, Michigan State University, East Lansing, Michigan; President, Physical Therapy Orthopaedic Specialists, Inc., Minneapolis

Beate Carrière, P.T., C.I.F.K.
Clinical Specialist and Student Coordinator, Department of Physical Medicine, Kaiser Permanente Hospital, Los Angeles

James R. Cropper, M.S., P.T.
Physical Therapy Supervisor, Clinton Memorial Hospital, Wilmington, Ohio

Brian Demby, M.D.
Radiologist, Southwest Memorial Hospital, Cortez, Colorado

Jeffrey J. Ellis, P.T., M.T.C.
Clinical Professor of Orthopedic Physical Therapy, Advanced Masters Program, Touro College, Dix Hills, New York; Physical Therapist, Department of Physical and Rehabilitation Medicine, Brookhaven Memorial Hospital, Patchogue, New York

Timothy W. Flynn, P.T., M.S., O.C.S.
Instructor of Continuing Medical Education, College of Osteopathic Medicine, Michigan State University, East Lansing, Michigan; Doctoral Candidate, Center for Locomotion Studies, Pennsylvania State University, State College, Pennsylvania

Wolfgang G. Gilliar
Adjunct Instructor of Physical Medicine and Rehabilitation, College of Osteopathic Medicine, Michigan State University, East Lansing, Michigan; Private Practice, Physical Medicine and Rehabilitation, San Mateo, California

John S. Halle, Ph.D., M.P.T.
Deputy Director, Army Physical Fitness Research Institute, U.S. Army War College, Carlisle Barracks, Pennsylvania

Gregory S. Johnson, P.T.
Founder and Director, Institute of Physical Art; Founder and Therapist, Steamboat Spine and Sports, Steamboat Springs, Colorado

Wade A. Lillegard, M.D.
Center for Sports Medicine, Duluth Clinic, Duluth, Minnesota

Mary E. Reid, M.D.
Orthopedic Staff and Spine Service Chief, Department of Surgery, Brooke Army Medical Center, Fort Sam Houston, Texas

Edward G. Stiles, D.O.
Adjunct Professor of Bio-Mechanics, Michigan State University College of Osteopathic Medicine, East Lansing, Michigan

Thomas K. Szulc, M.D.
Chief, Pain Services, North Shore University Hospital, Plainview, New York

Mark A. Tomski, M.D.
Clinical Assistant Professor of Rehabilitation Medicine, University of Washington, Seattle

Frank B. Underwood, M.P.T., E.C.S., Ph.D.
Assistant Professor of Physical Therapy, U.S. Army–Baylor University; Electromyographer, Department of Neurology, Brooke Army Medical Center, Fort Sam Houston, Texas

Foreword

Chest pain presents a diagnostic and therapeutic challenge to the practitioner. About 40% of patients presenting to the emergency room with chest pain have musculoskeletal problems of the chest. The ability to assess the biomechanical function of the chest wall assists the practitioner in making a diagnosis and developing a treatment plan.

This book discusses the thoracic spine and rib cage: its anatomy and biomechanics, its neurophysiology, and appropriate imaging studies for patients with pain. Organic problems of the viscera housed within the thoracic spine and ribs and organic pathology of the rib cage itself are identified. The appropriate structural diagnostic procedures and manual medicine treatment procedures for dysfunctions of the thoracic cage are emphasized.

This book will help the practitioner in the sifting and sorting of the diagnostic process for thoracic spine and rib cage pain, develop an appropriate differential diagnosis, and outline a manipulative medicine and exercise program for the presentation.

Philip E. Greenman

Preface

The human spinal region has been explored extensively in a wide variety of medical texts. The majority of the texts emphasize the lumbosacral region and, to a lesser degree, the cervical spine region. In comparison, very little has been written about the thoracic spine and the rib or costal cage in which it articulates. The purpose of this book is to provide a reference that the health care practitioner can readily use when evaluating this region for injury or dysfunction and screening for organic pathology, in providing appropriate and effective treatment, and in preventing recurrence of problems through patient-directed exercise programs.

It is hoped that this book will provide an excellent resource for any health care practitioner who confronts pain or dysfunction in the thoracic spine and rib cage. The book has been divided into four sections: essential principles, examination and differential diagnostic procedures, treatment, and clinical perspectives and concerns. This format is designed to take the reader systematically through the steps necessary to manage patients presenting with mid-back and chest wall pain or dysfunction, or pathology originating there but referred distally to another body region.

The first section presents the essential principles of anatomy, biomechanics, and neurophysiology in a clear and focused manner that allows for rapid synthesis of the material within the framework of patient care. The chapters on examination and differential diagnostic procedures guide the practitioner through a thorough examination that rules out organic pathology and clearly defines musculoskeletal dysfunction. The treatment chapters provide detailed instruction in various manual medicine manipulative treatment options to treat pain and dysfunction including muscle energy, mobilization, high-velocity thrust, and myofascial techniques. A separate chapter provides detailed injection and alternate treatment approaches. All treatment is provided with the patient as the key element in achieving long-term success; to that end, a chapter on thoracic spine exercise programs is included. The final section provides clinical presentations and examples of the treatment approaches previously provided and establishes clear guidelines for the appropriate use of therapeutic interventions.

The contributors are a multidisciplinary group who have provided a readable reference in their areas of expertise. It is hoped that this book will fill a void in the present literature and be immediately helpful for both the novice and experienced musculoskeletal practitioner.

Timothy W. Flynn

Acknowledgments

This book would not have been possible without the help and support of a number of people. It has been a great privilege working with the contributing authors, whose time and talent resulted in a thorough, practical, user-friendly medical text on a region of the body that is frequently overlooked. I will always be particularly indebted to Philip E. Greenman for his mentoring and constant educational stimulation. In addition, I feel fortunate to have learned from and taught with the late John Bourdillon, M.D., whose hands and words still influence me.

I extend my appreciation to Barbara Murphy of Butterworth-Heinemann for her encouragement and support of an idea conceived on a napkin 3 years ago, and to Michelle St. Jean-Richards, who inherited the project mid-stream and helped prepare it for production.

To Victor Powell, medical illustrator, I express my thanks for the many illustrations and frequent laughs. Additionally, I thank Raul, Robert, and the entire medical photography staff for their assistance.

Finally, I thank my wife Sue both for taking the time to model for a number of photographs and for her constant support throughout this endeavor. Last, but not least, I thank David and Phillip for putting up with an occasionally distracted father who often disappeared to the computer.

PART I
Essential Principles

Chapter 1

Regional Anatomy and Biomechanics

James R. Cropper

The thoracic region of the spine is a transitional zone between the cervical and lumbar regions. In the thoracic region, the vertebrae become gradually larger and more dense with increasing superincumbent load from superior to inferior [1–3]. The thoracic region of the spine consists of 12 vertebrae that have a characteristic form and yet a similar function to the vertebrae of the other spinal regions. Each region provides a balance of stability and mobility suitable to the function of that region. The thoracic region is the second least mobile of the spinal regions (after the pelvic girdle). The presence of the rib cage and the low ratio of intervertebral disc height to vertebral body height (1 to 5) account for the reduced mobility [3].

Osteology

Typical Thoracic Vertebra

Each thoracic vertebra consists of the following structures: body, costal demifacets, pedicles, laminae, articular facets, transverse processes, and a spinous process (Fig. 1.1). The anteroposterior and transverse dimensions of the body are almost equal, and the waist is somewhat hollow anteriorly and laterally [1, 3, 4]. The height of the body is slightly higher posteriorly than anteriorly, which contributes to the gentle kyphosis of the thoracic spine [3, 5]. Each body contains two pairs of costal demifacets posterolaterally, one set superior and one inferior,

for articulation with the rib heads (except T10, T11, and T12, which only have one pair) [1].

The two pedicles protrude directly posterior and are not divergent as in the cervical spine. This is because the spinal cord is smaller in the thoracic spine [1]. Located posteriorly, the laminae are higher than they are wide and overlap their neighbors like tiles on a roof [1, 4]. The superior articular facets are slightly convex and are oriented 60 degrees from the horizontal plane and 20 degrees from the frontal plane [3, 6]. The inferior facets are slightly concave and face anteriorly, slightly inferiorly, and medially to match the superior facets of the inferior joint partner [4] (Fig. 1.2).

The transverse processes attach to the vertebra at the junction of the pedicle and lamina and project laterally and slightly posteriorly [4]. Their spread laterally diminishes from T1 to T12, where the T12 transverse processes resemble those of L1 [2]. The spinous processes attach posteriorly and centrally at the junction of the left and right laminae. They project posteriorly and inferiorly to varying degrees. Whereas the degree of inferior projection is variable within and among subjects, the "rule of threes" [3, 7, 8] (Table 1.1) is helpful during palpation by describing the relationship of a vertebra's spinous process to its transverse process.

The thoracolumbar spine is an area of transition between the kyphotic thoracic spine and the lordotic lumbar spine. Stagnara et al. [9] measured the sagittal plane reciprocal angulation and noted the transitional vertebrae occurred from T10 to L2. The most

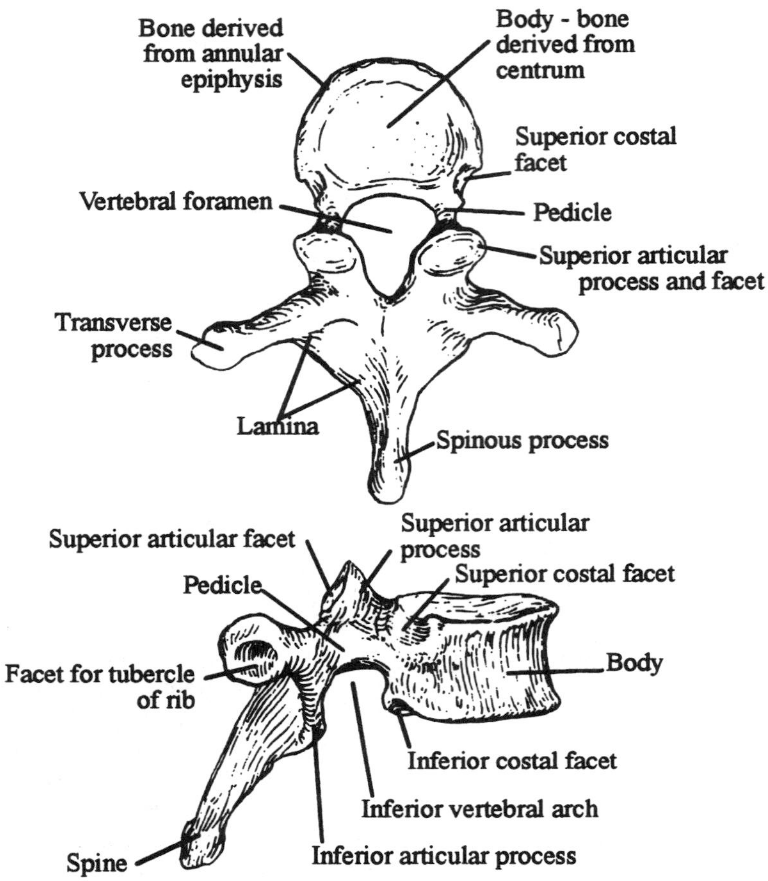

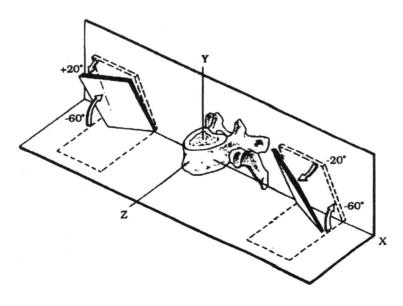

Bone derived
from annular
epiphysis

Body - bone
derived from
centrum

Superior costal
facet

Vertebral foramen

Pedicle

Superior articular
process and facet

Transverse
process

Lamina

Spinous process

Figure 1.1. A typical thoracic vertebra.

Superior articular facet

Superior articular
process

Superior costal facet

Pedicle

Facet for tubercle
of rib

Body

Inferior costal facet

Inferior vertebral arch

Spine

Inferior articular process

Figure 1.2. The superior articular facets are oriented 60 degrees from the horizontal plane and 20 degrees from the frontal plane. (Reprinted with permission from AA White, MM Panjabi. Clinical Biomechanics of the Spine. Philadelphia: Lippincott, 1990.)

Table 1.1. Rule of Threes

Vertebra	Spinous Process Level*
T1–T3	Same level
T4–T6	Half a level below
T7–T9	One whole level below
T10	One whole level below
T11	Half level below
T12	Same level

*Relative to the transverse process level.

frequent transitional segment was L1 (33%), followed by T12 (22%), and L2 (21%).

The Sternum

The sternum (Fig. 1.3) consists of three parts: a cranial portion called the manubrium, a body, and a caudal element called the xiphoid process [1]. It is slightly convex anteriorly and concave posteriorly. The manubrium is a triangle-shaped bone that is thick superiorly and thinner at its attachment with the body. The clavicles attach superolaterally at the clavicular notches. Laterally are the facets for attachment of the first ribs. The second ribs attach at the junction of the manubrium and the body. The suprasternal notch (or jugular notch) is on the superior surface of the manubrium. The body of the sternum is longer and flatter than the manubrium and is wider inferiorly than superiorly. The xiphoid process is the smallest and most variable component of the sternum. It is cartilaginous in youth and becomes partially ossified in adulthood.

The Ribs

The ribs are long, elastic, curved bones that form most of the thorax. They are made of highly vascular spongy bone encased in a thin layer of compact bone [1]. The medullary canal contains a large portion of red bone marrow. There are 12 pairs of ribs formed from the costal elements of each thoracic vertebra. All vertebrae have costal elements, but only

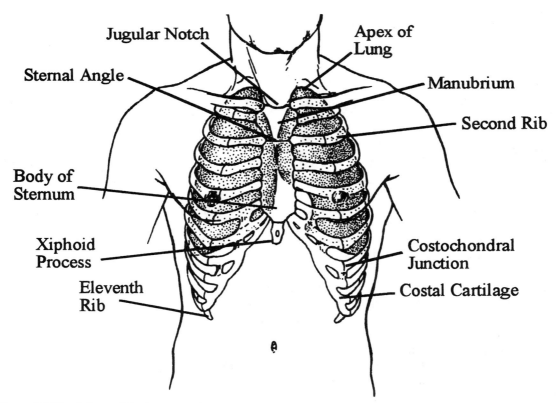

Figure 1.3. The skeleton of the thorax, anterior aspect.

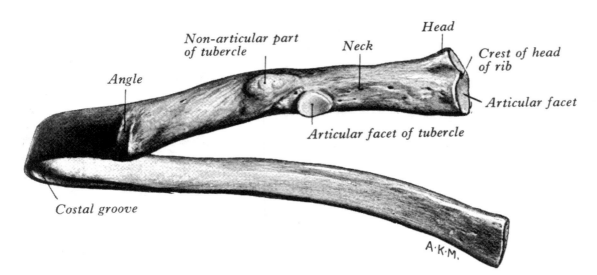

Figure 1.4. A typical rib. (Reprinted with permission from R Warwick, PL Williams. Gray's Anatomy [35th ed]. Edinburgh: Churchill Livingstone, 1973.)

in the thoracic spine do they normally find full expression. In the cervical spine, they become the anterolateral border of the transverse foramina. In the lumbar spine they become what we recognize as transverse processes (the lumbar accessory processes are the morphologically true transverse processes) [1].

The ribs are divided into two unrelated classifications: (1) true/false, and (2) typical/atypical [1, 3, 8]. Ribs 1 through 7 are true ribs, so named because their cartilage attaches directly to the sternum. The remainder are false ribs. The distal attachment of the false ribs is to the costochondral cartilage of their superior partner. Ribs 3 through 9 are typical ribs, whereas ribs 1, 2, 10, 11, and 12 are atypical. The typical ribs (ribs 3 through 9) share a common structure (Fig. 1.4). The head of the rib attaches to the costovertebral demifacets on the bodies of the vertebrae forming the costovertebral joints (Fig. 1.5). There are two articular facets on the head of each typical rib. The superior rib facet attaches to the costal semilunar demifacet of the vertebra above its level, whereas the inferior rib facet attaches to the costal semicircular demifacet of the numerically corresponding vertebra [1]. Between the facets on the head is a crest that attaches to the intervertebral disc and therefore has the potential for influencing disc mechanics and loads. Just distal to the head of a typical rib is the neck. The neck is a flattened portion of the rib that lies just an-

terior to the transverse process. Distal to the neck is a tubercle that has articular and nonarticular portions [1]. The articular (medial) surface of the tubercle attaches to the transverse process to form the costotransverse joint. The more lateral, nonarticular portion of the tubercle provides attachment for the lateral costotransverse ligament.

The next distal structure on a typical rib is the rib angle, which is located 5–6 cm from the tubercle and is a common palpation landmark. Distal to the rib angle, the shaft of the typical ribs begins its curved pathway [1]. The external surface of the shaft is smooth and convex and the internal surface is smooth with the costal groove for the intercostal nerve coursing along the lower border [1]. The superior surface of the shaft is rounded, whereas the inferior surface is sharp. The distal end of the typical rib is cup-shaped for attachment with the costochondral cartilage.

The atypical first rib (Fig. 1.6A) is small and flat and is the most curved of all of the ribs [1]. Its head is small and rounded, with only one joint surface for attachment to the superior circular costovertebral facet of T1. There are two shallow grooves on the superior surface of the rib separated by a small ridge. The posterior groove accommodates the subclavian artery and the lower trunk of the brachial plexus, whereas the anterior one is for the subclavian vein. The ridge between the two grooves pro-

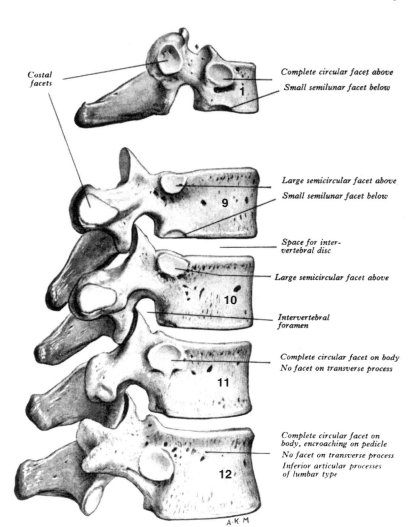

Costal
facets

Complete circular facet above

Small semilunar facet below

Large semicircular facet above

Small semilunar facet below

*Space for inter-
vertebral disc*

Large semicircular facet above

*Intervertebral
foramen*

Complete circular facet on body
No facet on transverse process

*Complete circular facet on
body, encroaching on pedicle*
No facet on transverse process
*Inferior articular processes
of lumbar type*

A·K·M

Figure 1.5. The first, ninth, tenth, eleventh, and twelfth thoracic vertebrae. Right lateral aspect. (Reprinted with permission from R Warwick, PL Williams. Gray's Anatomy [35th ed]. Edinburgh: Churchill Livingstone, 1973.)

vides attachment for the anterior scalene muscle. The undersurface of the first rib is smooth and contains no costal groove [1]. The first rib has no angle [8]. The inner curvature of the first rib largely defines the margin of the thoracic inlet. Its obliquity is accounted for by the presence of the apex of the lung in the base of the neck [1].

The atypical second rib (Fig. 1.6B) is longer and not as flat as the first rib, but the curve is similar [1, 3]. The demifacets of the head articulate with the costovertebral demifacets of T1 and T2. It is considered atypical because of its attachment to the junction of the manubrium and the body of the sternum [8]. Anatomists describe the second rib as either having no rib angle or a slight one [1, 8]. The costal

groove is primarily posterior on the undersurface of the rib and is poorly marked [1].

The atypical tenth rib would otherwise be typical except for its single costal facet attachment to T10 and none to T9. *Gray's Anatomy*, however, describes possible articulation with the T9–T10 intervertebral disc [1]. Attachment of the tenth rib to the T10 transverse process is variable [10]. The atypical eleventh and twelfth ribs are short and have no attachment directly or indirectly to the sternum. They have large heads with single facets attaching only to their corresponding vertebra. They have no neck or tubercle and do not attach to transverse processes. The eleventh rib has a small costal groove and a small angle, whereas the twelfth has neither [1]. Each has

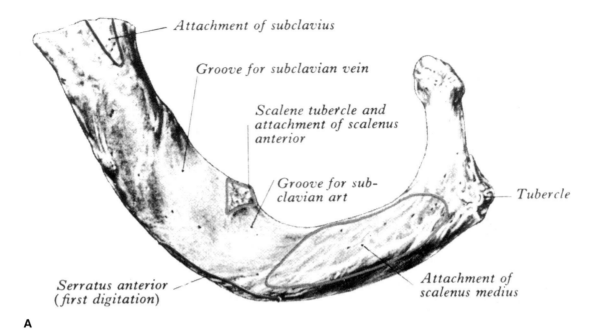

Attachment of subclavius

Groove for subclavian vein

Scalene tubercle and attachment of scalenus anterior

Groove for sub-clavian art

Tubercle

Serratus anterior (first digitation)

Attachment of scalenus medius

A

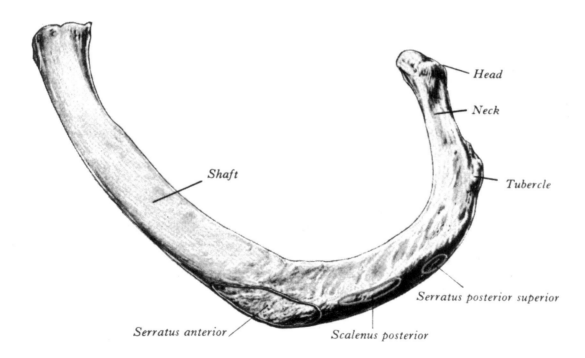

Head

Neck

Shaft

Tubercle

Serratus posterior superior

Serratus anterior

Scalenus posterior

B

Figure 1.6. A. The first rib. B. The second rib. (Reprinted with permission from R Warwick, PL Williams. Gray's Anatomy [35th ed]. Edinburgh: Churchill Livingstone, 1973.)

a cartilage cap on the distal end. Both ribs (rib 12 more than 11) are angled such that their inner surface faces upward and inward [1].

Arthrology

Intervertebral (Interbody) Joints

The mobility of the thoracic spine is relatively low compared with the other areas of the spine. This is partially attributable to the configuration of the intervertebral joints. The thoracic discs are thinner compared with the those in the lumbar spine. The ratio of disc height to vertebral body height is only 1 to 5 compared with 2 to 5 in the cervical spine and 1 to 3 in the lumbar spine [3]. However, some investigators report that the annulus fibrosus is stronger in this region than in other regions, which contributes to the ability of the thoracic spine to resist rotational stress [11]. The addition of the ribs further restricts mobility. The thoracic disc, as in other areas, is protected anteriorly and posteriorly by anterior and posterior longitudinal ligaments. In spite of all this protection, Wood et al. [12], presenting their study of thoracic magnetic resonance imaging (MRI) evaluation, report that only 32% of asymptomatic subjects (n = 90) had no anatomic disc abnormality. Furthermore, 24% had frank disc herniation, 42% had bulging discs, and 46% had annular tears. These findings refute the traditional notion that disc pathology in the thoracic spine is rare.

Facet Joint Structure

The facet joints (apophyseal joints) in the thoracic spine consist of conjoining superior and inferior articular processes of adjacent vertebrae. These processes are lined with hyaline cartilage. Facet joints are synovial and are therefore encased in a fibrous capsule lined with synovial tissue. The capsule, thin and loose, attaches just peripheral to the margins of the articular surfaces of the facets [1]. The joints are planar in structure [1]. The superior articular facets are slightly convex and are oriented 60 degrees from the horizontal plane and 20 degrees from the frontal plane [3, 6]. The inferior facets face anteriorly, slightly inferiorly, and medially to match the superior facets of the inferior joint partner [4].

The twelfth (sometimes the eleventh) thoracic vertebra is transitional in that the superior facets are oriented as typical thoracic facets, generally in the frontal plane, and the inferior facets are oriented as typical lumbar facets, generally in the sagittal plane.

Costovertebral Joint Structure

The costovertebral joints are formed by the joining of the heads of the ribs with the costal demifacets on the vertebral bodies of the thoracic vertebrae (Figs. 1.7 and 1.8). The joints are customarily classified as planar, although some are curved [1]. The costovertebral joints of the first, tenth (sometimes), eleventh, and twelfth ribs articulate with a single costal facet on their respective vertebral body [1, 12]. The remaining ribs attach to the costal facet of their correspondingly numbered vertebra, to the inferior costal demifacet of the vertebral body above, and to the intervertebral disc. The ligaments associated with the costovertebral joint are capsular, radiate, and intra-articular [1].

The capsule of each costovertebral joint attaches to each associated vertebra and intervertebral disc. The upper fibers pass into the intervertebral foramen to reach the back of the disc. The posterior fibers are continuous with the fibers of the costotransverse ligament.

The radiate ligaments (see Fig. 1.7) attach anteriorly to the bodies of the vertebra at rib level, to the one above, and to the intervening disc. The fibers fan out so that the superior fibers ascend to the level above, the inferior fibers descend to the corresponding vertebrae, and the middle fibers attach to the disc [1]. Even at the levels where the ribs attach with only one vertebra, the radiate ligaments ascend to the level above [1].

Only the costovertebral joints that articulate with two vertebrae have intra-articular ligaments. This ligament attaches from the crest on the rib head between the two demifacets to the intervertebral disc. It completely divides the joint [1] so that even though it is intra-articular, as with the cruciates in the knee, it is extrasynovial.

Costotransverse Joint Structure

The articular portion of the tubercle of ribs 1–10 articulates with the facet on the correspondingly numbered transverse process (see Fig. 1.8; see also Fig. 1.5). Ribs 11 and 12 have no costotransverse attach-

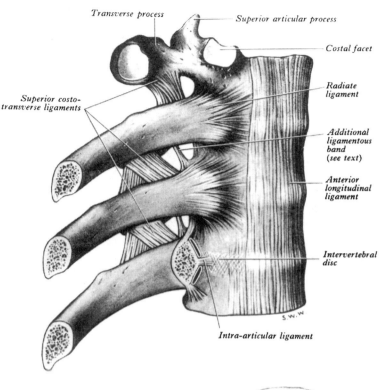

Transverse process

Superior articular process

Costal facet

Radiate ligament

Superior costo-transverse ligaments

Additional ligamentous band (*see text*)

Anterior longitudinal ligament

Intervertebral disc

S.W.W

Intra-articular ligament

Figure 1.7. The costovertebral joints, right anterolateral aspect. In the lowest joint shown, most of the radiate ligament and the anterior part of the head of the rib have been excised to show the two joint cavities and the intra-articular ligament between them. (Reprinted with permission from R Warwick, PL Williams. Gray's Anatomy [35th ed]. Edinburgh: Churchill Livingstone, 1973.)

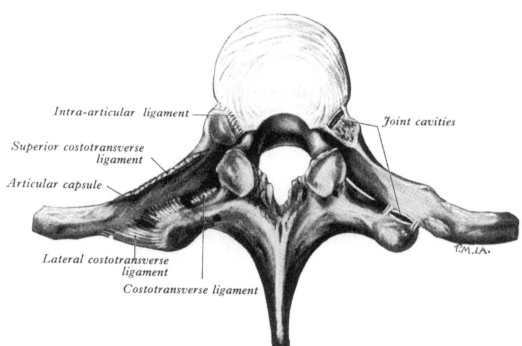

Intra-articular ligament

Joint cavities

Superior costotransverse ligament

Articular capsule

Lateral costotransverse ligament

Costotransverse ligament

T.M.IA.

Figure 1.8. The costovertebral joints, superior aspect. (Reprinted with permission from R Warwick, PL Williams. Gray's Anatomy [35th ed]. Edinburgh: Churchill Livingstone, 1973.)

ment. In the upper thoracic spine (T1–T5 or T6), the rib joint partner is convex and the transverse process partner is concave. The costotransverse joints in the lower thoracic spine are planar [1] (Fig. 1.9). The ligaments associated with the costotransverse joints are the costotransverse, the superior costotransverse, and the lateral costotransverse ligaments (see Figs. 1.7 and 1.8). The joints are synovial and therefore have a joint capsule.

The costotransverse ligament attaches the rib to the transverse process and occupies the costotransverse foramen; this area is the analog to the transverse foramen in the cervical spine. The ligament is rudimentary or missing from the eleventh and twelfth ribs [1].

The superior costotransverse ligament is divided into anterior and posterior layers [1]. The anterior layer runs from the crest of the neck of the rib up to the undersurface of the transverse process above. Laterally, the anterior layer is continuous with the internal intercostal membrane. It is crossed here by the intercostal vessels and nerve [1]. The posterior layer runs from the dorsal aspect of the associated rib and courses upward and medially to attach to the transverse process of the vertebra above. It is continuous laterally with the fibers of the external intercostal muscle.

Costochondral Junction

The costal cartilage is fitted into a depression in the distal end of each rib and secured by enveloping periosteum (which is continuous with the perichondrium) [1]. It can be a site of primary sprains or irritations (costochondritis), or secondary pain caused by rib cage dysfunction.

Costosternal Joint Structure

The costal cartilage of the first rib forms a synchondrosis with the manubrium [1]. The costal cartilage of the second rib joins with two demifacets at the junction of the manubrium and the body of the sternum, where there are two synovial joint cavities and an intra-articular ligament. The remaining true ribs attach into cavities in the sternum, forming synovial joints [1, 6]. These small joints are stabilized by broad, thin, radiate ligaments that blend with fibers from neighboring ribs and contralateral ribs. They also blend with insertional fibers from the pectoralis major muscle [1].

Ligaments

Anterior Longitudinal Ligament

The anterior longitudinal ligament (Fig. 1.10; see also Fig. 1.7) runs the length of the spine from the occipital bone to the sacrum. It is thicker and narrower in the thoracic region than in the cervical and lumbar regions. It is firmly attached to the intervertebral discs and the margins of the vertebral bodies anteriorly. It is also loosely attached to the middle of the vertebral body. This attachment is somewhat narrower than the attachment to the disc, but the fibers are thicker and fill the space between the body and the taut ligament.

Posterior Longitudinal Ligament

The posterior longitudinal ligament provides a smooth anterior wall for the vertebral canal. It is broad and nearly uniform in width in the cervical and upper thoracic regions but becomes more diamond-shaped in the lower thoracic and lumbar regions. It attaches to the intervertebral discs and the

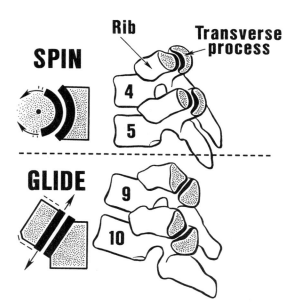

Figure 1.9. Configuration of the costotransverse joint surface.

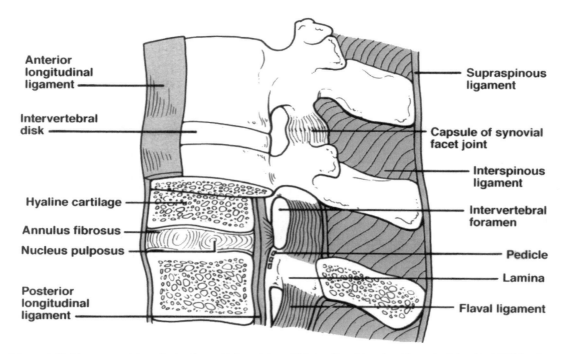

Figure 1.10. Ligaments of the spinal column. (Adapted from RW Bowling, P Rockar. Thoracic Spine. In JK Richardson, ZA Iglarsh [eds], Clinical Orthopaedic Physical Therapy. Philadelphia: Saunders, 1994;7–118.)

margins of the vertebral bodies. It does not attach to the middle of the vertebral bodies posteriorly to allow for emergence of the basivertebral veins.

Ligamentum Flavum

The ligamenta flava connect adjacent lamina in the interior of the spinal canal. They extend from the articular processes (where they blend with capsular fibers) to the central portion of the posterior arch, where the left and right ligaments blend leaving only a small opening for passage of small veins. Ligamentum flavum is composed of yellow, elastic fibers that tend to continually provide an elastic force that would keep each segment extended [1, 13].

Supraspinous and Interspinous Ligaments

The supraspinous ligament is a strong and fibrous connecting band between the apex of adjacent spinous processes. It is a continuation of the ligamentum nuchae and runs as far inferiorly as L4 (73%) (L3, 22%; L5, 5%) but not to the sacrum [13]. The fibers

unite with the fibers of the interspinous ligament. This ligament attaches between spinous processes from the root of the process inferiorly toward the apex of the superior process. It extends from the supraspinous ligament to the ligamentum flavum.

Intertransverse Ligaments

The intertransverse ligaments are rounded (in the thoracic spine) ligaments connecting adjacent transverse processes and are intimate with the fibers of the deep muscles of the back [1].

Myology

Often, as we evaluate patients with thoracic spine pain, we consider the large muscles of the spine and shoulder girdle as possible sources. We palpate for spasm and check for imbalance. We then palpate landmarks such as rib angles and transverse processes. At these times we may forget the many small muscles so intimately associated with the landmarks and so capable of producing signif-

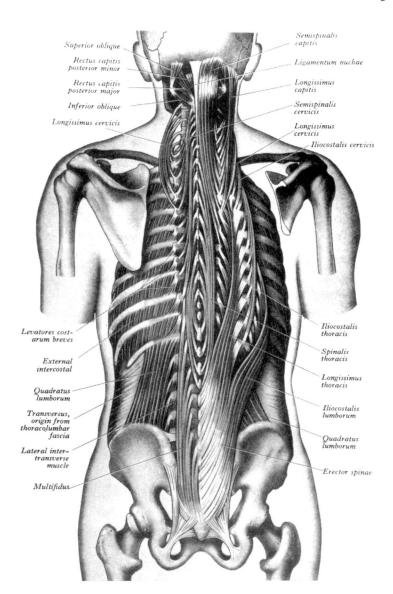

Superior oblique

Rectus capitis posterior minor

Rectus capitis posterior major

Inferior oblique

Longissimus cervicis

Semispinalis capitis

Ligamentum nuchae

Longissimus capitis

Semispinalis cervicis

Longissimus cervicis

Iliocostalis cervicis

Levatores cost-arum breves

External intercostal

Quadratus lumborum

Transversus, origin from thoracolumbar fascia

Lateral inter-transverse muscle

Multifidus

Iliocostalis thoracis

Spinalis thoracis

Longissimus thoracis

Iliocostalis lumborum

Quadratus lumborum

Erector spinae

Figure 1.11. Deep muscles of the spine. (Reprinted with permission from R Warwick, PL Williams. Gray's Anatomy [35th ed]. Edinburgh: Churchill Livingstone, 1973.)

icant pain. One must always remember, using the principles of layer palpation, to be mindful of all structures that can be palpated with a single press of the finger.

Iliocostalis Thoracis [1]

Constituting the thoracic portion of the iliocostalis muscle group (Fig. 1.11), the iliocostalis thoracis muscle starts from the upper borders of the angles of ribs 7–12 medial to the insertion of the iliocostalis lumborum. It ascends to the upper borders of the angles of ribs 1–6 and to the back of the transverse process of C7. It is innervated by the dorsal rami of the thoracic nerves. Its action is to extend the spine when working with its contralateral partner, and to bend the spine to the same side when working alone. Tissue texture changes and tenderness to palpation of this muscle at the rib angle is often pathognomonic for rib cage dysfunction, particularly the external rib torsion (see Chapter 8).

Longissimus Thoracis [1]

The longissimus thoracis muscle begins in the lumbar region (see Fig. 1.11) with fibers that are attached to the posterior surfaces of the transverse and accessory processes of the lumbar vertebra and to the middle layer of the thoracolumbar fascia. At this level it is blended with the iliocostalis lumborum. Its insertion is to the tips of the transverse processes of all thoracic vertebrae and to the lower nine or ten ribs medial to the angles. It is innervated by the dorsal rami of the thoracic nerves. Its action is to extend the spine when acting in unison and to bend the spine to the same side with unilateral contraction.

Spinalis Thoracis [1]

The inferior attachment of the spinalis thoracis (see Fig. 1.11) is by three or four tendons to the spines of T11, T12, L1, and L2. The tendons blend into a single muscle belly and then attach superiorly to the spinous processes of the upper thoracic vertebrae. The number of superior attachments varies from four to eight. It is innervated by the dorsal rami of the thoracic nerves. Its action is extension of the thoracic spine.

Semispinalis Thoracis [1]

The semispinalis thoracis, thin and fleshy, arises from the transverse processes of T6–T10 and attaches to the spinous processes of C6–T4. It is innervated by the dorsal rami of the thoracic spinal nerves. The semispinalis thoracis muscles act in unison by extending the thoracic spine and rotating to the opposite side with unilateral contraction.

Multifidus [1]

The multifidus is an extensive, fleshy muscle that fills the groove at the side of the spinous processes from the sacrum to C2 (see Fig. 1.11). In the thoracic spine, the multifidus arises from all of the transverse processes. The fasciculi ascend a variable number of vertebrae to attach to the entire length of a spinous process above. The more superficial fasciculi ascend three or four levels, whereas the deep-est fasciculi ascend to adjacent superior levels. The innervation in the thoracic area is from the dorsal rami of the thoracic spinal nerves. Its action is to extend the thoracic spine during bilateral contraction and to minimally rotate to the opposite side with unilateral contraction.

Rotatores Thoracis (Longus, Brevis) [1]

The rotatores muscles are most well developed in the thoracic spine (Fig. 1.12). They are the deepest of the transversospinalis muscles. They arise from the root of the transverse process and insert one or two levels (brevis or longus) above to the inferior and lateral surface of the lamina. They are innervated by the dorsal rami of the thoracic spinal nerves. As the name implies, the action of the rotatores is rotation of the appropriate segments, with extension being an accessory action.

Intertransversarii [1]

The intertransversarii are short muscles attaching between transverse processes in all regions but are well developed in the cervical spine. They exist in the thoracic spine only from T10–T11 to T12–L1. Whereas they consist of two slips in the cervical and lumbar regions, they have only one muscle belly in the thoracic region. They are innervated by the dorsal rami of the thoracic spinal nerves. Their function is bending the spine to the ipsilateral side. The multifidus, rotatores thoracis, and intertransversarii will often have tissue texture changes and tenderness to palpation in the presence of thoracic spine segmental dysfunction (see Chapter 8).

Levatores Costarum [1]

The levatores costarum muscles (see Fig. 1.11) arise from the ends of the transverse processes of C7 and all thoracic vertebrae except T12. The levatores costarum brevis muscles attach to the posterior and superior borders of the rib of the next lower level. At the four lower levels, the muscle divides into two fascicles, one of which (the levator costarum longus) descends to the second rib below. They are innervated by the lateral branches of the dorsal rami of the cor-

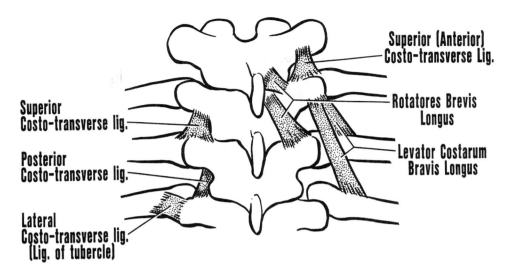

Superior (Anterior) Costo-transverse Lig.

Rotatores Brevis Longus

Levator Costarum Bravis Longus

Superior Costo-transverse lig.

Posterior Costo-transverse lig.

Lateral Costo-transverse lig. (Lig. of tubercle)

Figure 1.12. Short muscles of the thoracic spine.

responding thoracic spinal nerves. Their action is elevation of the ribs, but they may act as side benders and rotators of the thoracic segment when the rib is fixed (see Chapter 9).

Serratus Posterior Superior [1]

The serratus posterior superior muscle is thin and quadrilateral. Its origin is from the lower part of the ligamentum nuchae, from the spinous processes of C7–T2 (or T3), and from the supraspinous ligament. It attaches to the upper borders of ribs 2–5 a little lateral to their rib angles. Its action is rib elevation, but according to *Gray's Anatomy* [1], the context of the elevation is unclear. In other words, it does not seem to be a respiratory muscle. It is innervated by intercostal nerves 2–5.

Serratus Posterior Inferior [1]

The serratus posterior inferior is also thin and roughly quadrilateral (Fig. 1.13). Its origin is by a thin aponeurosis from the spinous processes of T11–L2 (or L3) and from the supraspinous ligament. The aponeurosis is blended with the lumbar portion of the thoracolumbar fascia. It inserts onto the lower four ribs just lateral to their angles. It is innervated

by the ventral rami of thoracic spinal nerves 9–12. Its action is to draw the ribs down and back.

Trapezius [1]

The trapezius muscle (see Fig. 1.13) is flat and triangular, extending over the back of the neck and the upper thorax. It is divided into upper, middle, and lower portions. The trapezius takes its proximal attachment from the medial one-third of the superior nuchal line of the occipital bone, the external occipital protuberance, the ligamentum nuchae, the spinous process of C7, and all thoracic spinous processes. The upper trapezius attaches distally to the posterior border of the lateral third of the clavicle. The distal attachment of the middle trapezius is to the medial margin of the acromion and to the superior lip of the crest of the spine of the scapula. The fibers of the lower trapezius attach into an aponeurosis that glides over the smooth surface of the root of the spine of the scapula, attaching ultimately in a tubercle at its apex.

The action of the upper trapezius when acting unilaterally, and when the scapula is fixed, is ipsilateral side-bending, extension, and contralateral rotation of the cervical spine. When acting bilaterally, it extends the neck. When the insertion is free to move, it participates with the levator scapula to elevate the

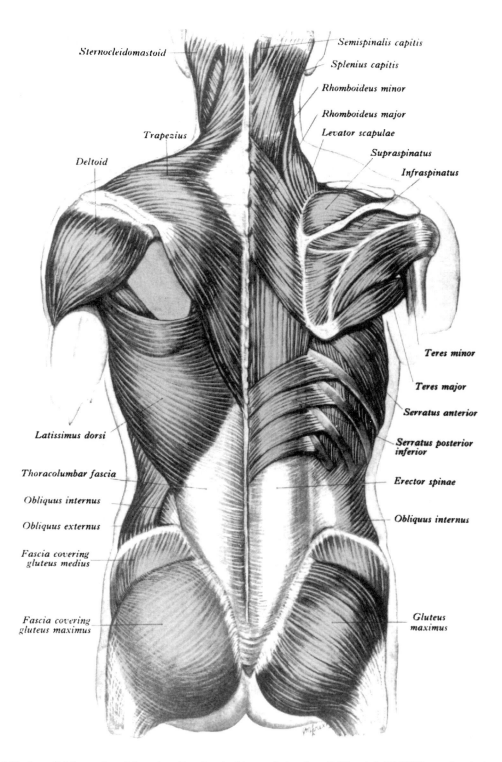

Figure 1.13. Superficial muscles of the spine. (Reprinted with permission from R Warwick, PL Williams. Gray's Anatomy [35th ed]. Edinburgh: Churchill Livingstone, 1973.)

scapula and with the lower trapezius in a force couple for upward rotation of the scapula. The action of the middle trapezius (with the rhomboids) is to retract the scapula. The lower trapezius, apart from participating in the force couple with the upper trapezius, is a scapular depressor and retractor.

The trapezius is innervated by cranial nerve XI (spinal accessory) and by the ventral rami of C3 and C4. However, the spinal nerve innervation is believed to be entirely for proprioception.

Levator Scapulae [1]

The proximal attachment of the levator scapulae muscle (see Fig. 1.13) is to the transverse processes of C1 and C2 and to the posterior tubercles of the transverse processes of C3 and C4. Its distal attachment is the medial border of the scapula between the superior angle and the root of the spine of the scapula.

The action of the levator scapulae muscle, in isolation from other muscles, is to elevate the scapula and rotate it downward. It works with the upper trapezius to provide elevation of the scapula without rotation. When the insertion is fixed, it will act unilaterally to provide ipsilateral side-bending and rotation of the neck. It is innervated by C3 and C4 spinal nerves and by C5 through the dorsal scapular nerve.

Anterior Scalene [1]

The anterior scalene muscle arises from the anterior tubercles of the transverse processes of C3–C6 and attaches to the scalene tubercle on the inner border of the first rib (see Fig. 1.6A). The subclavian vein passes anterior to the distal attachment and the subclavian artery passes posteriorly. When the first rib is fixed, the anterior scalene bends the cervical vertebrae to the same side and rotates them to the opposite side. When the cervical spine is fixed, the muscle elevates the first rib, acting as a secondary muscle of inspiration. It is innervated by branches from the ventral rami of C4–C6.

Middle Scalene [1]

The middle scalene is the largest and longest of the scalene muscles. Its proximal attachment is from the transverse processes of C2 (frequently C1) through C7. It attaches distally to the first rib in the space between the rib tubercle and the groove for the subclavian artery (see Fig. 1.6A). The action of the middle scalene is to bend the cervical spine to the same side when the first rib is fixed and to assist with elevation of the first rib when the cervical spine is fixed. It is innervated by branches from the ventral rami of C3–C8.

Posterior Scalene [1]

The smallest of the scalene muscles, the proximal attachment of the posterior scalene is from the posterior tubercles of the transverse processes of C4–C6. It attaches distally to the outer surface of the second rib (see Figure 1.6B). The action of the posterior scalene is to bend the lower part of the cervical spine posteriorly and to the same side. It is innervated by the ventral rami of C6–C8.

Internal and External Intercostals

The internal and external intercostal muscles fill the space between each pair of ribs (Fig. 1.14). The fibers of the internal intercostal muscle run diagonally toward the posterior as they descend from the superior to the inferior rib. The muscle is thicker anteriorly and thinner posteriorly [14]. The external intercostal fibers run in the opposite direction of the internal intercostal fibers and have reciprocal thickness in that they are thicker posteriorly and become thinner anteriorly. They are innervated by the intercostal nerves. Their actions are still not clearly understood despite considerable research. In a mathematical study about the action of intercostals of the upper thoracic spine, Saumarez [14] suggested that assigning the internal and external intercostals separate functions for inspiration and expiration is an oversimplification. The study suggests that the intercostal muscles are designed to provide optimal stability so the rib cage can withstand the pneumatic demands of respiration.

Transversus Thoracis [1]

The transversus thoracis muscle arises from the posterior surface of the lower one-third of the sternum,

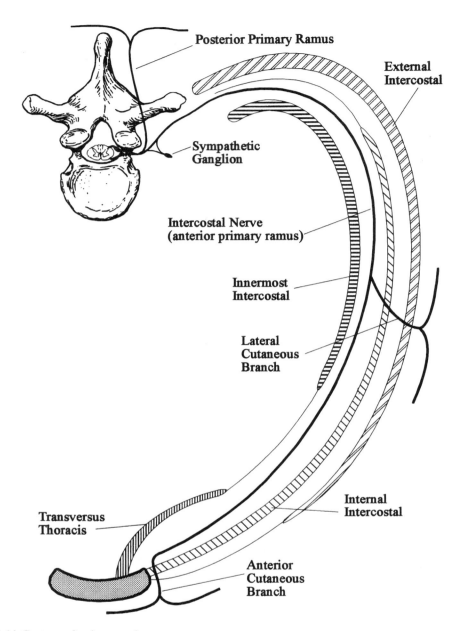

Figure 1.14. Contents of an intercostal space.

the posterior surface of the xiphoid process, and the costal cartilages of the lower three or four true ribs (Fig. 1.15). It fans out laterally and superiorly to attach to the lower borders and internal surfaces of ribs 2–6. It is innervated by adjacent intercostal nerves. Its action is to draw the costal cartilages down.

Pectoralis Major [1]

The pectoralis major muscle (Fig. 1.16) is a thick muscle with two portions: clavicular and sternocostal. The clavicular portion arises from the sternal half of the clavicle and is often distinctly

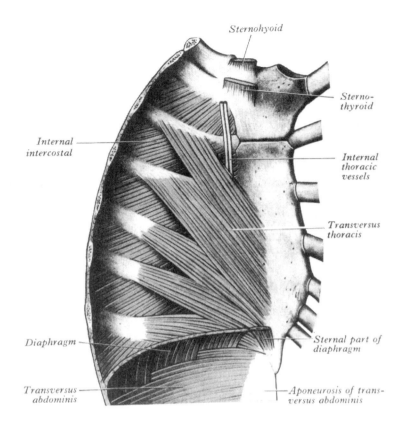

Sternohyoid

Sterno-thyroid

Internal intercostal

Internal thoracic vessels

Transversus thoracis

Diaphragm

Sternal part of diaphragm

Transversus abdominis

Aponeurosis of trans-versus abdominis

Figure 1.15. The transversus thoracis muscle. (Reprinted with permission from R Warwick, PL Williams. Gray's Anatomy [35th ed]. Edinburgh: Churchill Livingstone, 1973.)

separated from the sternocostal portion. The sternocostal portion of the muscle arises from the manubrium, half the breadth of the sternum as low as the attachment of the sixth or seventh costal cartilages; from the costal cartilages of all the true ribs (except occasionally the first and seventh); from the ventral extremity of the sixth rib; and from the aponeurosis of the external abdominal oblique muscle. The distal attachment of the muscle is into the lateral lip of the bicipital groove. The tendon forms anterior and posterior laminae.

The action of the pectoralis major muscle is most evident under resistance. Each portion of the muscle is capable of acting independently. The general action of the muscle working as a whole is to flex and internally rotate the humerus. The clavicular portion flexes the humerus and provides pure horizontal adduction. The sternocostal portion flexes the neutral or extended humerus, depresses the shoulder, and moves the abducted humerus in a diagonal toward the opposite hip. When the distal attachment is fixed with the humerus flexed, the pectoralis major will tend to pull the rib cage anteriorly, supe-

riorly, and laterally. When the distal attachment is fixed with the humerus in extension, the muscle will tend to pull the rib cage laterally and posteriorly. The muscle is innervated by the lateral and medial pectoral nerves (C5–T1).

Pectoralis Minor [1]

The pectoralis minor muscle (see Fig. 1.16) is a thin, triangular muscle arising from the anterior and superior surfaces of ribs 3, 4, and 5 (sometimes 2, 3, and 4) and the fascia of the external intercostal muscle. Its distal attachment is into the medial and superior surface of the coracoid process. The primary action of the muscle is to protract the scapula. It also participates in a force couple with the levator scapula and rhomboids to provide downward rotation of the scapula. When the distal attachment is fixed, the muscle will tend to elevate the third, fourth, and fifth ribs. The pectoralis minor muscle is innervated by the medial and lateral pectoral nerves (C6, C7, and C8).

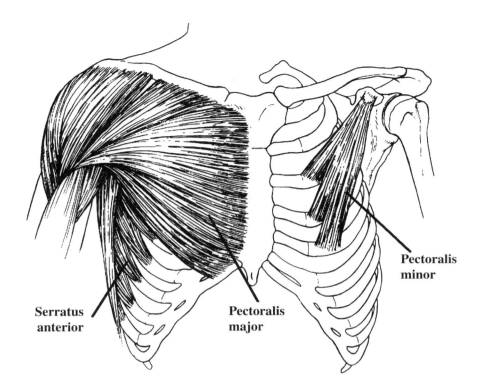

Figure 1.16. The pectoralis and serratus anterior muscles.

Serratus Anterior [1]

The serratus anterior muscle (see Fig. 1.16) arises from the outer surface and the superior border of the upper eight to ten ribs and the fascia of the associated external intercostal muscles. It courses close to the chest wall to attach into the anterior surface of the vertebral border of the scapula. Its action is to protract the scapula. The lower (and stronger) fibers participate in a force couple with the upper and lower trapezius to provide upward rotation of the scapula. When the scapula is fixed, contraction will tend to pull the ribs posteriorly. It is innervated by the long thoracic nerve (C5, C6, and C7).

Diaphragm [1]

The diaphragm, although the primary muscle of inspiration, has broad musculoskeletal attachments to the ribs and spine. Its fibers are grouped into three parts: sternal, costal, and lumbar. The sternal part arises from the back of the xiphoid process. The costal part arises from the internal surfaces of the costal cartilages and adjacent parts of the lower six ribs, interdigitating with the transversus thoracis. The lumbar part arises from two aponeurotic arches. The lateral arch envelops the quadratus lumborum, and the medial arch envelops the psoas major muscle. The lumbar part also arises from two crura that take their origin from the bodies and intervertebral discs of the first two (left crura) or three (right crura) lumbar vertebrae. The diaphragm is innervated by the phrenic nerve (C3, C4, and C5).

Thoracolumbar Fascia [1]

The thoracolumbar fascia covers the deep muscles of the back (Fig. 1.17). It begins anterior to the serratus posterior superior muscle. It is thin and fibrous in the thoracic spine, taking its origin from the spines of the thoracic vertebrae and attaching to the rib angles of all the ribs. It covers the extensor mus-

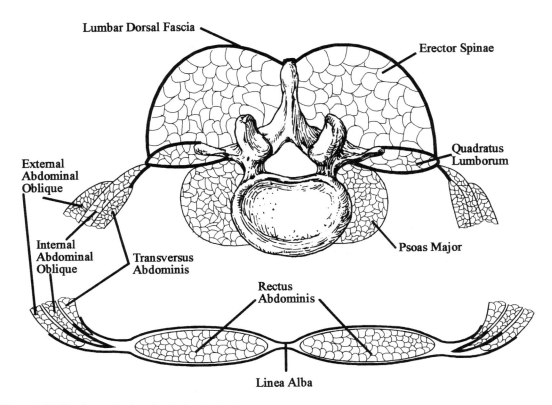

Figure 1.17. The thoracolumbar (lumbodorsal) fascia.

cles in the thoracic spine. In the lumbar spine it has three layers with extensive attachments.

Abdominal Muscles [1]

The abdominal muscles (see Fig. 1.17), having broad attachments to the ribs and to the thoracolumbar fascia, are important in the study and understanding of all regions of the spine. They provide support for the viscera, act as prime movers for spine motion, and act as postural muscles. The abdominal cavity may be viewed as a hydraulic chamber. The spine and pelvis provide the only rigid support for the chamber. With the diaphragm as the superior boundary and the pelvic floor as the inferior boundary, the abdominal muscles provide nearly all of the remaining support. When the abdominal muscles are strong and well toned, the abdominal cavity tends to be more cylindrical, helping to provide superior and inferior support for the lumbar spine [3]. When the abdominal muscles are weak and stretched, the cavity is

more spherical, providing less spine support. Abdominal muscle weakness has been shown to affect posture and spine health. As accessory muscles of expiration, the abdominal muscles have a direct action on the rib cage to pull it inferiorly.

The abdominal group consists of four muscles: the rectus abdominis, the external oblique, the internal oblique, and the transversus abdominis. The rectus abdominis arises from the crest of the pubis and from the ligamentous fibers forming the front of the symphysis pubis. It attaches into the fifth, sixth, and seventh costal cartilages and usually to the anterior end of the fifth rib. It is separated from its partner by the linea alba. Its action is to approximate the ribs and the pelvis. It is innervated by the ventral rami of the lower six or seven thoracic spinal nerves.

The external oblique arises by fleshy strips from the lower eight ribs that interdigitate with the attachments of the serratus anterior and latissimus dorsi. The fibers from the lower two ribs attach into the anterior half of the lateral lip of the iliac crest. The remaining fibers end in an aponeurosis that at-

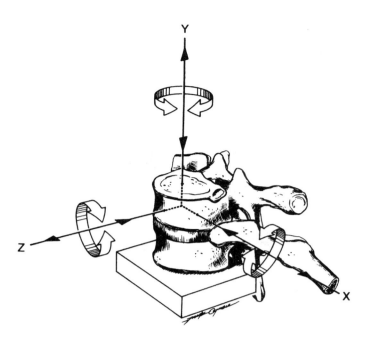

Figure 1.18. The right-handed orthogonal (90-degree angle) coordinate system. (Reprinted with permission from D Lee. Biomechanics of the thorax: A clinical model of in vivo function. Journal of Manual and Manipulative Therapy 1993;1:14.)

taches into the linea alba and inferiorly into the symphysis pubis and pubic crest. The posterior border of the muscle is free. The general fiber direction of the external oblique is inferior and anterior. The action of the external oblique is to approximate the hemithorax with the contralateral hemipelvis. The external oblique is innervated by the ventral rami of the lower six thoracic spinal nerves.

The internal oblique is internal to the external oblique and is thinner and less bulky. It arises from the lateral two-thirds of the inguinal ligament, the anterior two-thirds of the iliac crest, and from the thoracolumbar fascia. The posterior fibers arising from the iliac crest pass superiorly and laterally to attach to the inferior borders of the lower three or four ribs. The fibers arising from the inguinal ligament run inferiorly and medially across the spermatic cord (the round ligament in female subjects). The remaining fibers course superiorly and medially, forming an aponeurosis. The superior two-thirds of the aponeurosis splits to engulf the rectus abdominis and reunite at the linea alba. The lower third passes in front of the rectus to attach into the linea alba. The internal oblique works in synergy with the contralateral external oblique to provide combined trunk rotation and flexion (approximating hemithorax with contralateral hemipelvis). The internal oblique is innervated by the ventral rami of the lower six thoracic and first lumbar spinal nerves.

The transversus abdominis is the innermost of all the abdominal muscles and is so named because the fibers course mostly in the transverse plane. It arises from the lateral third of the inguinal ligament, the anterior two-thirds of the iliac crest, the thoracolumbar fascia, and the lower six costal cartilages. It attaches by way of an aponeurosis to the linea alba. The superior three-fourths pass behind the rectus abdominis, blending with the aponeurosis of the internal oblique. The inferior one-fourth passes anteriorly to the rectus abdominis. Its action is to pull the abdomen in so as to compress the contents. It is innervated by the ventral rami of the lower six thoracic and first lumbar spinal nerves.

Biomechanics

Coordinate System

The coordinate system we will use to describe the direction of spine motion is that used by White and Panjabi [6] (Fig. 1.18). It is the right-handed orthogonal (90-degree angle) coordinate system. Consider the human body in the anatomic position. The origin of the coordinate system is between the cornua of the sacrum. The X axis lies in the intersection of the frontal and horizontal planes. The positive X direction is to the left. The Y axis lies in the intersection of the sagittal and frontal planes. Its positive Y direction is up. The Z axis lies in the intersection of the sagittal and horizontal planes. Its positive Z direction is forward.

In describing the motions of the spine, we will consider the rotations about the axes and translations in the planes or in the direction that an axis points. Rotation in the clockwise direction is positive. The clockwise direction is determined by imagining yourself at the zero point of an axis and facing in its positive direction. The clockwise direction will be toward your right. Therefore, angles that are clockwise about the X axis (+ X) describe flexion. Angles that are clockwise about the Z axis (+ Z) describe right side-bending. Angles that are clockwise about the Y axis (+ Y) describe axial rotation to the left.

Biomechanical Models

There is a considerable amount of information in the literature concerning biomechanics of the cervical spine, the lumbar spine, and pelvis. White and Panjabi [6] and Kapandji [4] provide what is probably the most complete information on the biomechanics of the thoracic spine and rib cage. Several studies can be found in the literature based on three-dimensional mathematical models [14–17]. Andriacchi et al. [15] studied the effect of the rib cage on the thoracic spine and found that the rib cage (with sternum) increases stiffness 2.64 times in extension and 2.14 times in flexion. Removal of the sternum resulted in such a decrease in stiffness that it was nearly equal to the stiffness of the ligamentous spine alone. The load-bearing capability of the thoracic spine was also influenced by the addition of the rib cage. Compressive loads required to cause buckling of the spine increased three to four times with the addition of the rib cage.

Saumarez [14] reported that there is considerable movement of the spine and sternum independent of one another. This allows for motion of the spine without necessarily causing or requiring rib cage movement.

Panjabi et al. [17] performed in vitro analysis of the mechanical properties of the thoracic spine using fresh cadaver specimens. They obtained 396 load-displacement curves from 11 functional spinal units (FSUs) for three translations and three rotations about the X, Y, and Z axes. An FSU is defined as the smallest unit of the spine that still exhibits the biomechanical characteristics of the spine. It is composed of two adjacent vertebral bodies and the intervening ligamentous structures [18, 19].

A search for literature that presents an in vivo model of thoracic spine and rib cage biomechanics was disappointing. However, Lee [10] has proposed a clinical model of in vivo function of the middle and lower thorax that is an insightful and helpful tool for evaluating and understanding clinical findings.

Range of Motion

Range of motion for the thoracic spine is given in Table 1.2 and is graphically represented in Fig. 1.19.

Biomechanics of Thoracic Motion

Flexion

Flexion occurs in the sagittal plane during forward bending of the trunk and during the exhalation phase of respiration. It is rotation around the X axis in the positive direction (Fig. 1.20). Flexion of the FSU is coupled with anterior translation along the Z axis (0.5 mm) and very slight distraction (+Y axis translation). When translation was introduced along the Z axis, it was coupled with X-axis rotation (flexion) and slight compression (–Y-axis translation) [17]. During flexion, the articular facets of the superior vertebra glide upward and forward on the inferior partner. The conformation of the joint surfaces supports this motion.

Since Panjabi, Brand, and White [17] did not address osteokinematics of the ribs during flexion, Lee [10] provided the following clinical hypothesis (Fig. 1.21): During flexion, the superior segment of the FSU translates anteriorly, causing forward motion of the superior demifacet of the costovertebral joint. This motion facilitates anterior rotation of the rib by applying a pushing moment to the superior demifacet of the rib head. An analogy would be rolling a pencil between one's hands. In the middle thoracic spine, the joint configuration of the costovertebral joint is concave transverse process facet on convex rib facet. The anterior rotation of the rib at the costovertebral joint during flexion is therefore accompanied by superior glide of the costotransverse rib

Table 1.2. Limits and Representative Values of Ranges of Rotation of the Thoracic Spine

Interspace	Combined Flexion/Extension (± X-axis Rotation)		One Side Lateral Bending (Z-axis Rotation)		One Side Axial Rotation (Y-axis Rotation)	
	Limits of Ranges (degrees)	Representative Angle (degrees)	Limits of Ranges (degrees)	Representative Angle (degrees)	Limits of Ranges (degrees)	Representative Angle (degrees)
T1–T2	3–5	4	5	5	14	9
T2–T3	3–5	4	5–7	6	4–12	8
T3–T4	2–5	4	3–7	5	5–11	8
T4–T5	2–5	4	5–6	6	5–11	8
T5–T6	3–5	4	5–6	6	5–11	8
T6–T7	2–7	5	6	6	4–11	7
T7–T8	3–8	6	3–8	6	4–11	7
T8–T9	3–8	6	4–7	6	6–7	6
T9–T10	3–8	6	4–7	6	3–5	4
T10–T11	4–14	9	3–10	7	2–3	2
T11–T12	6–20	12	4–13	9	2–3	2
T12–L1	6–20	12	5–10	8	2–3	2

Source: Reprinted with permission from AA White, MM Panjabi. Clinical Biomechanics of the Spine. Philadelphia: Lippincott, 1990.

Thoracic Spine Motion

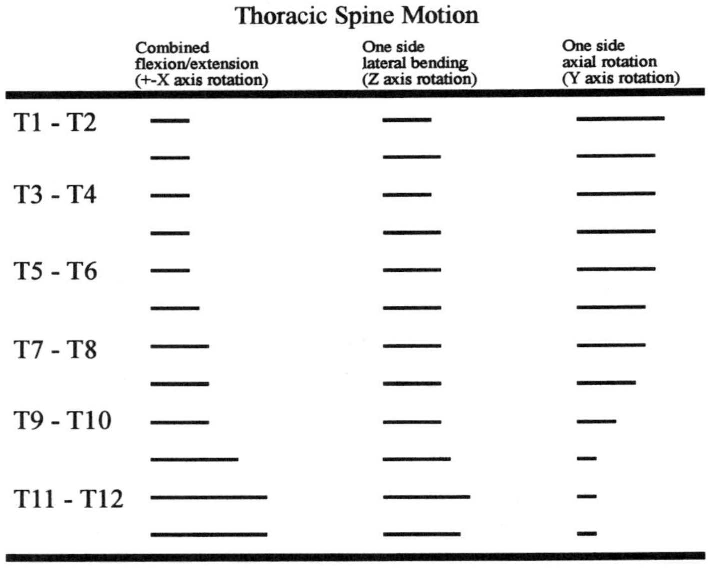

Figure 1.19. Rotatory ranges of motion in the thoracic spine about the traditional axes. (Adapted from AA White, MM Panjabi. Clinical Biomechanics of the Spine. Philadelphia: Lippincott, 1990.)

facet. In the lower thoracic spine, the ribs follow the motion in the sagittal plane but rotation does not tend to occur because of the planar conformation of the costotransverse joints. Furthermore, ribs 11 and 12 attach to only their corresponding vertebral body and do not have costotransverse joints.

Extension

Extension also occurs in the sagittal plane (Fig. 1.22) but in the negative (–X) direction. It occurs with backward bending, with elevation of both arms, and with the inspiration phase of respiration. It is

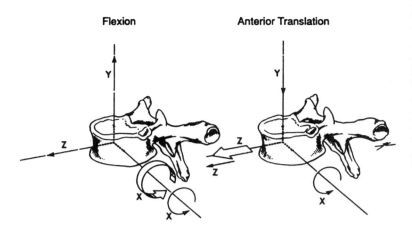

Flexion

Anterior Translation

Figure 1.20. Forward sagittal rotation around the X axis induces anterior translation along the Z axis and slight distraction along the Y axis. Anterior translation along the Z axis induces forward sagittal rotation around the X axis and slight compression along the Y axis. (Reprinted with permission from D Lee. Biomechanics of the thorax: A clinical model of in vivo function. Journal of Manual and Manipulative Therapy 1993;1:15.)

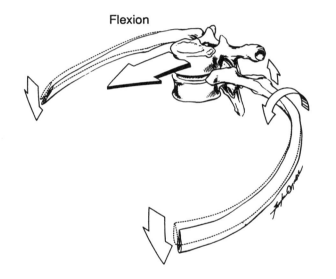

Flexion

Figure 1.21. The osteokinematic and arthrokinematic motion proposed to occur in the thorax during flexion. (Reprinted with permission from D Lee. Biomechanics of the thorax: A clinical model of in vivo function. Journal of Manual and Manipulative Therapy 1993;1:15.)

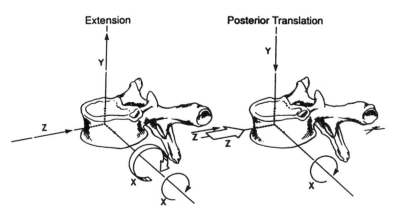

Extension

Posterior Translation

Figure 1.22. Backward sagittal rotation around the X axis induces posterior translation along the Z axis and slight distraction along the Y axis. Posterior translation along the Z axis induces backward sagittal rotation around the X axis and slight compression along the Y axis. (Reprinted with permission from D Lee. Biomechanics of the thorax: A clinical model of in vivo function. Journal of Manual and Manipulative Therapy 1993;1:17.)

Extension

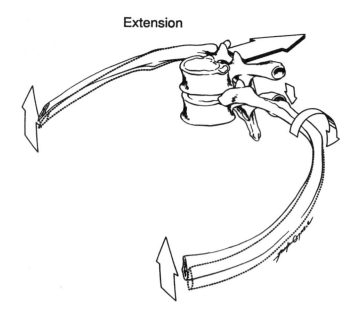

Figure 1.23. The osteokinematic and arthrokinematic motion proposed to occur in the thorax during extension. (Reprinted with permission from D Lee. Biomechanics of the thorax: A clinical model of in vivo function. Journal of Manual and Manipulative Therapy 1993;1:17.)

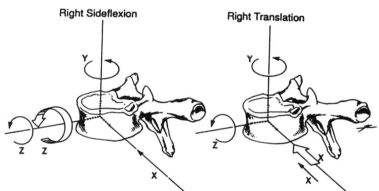

Figure 1.24. Right side flexion (side-bending) around the Z axis induces left rotation around the Y axis and right translation along the X axis. Right lateral translation along the X axis induces right side flexion around the Z axis and left rotation around the Y axis. (Reprinted with permission from D Lee. Biomechanics of the thorax: A clinical model of in vivo function. Journal of Manual and Manipulative Therapy 1993;1:17.)

coupled with posterior translation along the Z axis (–Z direction) of about 1 mm and with very slight distraction. When posterior translation was introduced to the superior segment of the FSU in the experimental model, posterior rotation about the X axis was coupled with slight compression [17]. The inferior facets of the superior joint partner glide posteriorly and inferiorly.

The clinical hypothesis [10] concerning rib osteokinematics during middle thoracic extension is that the posterior translation of the superior segment of the FSU creates a force that facilitates posterior rotation of the rib head by applying a pulling moment to the superior demifacet of the rib head (Fig. 1.23). The accompanying motion of the rib at the costotransverse joint is inferior glide. In the lower

thoracic spine, the ribs follow the motion in the sagittal plane, but rotation does not tend to occur because of the planar conformation of the costotransverse joints.

Side-Bending

Side-bending of the thoracic spine occurs in the frontal plane (Fig. 1.24). Rotation about the Z axis is coupled with contralateral rotation about the Y axis and ipsilateral translation along the X axis [17]. Translation forces applied to the superior FSU partner are coupled with ipsilateral side-bending along the Z axis and contralateral rotation around the Z axis [17]. If one takes a problem-solving approach to understanding these mechanics but considers only

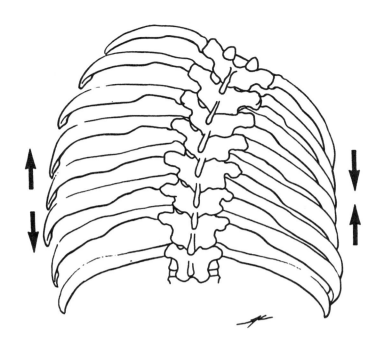

Figure 1.25. As the thorax side-bends to the right side, the ribs on the right approximate and the ribs on the left separate at their lateral margins. The costal motion appears to stop first. The thoracic vertebrae then continue to side-bend slightly to the right side. (Reprinted with permission from D Lee. Biomechanics of the thorax: A clinical model of in vivo function. Journal of Manual and Manipulative Therapy 1993;1:18.)

the vertebrae without the ribs, contralateral Y-axis rotation is hard to explain. Looking at the facet joints alone, with their orientation of 30 degrees from the frontal plane, side-bending should be coupled with ipsilateral rotation. However, if we apply Lee's clinical hypothesis [10], these mechanics become clear.

As side-bending occurs, the ribs on the ipsilateral side of the bend approximate before the joint motion is completed (Fig. 1.25). This stops rib motion, but the vertebrae continue. Remember that the configuration of the costotransverse joints in the middle thoracic spine is convex rib facet on concave transverse process facet. As the transverse process ipsilateral to the side-bending attempts further motion in an inferior direction, the rib facet is forced superiorly. This creates an anterior (internal) rotation moment at the rib because of the concave structure of the transverse process joint partner. The anteriorly rotating rib head forces the superior vertebra forward at the costovertebral joint.

Meanwhile, on the contralateral side, the ribs distract during the side-bending. They reach the limit of their passive restraints (intercostals) quickly because of the long lever arm. These ribs, now stabilized distally, are forced inferiorly at the costotransverse joint as the transverse process continues motion in the superior direction. A posterior (external) rotation moment is created because of the costotransverse joint configuration. The posteriorly rotating rib head forces the superior vertebra backward at the costovertebral joint. The result of the ipsilateral ribs rotating anteriorly and the contralateral ribs rotating posteriorly is a coupling action that facilitates contralateral rotation of the superior vertebra of the FSU (Fig. 1.26).

In the lower thoracic spine, the ribs do not appear to direct the rotation of the superior segment of the FSU by rotation at the costovertebral joint. However, as the side-bending occurs and the ribs approximate, the lower thoracic ribs (excluding ribs 11 and 12) will glide superiorly and posteriorly along the plane of the costotransverse joint. The transverse process of the vertebra at rib level will move inferiorly and anteriorly ipsilaterally, and the contralateral rib will move superiorly and posteriorly, hence, rotation in the opposite direction from the side-bending.

Rotation

Panjabi et al. [17] reported that Y-axis rotation is coupled with contralateral Z-axis rotation and contralateral X-axis translation (Fig. 1.27). However, the coupling observed clinically does not include contralateral but rather ipsilateral Z-axis rotation. For instance, it can be easily shown in the clinic that right rotation (introduced first) is coupled with right

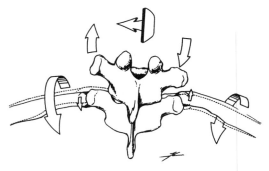

Figure 1.26. The superior glide of the right rib at the costo-transverse joint induces anterior rotation of the same rib because of the convexoconcavity of the joint surfaces. The inferior glide of the left rib at the costotransverse joint induces posterior rotation of that rib. This bilateral costal rotation in opposing directions tends to drive the superior vertebra into left rotation. (Reprinted with permission from D Lee. Biomechanics of the thorax: A clinical model of in vivo function. Journal of Manual and Manipulative Therapy 1993;1:18.)

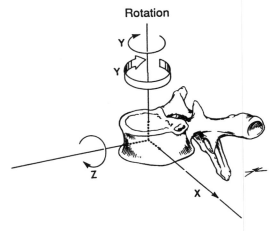

Figure 1.27. Right rotation around the Y axis induces left side flexion around the Z axis and left translation along the X axis. (Reprinted with permission from D Lee. Biomechanics of the thorax: A clinical model of in vivo function. Journal of Manual and Manipulative Therapy 1993;1:19.)

side-bending. Lee [10] suggested that this conflict of observations could be a result of the differences of the in vitro and in vivo anatomic situation. Panjabi et al. [17] cut the ribs 3 cm distal to the costotransverse joints, eliminating the biomechanical influences of the costal cartilages and the sternum. Andriacchi et al. [15] documented the significant stabilizing contribution of the sternum to the rib cage and thoracic spine. Again, Lee [10] proposed a

clinical hypothesis to explain the clinical observation of ipsilateral coupling of side-bending with rotation in the middle thoracic spine.

To illustrate, we will consider right rotation of the middle thoracic spine. The superior segment of the FSU rotates to the right and translates left (Fig. 1.28). The result on the rib is posterior rotation of the right rib and anterior rotation of the left rib. The effect of the translation is that the superior segment will pull the right rib with it and push the left rib away. The rib motion causes the costovertebral and costotransverse ligaments to become taut. Lee further suggested that the superior segment must tilt to the right to release tension on the (superior) costotransverse ligament and allow further rotation.

I would suggest a slight modification to the clinical hypothesis here. The superior costotransverse ligament has two layers [1] (see Fig. 1.7). The anterior layer runs superiorly and laterally, originating from the crest of the neck of the rib and attaching to the undersurface of the transverse process above. The posterior layer originates from the dorsal surface of the neck of the rib and runs superiorly and medially to attach to the transverse process above. Therefore, during the translation activity suggested by Lee [10], fibers of the anterior layer would become taut on the right, whereas the fibers of the posterior layer become taut on the left side.

As previously stated, right rotation is accompanied by posterior rotation of the right rib and anterior rotation of the left rib because of the action at the costovertebral joint. Since the posterior layer of the superior costotransverse ligament attaches to the dorsal surface of the neck of the rib, it acts like a winch, pulling the right transverse process of the superior vertebra down as that rib rotates posteriorly and glides inferiorly at the right costotransverse joint. Likewise, the left rib releases its posterior layer of the superior costotransverse ligament as it rotates anteriorly and glides superiorly at the left costotransverse joint, allowing the left transverse process of the superior segment to move superiorly. Finally, as Lee [10] pointed out, the orientation of the facet joints in the middle thoracic spine easily allow (even facilitate) right side-bending with right rotation.

Rotation in the lower thoracic spine follows the same mechanics as in the middle except that rotation flexibility is greater in the lower. This is probably because of the reduction of bony attachments of

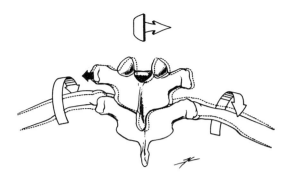

Figure 1.28. As the superior thoracic vertebra rotates to the right, it translates to the left. The right rib posteriorly rotates and the left rib anterior rotates as a consequence of the vertebral rotation. (Reprinted with permission from D Lee. Biomechanics of the thorax: A clinical model of in vivo function. Journal of Manual and Manipulative Therapy 1993;1:19.)

ribs 11 and 12 and because the planar costotransverse joints in the lower thoracic spine (oriented from posterior superior to anterior inferior) allow some anteroposterior gliding of the transverse process during trunk rotation and not primarily rib rotation as in the middle thoracic spine.

Respiration

We have been told that upper rib motion during respiration is similar to that of a pump handle and lower rib motion is similar to a bucket handle. The axis for rib motion is described by a line running between the costotransverse joint and the costovertebral joint through the neck of the rib. In the upper thoracic spine, this line is oriented toward, but not in, the frontal plane. The upper ribs therefore elevate and depress in a diagonal plane where the anterior end of the rib moves mostly in the sagittal plane but some in the frontal plane. The axis for lower rib rotation (excluding ribs 11 and 12) lies more toward the sagittal plane. The motion of the lower ribs is therefore in a diagonal that is primarily toward the frontal plane at the anterior end.

The clinical significance of these distinctions is that, in order to increase the volume of the thorax for inspiration, the rib cage must move generally up and out at all levels. All ribs, then (except ribs 11 and 12), have both pump handle and bucket handle components to their motion. This is important to remember when addressing respiratory dysfunctions of the rib cage (see Chapter 9).

References

1. Warwick R, Williams PL. Gray's Anatomy (35th ed). Edinburgh: Churchill Livingstone, 1973.
2. Bowling RW, Rockar P. Thoracic Spine. In Richardson JK, Iglarsh ZA (eds), Clinical Orthopaedic Physical Therapy. Philadelphia: Saunders, 1994;7–118.
3. DiGiovanna EL, Schiowitz S. An Osteopathic Approach to Diagnosis and Treatment. Philadelphia: Lippincott, 1991.
4. Kapandji IA. The Physiology of the Joints. Vol. 3. The Trunk and Vertebral Column. New York: Churchill Livingstone, 1974.
5. El-Khoury GY, Whitten CG. Trauma to the upper thoracic spine: Anatomy, biomechanics, and unique imaging features. AJR 1993;160:95–102.
6. White AA, Panjabi MM. Clinical Biomechanics of the Spine. Philadelphia: Lippincott, 1990.
7. Greenman PE. Principles of Manual Medicine. Baltimore: Williams & Wilkins, 1989.
8. Bourdillon JF, Day EA, Bookhout MR. Spinal Manipulation. Oxford: Butterworth-Heinemann, 1992.
9. Stagnara P, De Mauroy JC, Dran G et al. Reciprocal angulation of vertebral bodies in a sagittal plane: Approach to references for the evaluation of kyphosis and lordosis. Spine 1982;7:335–342.
10. Lee D. Biomechanics of the thorax: A clinical model of in vivo function. Journal of Manual and Manipulative Therapy 1993;1:13–21.
11. Malman DJ, Pintar FA. Anatomy and clinical biomechanics of the thoracic spine. Clin Neurosurg 1992;38: 296–324.
12. Wood KB, Garvey TA, Gundry C, Heithoff K. Thoracic MRI evaluation of asymptomatic individuals [abstract]. Presented at the Eighth Annual Meeting of the North American Spine Society. San Diego, 1993.
13. Anderson JE. Grant's Atlas of Anatomy. Baltimore: Williams & Wilkins, 1983.
14. Saumarez RC. An analysis of possible movements of human upper rib cage. J Appl Physiol 1986;60:678–689.
15. Andriacchi T, Schultz A, Belytschko T et al. A model for studies of mechanical interactions between the human spine and rib cage. J Biomech 1974;7:497–507.
16. Ben-Haim SA, Saidel GM. Mathematical model of chest wall mechanics: a phenomenological approach. Ann Biomed Eng 1990;18:37–56.
17. Panjabi MM, Brand RA, White AA. Mechanical properties of the human thoracic spine. J Bone Joint Surg [Am] 1976;58:642–652.
18. Panjabi MM, Hausfeld JN, White AA. A biomechanical study of the ligamentous stability of the thoracic spine in man. Acta Orthop Scand 1981;52:315–326.
19. Panjabi MM, Thibodeau LL, White AA. What constitutes spinal instability? Clin Neurosurg 1988;34:313–339.
20. Saumarez RC. An analysis of action of intercostal muscles in human upper rib cage. J Appl Physiol 1986; 60:690–701.

Chapter 2

Neurophysiologic Aspects of the Thoracic Spine and Ribs

Wolfgang G. Gilliar

WEAREMORECONNECTEDTHANWEHAVEBEENLEDTOBELIEVE

The physician should speak of that which is invisible. What is visible should belong to his knowledge, and he should recognize illnesses, just as anyone who is not a physician can recognize them from their symptoms. But this is far from making him a physician; he becomes a physician only when he knows that which is unnamed, invisible, and immaterial, yet has its effect.

— Paracelsus

The primary function assigned to the thoracic region of the spine, which is sandwiched between the more mobile cervical and lumbar regions, is generalized stability. Yet within that structural stability—because of the three-joint complex of ribs and thoracic vertebrae—occur small rhythmic movements with each respiratory cycle. This requires precise coordination and a smooth integration within and between the structures involved—that is, at the local ("peripheral" or "infraspinal"), spinal cord, and supraspinal levels. The receptors of the joints, capsules, muscles, and their reflexes in the thoracic spine do not differ from other spinal regions. The involvement of the sympathetic nervous system, originating from the thoracolumbar segments, and its associated reflexes, however, confer a distinct uniqueness to the discussion of the thoracic spine.

This chapter seeks to strike a balance between a broad overview and pertinent details of the neurophysiologic aspects of the thoracic spine and ribs.

From Structure to Function

The anatomic uniqueness of the thoracic spine has been covered in detail in Chapter 1. To set the stage and present the neurophysiologic principles within a "larger picture," Fig. 2.1 has been composed. Movement is governed by the facet joint inclinations, and in the thoracic spine, at least in the upper portions, motion in all three planes is relatively restricted. The blood supply and relatively small diameter of the thoracic spinal canal result in the area T4–T9 being called the "critical zone." There are 12 thoracic spinal nerves exiting the spinal foramina, with the individual spinal nerve being assigned its "number" according to the corresponding vertebra above. A comparison of various cross-sections of the spinal cord reveals a prominently enlarged C8 spinal segment, which is because of upper extremity fibers. The thoracic cross-sections are comparatively small. Within the cross-section of a particular thoracic spinal segment there is a prominent aggregate of gray matter nuclei collections in the so-called Clarke's column (Fig. 2.2). These aggregates of nuclei are important for sympathetic nervous system connections.

The presentation below pursues a logical sequence, starting with the peripheral receptors of joints and muscles, followed by a discussion of interneuronal networks. This is followed by a brief overview of muscle physiology. Relevant aspects of the sympathetic nervous system and its reflex circuits

31

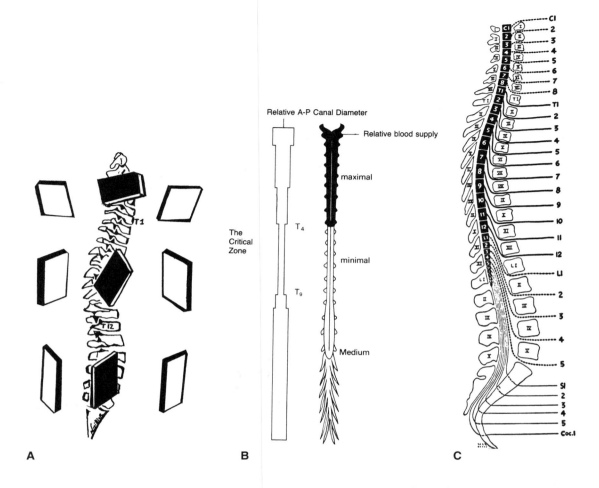

Figure 2.1. Composite overview of the various spinal and neural elements pertaining to the thoracic spine (not drawn to scale). A. Facet orientation governs the plane of motion. For the thoracic spine, the facet is inclined forward (60 degrees about the X axis) and is rotated (20 degrees about the Y axis). From an anterior view, the facet surfaces here drawn at either side of the spine "open" toward the observer. The facet orientation in the lumbar spine is almost vertical (X axis) with the surface being rotated "away" by 45 degrees (Y axis). B. In the thoracic spine, the critical zone (T4–T9) is an area in which the canal space and the free space between the spinal cord and the borders of the spinal canal are minimal. Despite the small size of the thoracic spinal cord, the relative free space is still minimal in the critical zone. The blood supply in that region is less than that elsewhere in the spinal cord. These factors contribute to the catastrophic nature of thoracic disc disease and clinical instability in the thoracic spine. (Reprinted with permission from AA White, MM Panjabi. Clinical Biomechanics of the Spine. Philadelphia: Lippincott, 1978.) C. The spinal cord segments with reference to the bodies and the spinous processes of the vertebrae. The thoracic spinal nerves exit "below" their respective intervertebral disc, that is, the T1 nerve root leaves the foramen between the first and second thoracic vertebrae. (Reprinted with permission from MB Carpenter. Core Text of Neuroanatomy [2nd ed]. Baltimore: Williams & Wilkins, 1978.) D. Selected spinal cord segments at different levels showing the variation in the size, shape, and topography of gray and white matter. Note that the gray columns are maximal in the cervical and lumbar enlargements, since they are associated with the larger nerves innervating their respective extremities. In the thoracic spinal cord segments, there is a prominent but small lateral horn that contains the intermediolateral cell column, which gives rise to preganglionic sympathetic efferent fibers. (Reprinted with permission from MB Carpenter. Core Text of Neuroanatomy [2nd ed]. Baltimore: Williams & Wilkins, 1978.) E. Conceptual overview of the various structures innervated by the sympathetic nervous system. (Reprinted from F Cervero. Visceral and Spinal Components of Viscero-Somatic Interactions. In MM Patterson, JN Howell [eds], The Central Connection: Somatovisceral/Viscerosomatic Interaction. Indianapolis: American Academy of Osteopathy, 1992;77–85.)

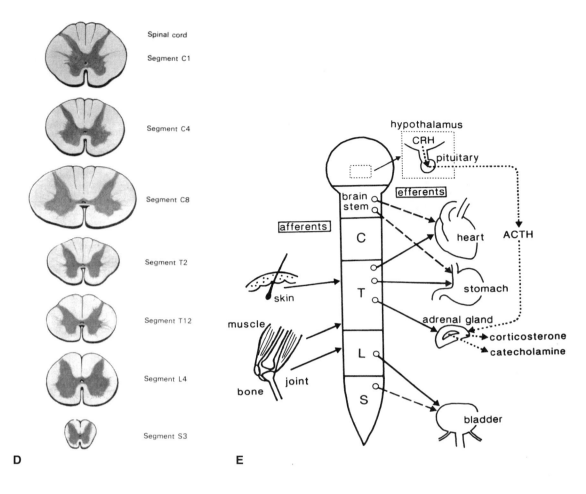

D   E

are then addressed. The chapter then presents recent notions of nociception and pain. The concepts of somatic dysfunction and the "facilitated segment" will conclude the discussion as the theoretical considerations presented are tied into clinical applications.

From Receptor to Monosynaptic Reflex

The function of the varied sensory organs of reception is to convert stimuli from the external and internal environment into impulses that, once carried to the central nervous system, will initiate voluntary or involuntary responses [1].

Within the context of the topic at hand, a functional categorization of the varied receptors will suffice (Table 2.1).

The superficial sensitivity, together with the proprioceptive sensation (receptors in muscles, joints,

ligaments, fascia, etc.) and the pain sensibility within the body constitutes the somatovisceral senses [2] (Figure 2.3).

Joint Receptors

The seminal work by Freeman and Wyke [3] and Wyke [4–6] has provided extensive and insightful information about the various receptors in the apophyseal joints (facet joints; or also known as the zygapophyseal joints). Joint receptors are present in all synovial joint capsules, including those of the thoracic spine. There are four categories of joint receptors, the first three of which represent mechanoreceptors and the last representing nociceptors. The receptor types differ in their structural composition, distribution, innervation pattern, threshold of activation, and adaptability. Further-

SPINAL CORD

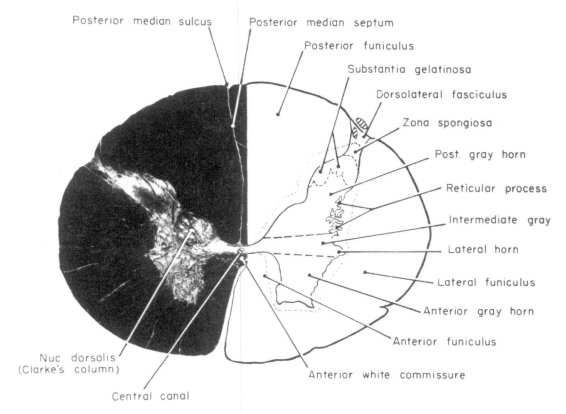

Figure 2.2. Section through a lower segment of adult human spinal cord demonstrating the subdivisions of the gray and white matter. Note the prominence of Clarke's column (nucleus dorsalis), the neuro-anatomic representation of the prominence of the sympathetic nervous system in the thoracic spine. (Reprinted with permission from MB Carpenter. Core Text of Neuroanatomy [2nd ed]. Baltimore: Williams & Wilkins, 1978.)

more, they differ in their effect on static and dynamic reflex controls of the striated muscles, both under normal and pathologic conditions [7] and either in pain suppression or pain evocation. The morphology and function of the individual receptors are presented in Table 2.2.

Once stimulated, the information initiated at the facet joint (or the paraspinal muscles, but not the extremity muscles) is carried through the appropriate afferent fibers to the associated dorsal rami rather than the ventral rami. The type I joint receptors, controlling primarily the outer layers of the joint capsule, have been found to inhibit impulses arising from pain receptors (nociceptors, type IV fibers). Type II fibers, located more deeply in the fibrous joint capsule, are rapidly adapting mechanoreceptors and transmit information relatively fast because of

their medium myelin thickness. They transitorily inhibit the nociceptive activity of the joint capsule. The type III receptors, resembling the structure of the Golgi tendon organs (discussed below), are innervated by large myelinated fibers, ensuring fast transmission speed. It is assumed that they have a function similar to the Golgi tendon organ as well. They adapt slowly and have an inhibitory effect on motoneurons [3]. The type IV receptors, or nociceptors, are thinly myelinated or nonmyelinated free nerve endings. Any abnormal stimulus can cause the nociceptor to fire, including abnormal constant pressure on the joint capsule, chemical irritation, or any significant disruption surrounding the joint and its structures. It is interesting to note that these receptors have been found to have reflexogenic effects on the respiratory and cardiovascular systems.

Table 2.1. Receptor Types in the Neuromusculoskeletal System

Proprioceptive receptors	
Joint capsule	Mechanoreceptors (type I, II)
	Nociceptors (type IV)
Skeletal muscle	Intrafusal muscle fibers
	Golgi tendon organs
Tendon	Mechanoreceptors (type III)
	Golgi tendon organs
	Nociceptors (type IV)
Ligament	Mechanoreceptors (type III)
Articular fat pad	Mechanoreceptors (type II)
	Nociceptors (type IV)
Exteroceptive receptors	
Skin	Krause's end bulb
	Meissner's corpuscles
	Merkel's discs
	Pacinian corpuscle
	Ruffini's end-organ
Visceral receptors	
Viscera	Visceroreceptive receptors (detection of distension)
	Receptors in smooth muscle (spasms)

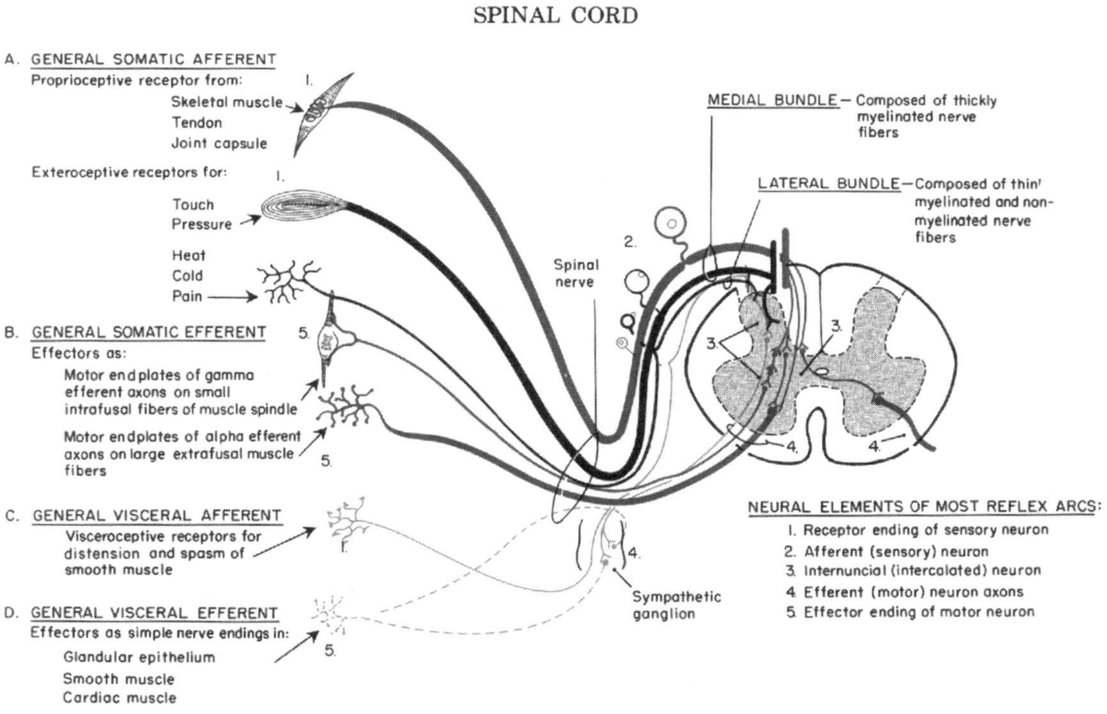

SPINAL CORD

Figure 2.3. Diagrammatic representation of the various functional components in a thoracic spinal nerve. Numbers in the diagram correspond to neural elements that form reflex arcs. (Reprinted with permission from MB Carpenter. Core Text of Neuroanatomy [2nd ed]. Baltimore: Williams & Wilkins, 1978.)

Table 2.2. Comparison of the Four Joint Receptor Types

Type	Morphology	Location	Parent Nerve Fibers	Behavioral Characteristics	Function
I	Thinly encapsulated globular corpuscles (100 × 40 μm) in clusters of 3–8	Fibrous capsulae of joint (superficial layers)	Small myelinated (6–9 μm)	Static and dynamic mechanoreceptors: low threshold, slowly adapting	Tonic reflexogenic effects on neck, limb, jaw, and eye muscles. Postural and kinesthetic sensation. Pain suppression.
II	Thickly encapsulated conical corpuscles (280 × 100 μm) singly or in clusters of 2–4	Fibrous capsulae of joint (deeper layers). Articular fat pads	Medium myelinated (9–12 μm)	Dynamic mechanoreceptors: low threshold, rapidly adapting	(a) Phasic reflexogenic effects on neck, limb, jaw, and eye muscles (b) Pain suppression
III	Fusiform corpuscles (600 × 100 μm) usually singly, also in clusters of 2–3	Ligaments, also in related tendons	Large myelinated (13–17 μm)	Mechanoreceptor: high threshold, very slowly adapting	—
IV	Three-dimensional plexus of unmyelinated nerve fibers	Entire thickness of fibrous capsulae of joint. Walls of articular blood vessels. Articular fat pads	Very small myelinated (2–5 μm), and unmyelinated	Nociceptor (pain-provoking): high threshold, non-adapting	(a) Tonic reflexogenic effects on neck, limb, jaw, and eye muscles (b) Evocation of pain (c) Respiratory and cardiovascular reflexogenic effects

Source: Reprinted with permission from MAR Freeman, BD Wyke. The innervation of the knee joint. An anatomical and histological study in the cat. J Anat 1967;101:505–512.

Innervation of the Joint Capsule

The joint capsule is innervated by the dorsal rami of the spinal nerve. As presented by Auteroche [8], one articular ramus of a nerve root contributes to more than one segmental joint capsule in the form of collaterals. Thus, the joint capsules are innervated plurisegmentally. Figure 2.4 provides a diagrammatic overview of the nerve supply to the joints, tendons, paravertebral muscles, and periosteum in a thoracic spinal section.

Muscle Receptors

The three major muscle sensory receptors activated during movement are the primary and secondary muscle spindles and the Golgi tendon organ (GTO). During movement different joint and cutaneous receptors are stimulated in unison and become involved in the flexor reflex afferent system. This section first describes the three different muscle receptors, followed by a discussion of interneuronal networks.

Muscle Spindle

The muscle spindle (Fig. 2.5) is primarily a stretch receptor composed of small, so-called *intrafusal* muscle fibers and enclosed by a connective tissue capsule. The information from the spindle is passed on to the associated primary afferent fiber of the type Ia. Muscles responsible for fine movement reveal the greatest spindle density.

Located within the muscle proper—for distinction purposes, the fibers of which are called *extra-*

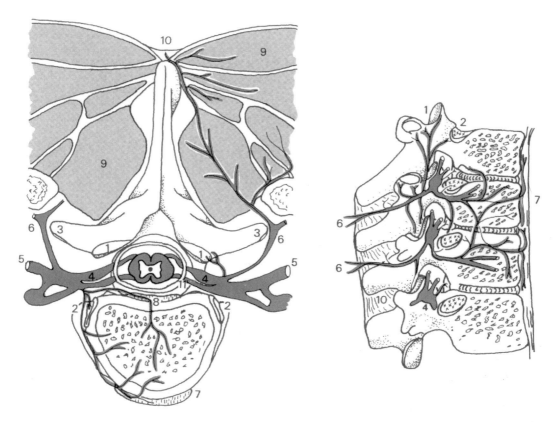

Figure 2.4. The nerve supply of the various joints, muscles and ligaments, and periosteum in the thoracic spine region (Reprinted with permission from J Dvorak, V Dvorak. Manual Medicine–Diagnostics [2nd ed]. New York: Thieme, 1990.) 1 = apophyseal joint; 2 = costovertebral joint; 3 = costotransverse joint; 4 = spinal ganglion; 5 = ventral ramus of spinal nerve; 6 = dorsal ramus of spinal nerve; 7 = anterior longitudinal ligament; 8 = posterior longitudinal ligament; 9 = paravertebral musculature; 10 = interspinous ligament; 11 = ventral ramus of the spinal nerve.

fusal—the spindles are arranged in parallel to these extrafusal muscle fibers. The connective tissue capsule of the spindle attaches to the connective tissue of the stroma of the muscle, while some of the intrafusal muscle fibers penetrate the capsule so as to attach directly to adjacent extrafusal muscle fibers.

The central portion of the spindle, representing the sensory endings, is composed of two groups of collections of intrafusal muscle fibers, namely the nuclear bag and the nuclear chain. There are about twice as many nuclear chain fibers as bag fibers. Because of their being arranged in parallel to the extrafusal fiber counterparts, an induced muscle stretch will result in the stretch of the central portion of the spindle, which then will lead to excitation of the sensory afferent nerve endings. In contradistinction to this noncontractile central portion of the spindle, there are contractile elements aggregated at the polar ends of the intrafusal muscle fibers. These contractile portions of the spindle's polar ends can be induced to contract and thus bring tension to the spindle, especially in a state when it would otherwise have shortened concomitantly with the contraction of the surrounding muscle (see the discussion of the gamma system below).

Spindle Innervation and Function

Muscle Spindle—Sensory Innervation

The sensory innervation at the spindle level is obtained via two sensory ending systems. The primary endings, which will transmit information to type Ia fibers, coil around the central region of the nuclear bag and chain

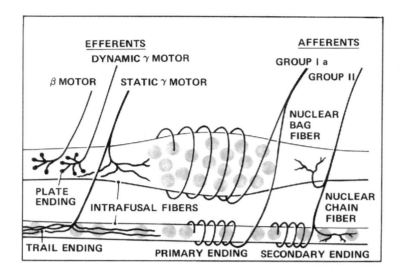

Figure 2.5. Diagrammatic representation of the intrafusal muscle fiber within the muscle spindle and related nerve endings. (Reprinted with permission from S Gilman, S Winans Newman. Manter and Gatz's Essentials of Clinical Neuroanatomy and Neurophysiology [7th ed]. Philadelphia: FA Davis, 1990.)

fibers. The secondary endings spiral around the areas adjacent to the central portion of the intrafusal fiber, primarily on the chain and bag fibers. The information from the secondary endings is transmitted via type II fibers, which are usually smaller in size than the type Ia fibers of the primary endings. The primary and secondary endings not only differ in their spatial arrangement, but there is a noted functional difference in response to a stretch in muscle as well. Whereas both endings are affected by prolonged, slow muscle stretch (static stretch), the primary endings are extremely responsive to dynamic stretch situations, that is, to the rate of change in muscle length.

Spindle Motor Innervation: Efferent Information

Each spindle receives at the contractile polar region (both the nuclear bag and the chain fiber) its efferent innervation from gamma motoneurons and skeletofusimotor fibers [9]. The latter fibers represent collaterals of motor axons connecting alpha motoneurons to extrafusal muscle fibers [9, 10].

The dynamic and static fusimotor systems can be controlled independently of each other by stimulation of different supraspinal structures [11]. It is suggested [12] that under a very controlled experimental set-up, fusimotor fibers to relaxed human skeletal muscles do not subject the spindles to significant background drive.

The Golgi Tendon Organ

The GTO ends freely between the collagenous fibers of the tendons and is primarily located at the muscle-tendon junction. In contradistinction to the muscle spindle, the GTO is arranged in series with the extrafusal muscle fibers. The afferent fiber connected with the GTO is the type Ib fiber. The fiber's terminals have a high threshold to externally applied muscle stretch. The usual stimulus to type Ib fibers is contraction of the extrafusal muscle fibers. Yet, as pointed out by Houk et al. [13], the active force required to fire a GTO is rather small and a GTO may even fire in response to contraction of a single in-series fiber. On the other hand, passive stretch of the muscle does not cause the GTO to fire quickly, because the fascial tissues surrounding the muscle fascicles accept the passive tension produced by the stretch [12].

Interneurons, or Beyond the Monosynaptic Stretch Reflex

Customarily the spinal cord has been likened to a simple relay station providing nothing more than mere connecting points between incoming messages and more-or-less "filtered" outgoing impulses. The simplest of such a relay circuit is exemplified by the monosynaptic reflex. There, the alpha motoneuron is directed to fire directly in response to the one-on-

one incoming impulses from its corresponding type Ia fiber (Fig. 2.6). Most reflexes, however, are routed through polysynaptic connections in a myriad of interneurons. Much of the information presented in this section is obtained from a superb and extremely readable review by Davidoff [12].

The majority of the spinal interneurons receive a wide and diverse convergence of inputs from several different peripheral sources, as well as supraspinal sources. The reflex apparatus and descending fiber systems apparently make use of many of the same spinal segmental neurons in interconnected ways [12].

The discussion at hand concentrates on three types of interneurons, namely the Renshaw cells, the type Ia inhibitory interneurons, and the interneurons mediating group I nonreciprocal inhibition.

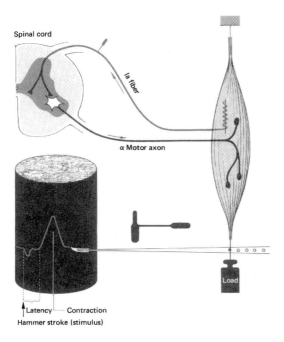

Figure 2.6. The reflex arc of the monosynaptic stretch reflex. Note the latency period between the hammer stroke to the tendon and the deflection induced by muscle contraction. The sensation of stretch is transmitted via the Ia fibers to the spinal cord so as to induce the reflex via the alpha motoneurons emanating from the anterior horn cell. (Reprinted with permission from RF Schmidt. Fundamentals of Neurophysiology. New York: Springer, 1985.)

Renshaw Cells: Recurrent Inhibition

Renshaw cells are responsible for recurrent inhibition (Fig. 2.7). Collateral axon branches arising from the alpha motoneuron send information to the neighboring Renshaw cell, which in turn directs inhibitory signals back to the sender alpha motoneuron as well as to other alpha motoneurons in close proximity. Renshaw cells also inhibit gamma motoneurons, type Ia inhibitory interneurons, and other Renshaw cells [14, 15].

Type Ia Inhibitory Interneurons: Reciprocal Inhibition

Reciprocal inhibition of antagonist muscles is mediated by type Ia inhibitory interneurons (Fig. 2.8). Induced stretch to the spindle in the agonist muscle increases the agonist motoneuron discharge via the segmental reflex arc. At the same time motoneurons of the antagonist muscles are inhibited by way of the type Ia inhibitory interneurons.

Again, carefully controlled experimental studies point in the direction of a delicately developed system in which type Ia afferents inhibit certain alpha motoneurons that are not strict mechanical agonists [16].

Interneurons Mediating Group I Nonreciprocal Inhibition: The Golgi Tendon Organ Connection

It has been the long-held notion that type Ib afferents from a particular muscle are specifically concerned with local force ("tension") feedback to that muscle (the previous name designation plays reference to that notion: they were previously called the Ib inhibitory interneurons). This has been found to be untrue [12] (Fig. 2.9).

Instead of being exclusively "assigned" to type Ib afferent fibers, the associated interneurons receive an equal amount of input from group Ia muscle spindle afferents [17]. This means that these interneurons are excited in a parallel fashion by both the type Ia and type Ib afferents, which prompted the creation of the rather simple designation "interneurons mediating group I nonreciprocal inhibition" [18–21].

Davidoff [12] stated that such complex connections are necessary components for coordination because some muscles have more than one action, and some

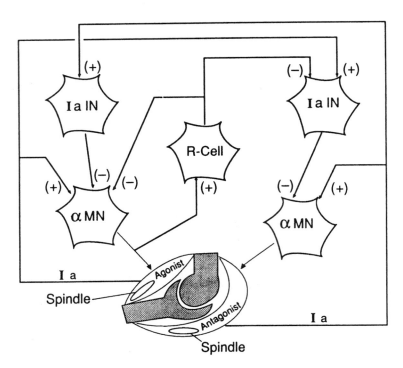

Figure 2.7. The Renshaw circuit. Note that the Renshaw cell assumes an integral part in recurrent inhibition: the alpha motoneuron discharge excites the Renshaw cell (through collaterals), which in turn forwards inhibitory signals back to the sending alpha motoneuron (recurrent inhibition), and also to the Ia inhibitory neurons. Thus, it appears that the Renshaw cells back the activity of the most active members of a synergy group while inhibiting others. (IN = interneuron; MN = motoneuron.) (Reprinted with permission from MB Glenn, J Whyte. The Practical Management of Spasticity in Children and Adults. Philadelphia: Lea & Febiger, 1990.)

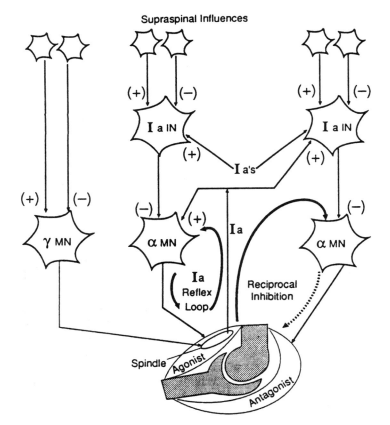

Figure 2.8. The gamma fusimotor system, with the associated stretch reflex component and reciprocal inhibition. Note the supraspinal influences, which have both excitatory and inhibitory effects upon the Ia interneurons, depending on the different situations. (IN = interneuron; MN = motoneuron.) (Reprinted with permission from MB Glenn, J Whyte. The Practical Management of Spasticity in Children and Adults. Philadelphia: Lea & Febiger, 1990.)

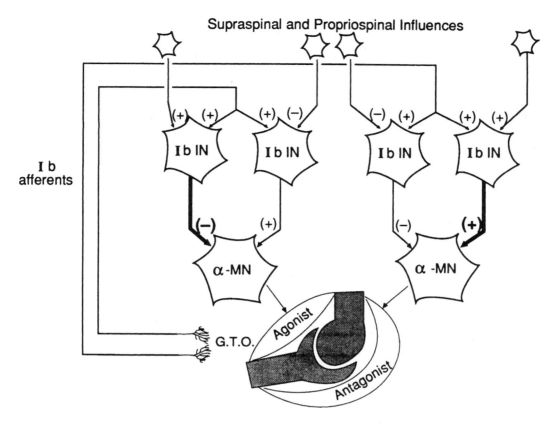

Figure 2.9. The agonist-antagonist interaction and the influences of the Ib afferents and interneurons. (IN = interneuron; MN = motoneuron; GTO = Golgi tendon organ.) (Reprinted with permission from MB Glenn, J Whyte. The Practical Management of Spasticity in Children and Adults. Philadelphia: Lea & Febiger, 1990.)

muscles work at more than one joint. This leads to the logical extension that to be able to maintain complex movements and movement patterns, the "system" must have a sufficiently high level of plasticity that allows for variation on the one hand while at the same time ensuring that routine events take place "automatically."

Interneuron Connections

In addition to intersegmental and intrasegmental interneuronal connections, supraspinal fiber influences have a major impact on the interneurons. Again, the interneurons are more than mere intercalated stations to subserve one-to-one relay stations.

The convergence of afferent and descending input on interneurons has two significant consequences [12]. First, transmission through the interneurons is determined not only by the excitatory input from a particular set of primary afferents (e.g., type Ia afferents), but is also a function of the summation of excitatory and inhibitory inputs converging from other afferent and descending fibers [21, 22]. Second, a stereotyped reflex, the same reflex circuit activated by excitation of a particular set of peripheral receptors, does not always bring about the same stereotyped reflex responses because of the extensive convergence from descending and afferent inputs [12].

Interneuron Presynaptic Inhibition

In recent studies, it has become apparent that reflex actions can be modified in either direction—that is, either enhanced or reduced. There seem to exist finely tuned spinal input-output patterns that are a function of which types of afferent fibers are stimulated and which other afferent fibers receive primary afferent depolarization (PAD)—the process by which inhibition is brought about [12, 23]. Activity in group I, primarily the group Ib afferents, is reported to lead to PAD in type Ia fibers, but not vice versa, that is, little or no PAD of type Ia origin is produced in type Ib afferents [12]. Furthermore, PAD of muscle proprioceptors can be induced by activation of pathways descending from a variety of supraspinal structures [24, 25].

In summary, the "system" seems to be set up so as to optimize the spinal cord reflex apparatus both under conditions when muscle spindle–determined position feedback is critical or under conditions where GTO-determined tension feedback is paramount [12].

Long-Latency Responses

Laboratory studies have demonstrated that in addition to the short-latency monosynaptic responses [26, 27], there are additional responses with longer latencies. These long-latency responses also appear to be significantly more potent than the monosynaptic response [26–29].

Even though not conclusively proven in the presently available research studies, it appears that the source of the afferent input for the long-latency responses can be attributed to the muscle spindle [30, 31], especially when sudden stretch is induced in an already isometrically contracting muscle (12). The information appears to be relayed through long-loop neural pathways to supraspinal structures [28, 32–35]. It is suggested that a transcortical reflex is involved [32, 36–38] in which motoneurons are stimulated to fire at the level of the sensorimotor cortex, thus generating late muscle responses [39]. The exact source of afferent input for and the specific role or roles of the long-latency reflex, particularly in relation to manipulative procedures, have not been conclusively identified.

From Spinal Cord to Effector Organ: Anterior Horn: Alpha, Beta, Gamma Motoneurons

Once the information in the spinal cord has been "sorted out" and is ready for transmission, there are essentially three motoneuron pathways: the alpha, beta, and gamma motoneurons. The least known of these three are the beta motoneurons, which inner-

vate both the intrafusal and extrafusal muscle fibers. The beta fibers receive input from both group Ia and II afferent fibers [10]. Yet the significance of this potentially important beta motoneuron feedback system has not been elucidated [12].

The alpha motoneuron has been called by Sherrington [40] the "final common path." Located in the anterior horn of the spinal gray matter are the cell bodies of the alpha motoneuron, which supplies the skeletal muscles. It should be noted here that the Bell-Magendie law, a long-standing neuroanatomic tenet, states that the dorsal root comprises solely primary afferent fibers and the ventral root solely efferent fibers of various sorts [41]. However, it now appears that, based on studies in cats and preliminary findings in humans, a number of the ventral root fibers are finely myelinated or unmyelinated primary afferents. This may be, at least in part, responsible for the persistence of or the return of pain after dorsal root ablation [41].

Alpha motoneurons are bundled together in groups, separated through interneurons. The topical organization is such that the neurons supplying the axial musculature find their cell bodies located more medially, whereas those for the limbs are located more laterally (Fig. 2.10).

Synaptic contacts on alpha motoneurons arise from a variety of sources and include type Ia afferent fibers from primary spindle endings; group II axons from secondary spindle endings; descending reticulo-, vestibulo-, rubro-, and corticospinal fibers; and excitatory and inhibitory interneurons, which form the majority of synaptic connections [12].

Whereas in the past it has been thought that the only determinant of alpha motoneuron discharge was the summation of the many asynchronous postsynaptic potentials coming from segmental and descending sources, it is now realized that the resting excitability and the response properties of alpha motoneurons depend on specialized intrinsic membrane properties [42]. This is an important concept, the ramifications of which can only be surmised at this time.

The third motoneuron pathway—that composed of the gamma interneurons—is described in the next section.

Alpha and Gamma Motoneurons: Coactivation

The gamma motoneurons, which innervate the contractile portion of the muscle spindle, have

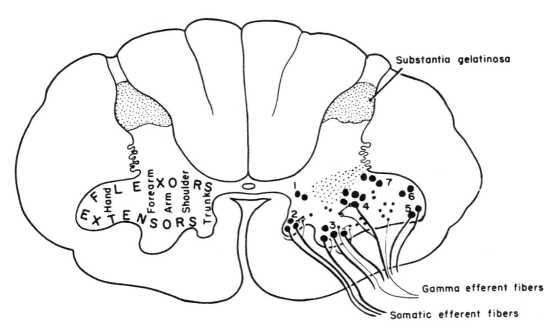

Figure 2.10. Motor nuclei location in the anterior gray horn of a lower cervical segment of the spinal cord. The general organization is such that the flexor muscle groups are arranged posteriorly, whereas the extensor groups are more anterior in the anterior gray horn. The nuclei of the trunk muscles are most medial, while the nuclei of the hand muscles are most lateral. Motor nuclei indicated on the right are: 1 = posteromedial; 2 = anteromedial; 3 = anterior; 4 = central; 5 = anterolateral; 6 = posterolateral; and 7 = retroposterolateral. Note the collaterals from somatic efferent axons that return to gray matter and synapse on small, medially placed Renshaw cells. Smaller cells appearing as the dotted zone in the intermediate gray zone indicate the area of the internuncial neuron pool. (Reprinted with permission from MB Carpenter. Core Text of Neuroanatomy [2nd ed]. Baltimore: Williams & Wilkins, 1978.)

been found to work in conjunction with the alpha motoneuron. A good number of different segmental and descending neuronal pathways evoke parallel effects in the alpha and gamma motoneurons that supply a given muscle or a group of synergistic muscles [43]. Alpha and gamma motoneurons innervating extrafusal and intrafusal muscle fibers in the same muscles receive a largely congruent synaptic input from group II afferents, flexor reflex afferents (FRAs) (Fig. 2.11), inhibitory interneurons, and supraspinal structures [12]. This "coactivation" of both the alpha and gamma systems ensures that the spindle remains at "tension" at all times—that is, it must be in a "loaded" situation, even when the surrounding muscle is shortened. Otherwise the spindle would, because of its parallel arrangement within the muscle and in the absence of any polar stretch, simply shorten every time the muscle shortens. (One may recall picking up a near-empty beer stein while thinking it was still full and spilling it.)

At this juncture, a logical extension of the above topic would be a detailed review of somatic reflexes. This discussion is beyond the scope of this chapter, so standard physiology texts should be consulted.

Classification of reflexes can be based on many a specific category (none of which can be all-encompassing, however), such as the type of stimulus and its response (somatosomatic, somatovisceral, viscerosomatic, and viscerovisceral), the number of synapses, levels of central nervous system involvement, and the type of pathologic condition present (upper motor neuron lesion, for instance). The simplest reflex is the monosynaptic, or muscle-stretch reflex. All the other known reflexes involve at least two synapses (inhibition of antagonists) or are polysynaptic (flexor withdrawal, crossed extensor reflex, etc.).

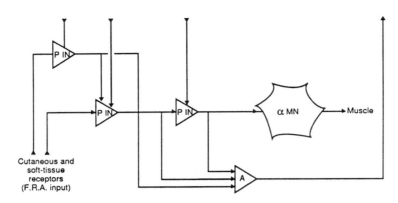

Figure 2.11. Flexor reflex afferent (FRA) pathways. P IN refers to propriospinal interneurons, which, because of their long ascending *and* descending axons, functionally interconnect the spinal cord horizontally (segmentally) and longitudinally. The P INs harmonize spinal afferent signals with intrinsic spinal activities so as to relay "the message" to the forebrain. They contribute to the propriospinal reflex mechanisms.

If two activated reflex systems occur at the same time, the one that is of more importance to the survival of the subject switches off the other. In general, protective reflexes (those that protect the organism from injury—i.e., response to irritation or pain) have a greater survival value than do postural reflexes [44]. The protective reflex is said to be prepotent to the postural reflex. However, it has not been conclusively shown what a reflex's long-term effects are when it is maintained for prolonged periods of time while it "overtakes" another. The somatovisceral and viscerosomatic reflex patterns and their clinical significance are addressed further below.

Skeletal Muscle Pathophysiology

Slow Twitch (Type I) and Fast Twitch (Type II) Fibers

Human skeletal muscle is responsible for the movement of the skeleton and organs such as the globe of the eye and the tongue [45]. Muscle is composed of contractile and connective tissue elements. The endomysium, a delicate connective tissue surrounding and thus separating the individual muscle fibers, is made up of reticulin fibers. Individual muscle fibers are grouped together within so-called fascicles, with the loose surrounding connective tissue called perimysium. Many fasciculi make up the muscle proper, which in turn is clad by an outer and dense connective tissue called the epimysium. Connective tissue of skeletal muscle also contains elastin fibers, which are more common in muscles attached to soft tissues (e.g., tongue, face). The connective tissue component of skeletal muscle has the mechanical function of controlling the degree of extension and contraction of the muscle and is involved in the generation of "stiffness" [1]. Three types of skeletal muscle can be differentiated simply on the basis of "color": red, white, and intermediate. They differ not only in their gross appearance, but also in the mode of energy metabolism, from aerobic through an intermediate type to anaerobic. The "red" muscles are also known as slow twitch muscles or the tonic or postural muscles, whereas the "white" muscles are referred to as fast twitch muscles or phasic muscles. Their differences are juxtaposed in Table 2.3. Functionally, it is important to remember that muscles concerned primarily with posture (type I fibers) tend to shorten in response to a functional disturbance, whereas the phasic muscles tend to become weak in response to a functional disturbance [7]. For example, it is a well-known clinical observation that the tonic hamstring muscles frequently are "tight" in response to some disturbance or dysfunction, they have shortened; yet we talk about the phasic abdominal muscles as weak rather than shortened when they become dysfunctional.

Autonomic Nervous System

Of great clinical interest in the past, especially in the osteopathic literature, have been interactions between somatic and visceral organs. In this discussion of the thoracic spine and the associated neurophysiologic considerations, the sympathetic nervous system and its participation in the various reflex components takes on a central role (Figs. 2.12 and 2.13). In contradistinction to the somatic nervous system, which

Table 2.3. Comparison of Tonic (Slow Twitch) and Phasic (Fast Twitch) Muscles

Flexion	Slow Twitch (I)	Fast Twitch (II)
Function	Tonic postural	Phasic
Twitch speed	Slow	Fast
Metabolism/enzymes	Oxidative	Glycolytic
Myosin ATPase	Low activity	High activity
Fatigability rate	Slow	Rapid
"Color"	Red	White
Capillary density	High	Low
Spindle number	High	Moderate
Innervation	α_2 motor neuron	α_1 motor neuron
Reaction to functional disturbance	Shortening	Weakening

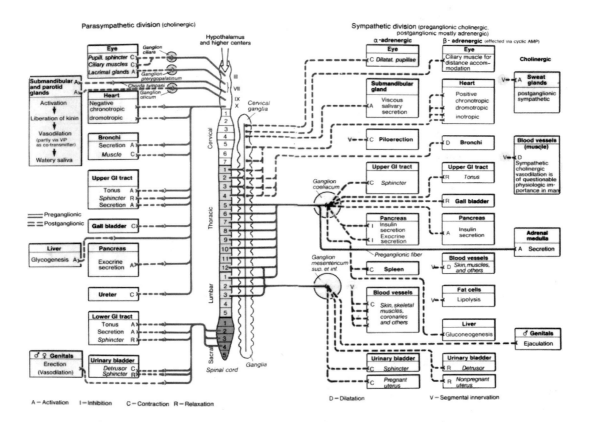

Figure 2.12. The functional organization of the autonomic nervous system, with the sympathetic division represented on the right side of the diagram and the parasympathetic division on the left side. Of interest is the segmental innervation (identified by "V") of the blood vessels of muscle, skin, coronaries, and "others." (Reprinted from A Despopolous, S Silbernagl. Color Atlas of Physiology [4th ed]. New York: Thieme, 1991.)

deals with the "outside motor system," the autonomic nervous system (ANS) is the functional division of the peripheral nervous system that encompasses the innervation of cardiac muscle and glands. It is thus responsible for the innervation of all of the body's effector organs excluding the skeletal muscles [44].

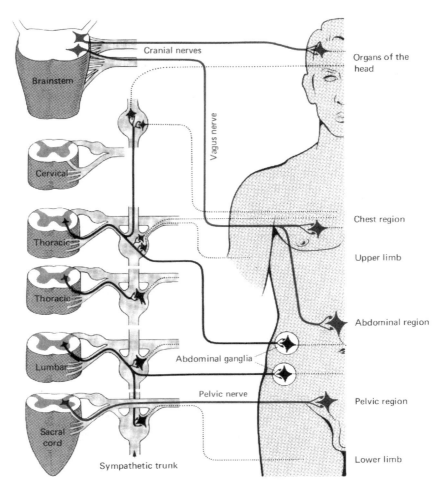

Figure 2.13. Origins of the sympathetic (thoracolumbar spine) and the parasympathetic (cervicosacral spine) neurons, and the regions of the body they innervate. (Reprinted with permission from RF Schmidt. Fundamentals of Neurophysiology. New York: Springer, 1985.)

Although by its original definition, the ANS consists of motor fibers only (general visceral efferents), the sensory fibers (general visceral afferents) accompanying the motor fibers to the viscera are integrally related, both anatomically and functionally, with the motor fibers and must be considered to be part of the ANS [43].

The ANS, functioning at the subconscious level, integrates all "internal" functions but does not do so independently, because it is in constant communication with the somatic motor system (Fig. 2.14). Thus, the autonomic and somatic system may best be viewed as a functionally married system. Neuroimmunologic interactions will not be addressed

here; rather, see the concise review presented by Ader et al. [46].

Unlike the somatic motor system, however, the peripheral autonomic system carries the electrical impulses to the related effector organs via a two-neuron chain [45]. The ANS has been divided into sympathetic and parasympathetic branches. Even though the internal organs as a rule receive their ANS input from both subsets, the sympathetic nervous system (SNS) will be discussed here in more detail and at the relative exclusion of the parasympathetic nervous system (PNS).

The thoracolumbar SNS fibers arise in the intermediolateral gray column (forming the lateral horn)

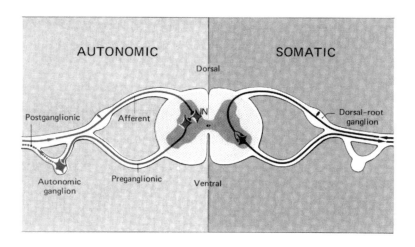

Figure 2.14. The autonomic reflex arc (polysynaptic, left side) in comparison with the somatic reflex arc (monosynaptic, right side). (IN = interneuron.) (Reprinted with permission from RF Schmidt. Fundamentals of Neurophysiology. New York: Springer, 1985.)

of the 12 thoracic and first two lumbar spinal segments (Fig. 2.15). In contrast, the PNS outflow fibers arise in cell bodies located in cranial and sacral levels.

Sympathetic Nervous System: A Brief Overview

The preganglionic SNS fibers, which originate in the intermediolateral gray column, after leaving the spinal cord course along the motor fibers through the ventral roots, where they split off to form the white communicating rami (see Fig. 2.13). They continue on to reach the chain ganglia of the sympathetic trunks. There are only a total of 14 white communicating rami on each side of the body.

In addition to these paired ganglia, there have been identified unpaired ganglia in the abdominal and pelvic regions. The preganglionic fibers of these unpaired ganglia pass right through the sympathetic trunk ganglia.

An important "safety factor" that guarantees ganglionic transmission is established by an intricate set of diverging and converging connections within the ganglia (see Fig. 2.15). Reflex regulation in the ANS is not unlike that of the somatic nervous system. The SNS and PNS function individually yet act reciprocally, just as the agonist and antagonist systems do.

Visceral reflex circuits are always polysynaptic. Visceral afferent fibers enter through the dorsal root ganglion and with a consistent pattern of central termination throughout the spinal cord with

areas of projection in laminae I and V but sparing the intermediate dorsal horn (laminae II, III, and IV) (Figure 2.16). The joint afferents terminate in lamina I and also some of the deeper layers (V–VII). Interestingly, some dorsal horn neurons are not driven by visceral afferent fibers and can only be excited from their somatic receptive fields [47]. Other cells have, in addition to their somatic input, an excitatory visceral drive (viscerosomatic neurons), which leads to the conclusion that the effects of visceral stimulation can only be mediated through convergent signals via somatosensory pathways [47].

Researchers from the basic sciences convened in 1989 at the American Academy of Osteopathy's International Symposium to present a state of the art update on the theme of "The Central Connection: Somatovisceral/Viscerosomatic Interaction." Again, although the temptation to present more detailed information of that symposium is great, the constraints of space allow only a synoptic overview.

Reflexes Between the Somatic and Visceral Systems

Interactions between the somatic and visceral organs are usually expressed as pathophysiologic changes in somatic structures brought about by reflexes triggered from internal organs [47] (Fig. 2.17). Some of these reflexes can persist beyond the time course of the original stimulus and can produce effects disproportionate to the stimulus intensity, leading to chronic changes [2, 47].

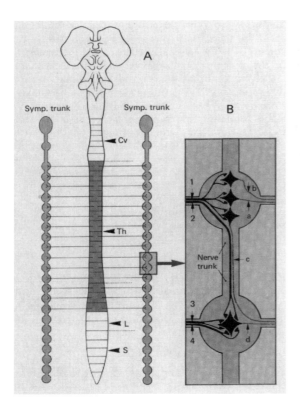

Figure 2.15. The sympathetic trunks. A. Position of the left and right sympathetic trunks in relation to the spinal cord and brain stem. The ganglia depicted are drawn oversize in reference to the spinal cord segments (the lumbar and sacral regions of the cord are too long compared with the sympathetic trunks). (Cv = cervical cord; Th = thoracic cord; L = lumbar cord; S = sacral cord. B. Divergence (1 onto a, b, and c) and convergence (2, 3, and 4 onto d) of preganglionic axons onto postganglionic neurons in the sympathetic trunk ganglia. (Reprinted with permission from W Jaenig. The Autonomic Nervous System. In RF Schmidt [ed], Fundamentals of Neurophysiology [3rd ed]. New York: Springer, 1985.)

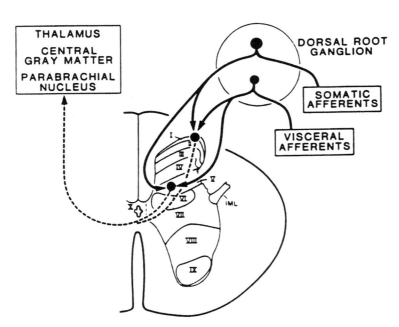

Figure 2.16. The representative areas of contribution to the dorsal horn from the somatic and visceral afferents. Notably involved are laminae I and V. (Reprinted with permission from F Cervero. Visceral and Spinal Components of Viscero-Somatic Interactions. In MM Patterson, JN Howell [eds], The Central Connection: Somatovisceral/Viscerosomatic Interaction. Indianapolis: American Academy of Osteopathy, 1992;77–85.)

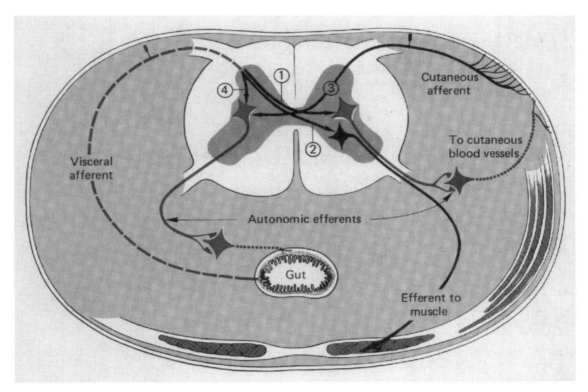

Figure 2.17. The synaptic connections joining the autonomic and somatic efferents and somatic and visceral afferents in the spinal cord to form the various reflex arcs: 1 = viscerocutaneous reflex; 2 = viscerosomatic reflex; 3 = cutaneovisceral reflex; 4 = intestinointestinal reflex. Interneurons in the spinal cord have been omitted for simplicity. (Reprinted with permission from RF Schmidt. Fundamentals of Neurophysiology. New York: Springer, 1985.)

A viscerosomatic reflex (Fig. 2.18) is the result of afferent stimuli arising from a visceral dysfunction, where impulses from visceral receptors are transmitted to the dorsal horn of the spinal cord, synapsing with interconnecting neurons [48]. After central processing at the spinal cord level—through convergence, divergence, facilitation, and suppression—the resultant "net" efferent information will be reflected in sensory and motor changes in the somatic tissues [48]. Cervero [47] further stated that there appear to exist different groups of neurons within the spinal cord that respond in different ways to the same kind of stimulus. This may be yet another indication of the hitherto unappreciated plasticity of such neurons. There are differences in neuronal response as well. Some neurons may respond quickly to any noxious stimulus, whereas other neurons do not react unless subjected to strong noxious stimuli, which may occur possibly in a pathologic condition lasting for hours or days before they can express any changes [47].

The following synopsis of the various reflex patterns is based mainly on the concise conclusions forwarded by Cervero [47].

Viscerovisceral Reflexes

Viscerovisceral reflexes are local reflexes. A noxious stimulus can trigger a number of reflexes entirely mediated by peripheral components of the nervous system and contained at a local level. The associated changes, either in the peripheral branches of the primary afferent fibers or changes in motility or secretion, can subsequently alter the peripheral environment of the sensory organs that innervate the internal organs. This cycle then can continue, leading to further peripheral and central changes. Thus, sympathetic efferents to the intestine are also excited by the visceral afferents from the intestine itself (see Fig. 2.17).

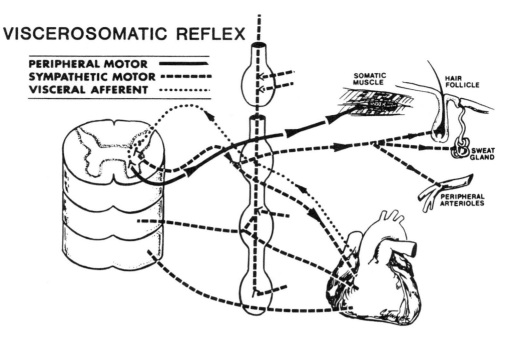

VISCEROSOMATIC REFLEX

PERIPHERAL MOTOR ━━━━
SYMPATHETIC MOTOR ▪▪▪▪▪▪▪
VISCERAL AFFERENT ••••••••

SOMATIC MUSCLE

HAIR FOLLICLE

SWEAT GLAND

PERIPHERAL ARTERIOLES

Figure 2.18. Schematic representation of the viscerosomatic reflex organization. The reflex, in this example, is initiated at the heart and transmitted through the visceral somatic afferent system, and impulses are then relayed back from the spinal cord to the respective effector organ, via reflex action, through either the sympathetic motor efferents, the peripheral motor efferents, or both. (Reprinted with permission from MC Beal. Viscerosomatic Reflexes. In MM Patterson, JN Howell [eds], The Central Connection: Somatovisceral/Viscerosomatic Interaction. Indianapolis: American Academy of Osteopathy, 1992;19–27.)

Viscerosomatic Reflexes

With viscerosomatic reflexes, some changes in internal environment have been allowed in one of the viscera (or induced in controlled laboratory situations). The stimuli for such changes, which also can be associated with pain production, include inflammatory processes, obstruction or enlargement of a viscus, rupture, ischemia, or chemical irritation [49].

When visceral afferents are stimulated, one may clinically observe reddening of the skin area (viscerocutaneous reflex). One may also see accompanying "tightness" of abdominal muscles (viscerosomatic reflex). This clinical observation leads to the conclusion that the visceral afferents of the intestines are connected to (1) autonomic efferents to the cutaneous blood vessels, and (2) autonomic efferents to the abdominal muscles, which establishes the viscerosomatic reflex [50].

It is again emphasized that these spinal reflexes are under a considerable amount of supraspinal modulation and control. Their functional substrate is the convergence of visceral and somatic afferent fibers onto spinal motoneurons [47].

Somatovisceral Reflexes

Somatic nerve stimulation can regulate various visceral functions that are reflex in nature [51]. Studies confirm the notion that not only do they differ in the effects from one organ to another, but one site of somatic stimulation also differs from another [51]. The responses can vary from general (cardiac, adrenal function) to specific segmental organization (gastric, vesicle) [51]. It has also been shown that some hormones are reflexly regulated by stimulation of somatic nerves.

Positive Feedback Loops

Positive feedback loops (Fig. 2.19) are feedback loops between the spinal cord and the brain stem.

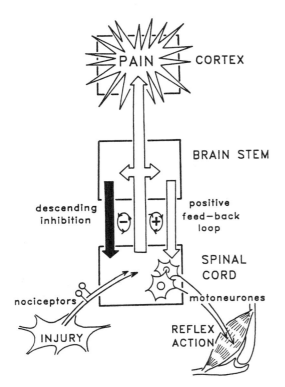

Figure 2.19. The various components of viscerosomatic interactions, including supraspinal, spinal, and peripheral ("infraspinal") structures. (Reprinted with permission from F Cervero. Visceral and Spinal Components of Viscero-Somatic Interactions. In MM Patterson, JN Howell [eds], The Central Connection: Somatovisceral/Viscerosomatic Interaction. Indianapolis: American Academy of Osteopathy, 1992;77–85.)

The reflexes are long lasting, mediated by a positive feedback loop between spinal and supraspinal (brain stem) areas involved in modulation of visceral and somatic sensorimotor integration. The main consequence of the activation of these loops is the maintenance of a state of high excitability with viscerosomatic systems, which will evoke long-lasting changes in somatic and visceral reflexes [51].

Nociception and Pain

Pain is an unpleasant sensory impression accompanied by awareness of a disagreeable experience. It is the reaction to the message that damage to the organism either has already occurred or is about to occur (nociception) [2]. Identification of the cause may be difficult and less important to some authors than the recognition of the effect [2].

Within the context of this discussion a brief review of recent research data is presented to demonstrate that (1) pain is not an independent sensation; (2) joint inflammation and possibly mechanical factors sensitize and activate nocicensors, and (3) pathophysiologic increases in nocicensor activity can lead to central sensitization [52].

The "old" gate theory presented by Melzack and Wall [53] suggested that while the thick myelinated afferent fibers inhibit ascending neurons of the nociceptive system ("gate closed"), the fine nociceptive afferents activate the afferent fibers ("gate open"). This view had to be modified in part and broadened to better explain the rationale for therapeutic interventions such as physical therapy and electrical stimulation [50, 52].

Both the nociceptive and mechanoreceptive fibers enter the gray matter of the spinal cord through the dorsal root in the posterior horn (Fig. 2.20; also see Fig. 2.16). In the spinal cord, the nociceptive fibers divide into many collateral branches. Some of these branches project directly through the gray matter to the basal nuclei (laminae IV and V). They also travel through the lateral spinothalamic tract and reach the limbic system, where the actual perception of pain occurs (see Fig. 2.20).

Based on the extensive work done by Schmidt et al. [52], some of their conclusions are presented here directly (Figs. 2.21 and 2.22).

1. All the parts of the nociceptive system may be modified in their function by pathophysiologic processes.
2. Joint pain is a consequence of activity in the nociceptive system, but not every activation of this system leads to conscious pain sensations.
3. Sensory, emotional, vegetative, and motor components contribute to the sensation and evaluation of pain.
4. Pathophysiologic processes may modify all pain components.
5. Joint inflammation sensitizes all fine afferents, and, in particular, the "sleeping" nociceptors "wake up."
6. The pathophysiologic increase in nocicensor activity leads to central sensitization.
7. The receptive fields of the neurons are not restricted to the joint but spread out much further. Because of the mechanism of convergence on these neurons, it is possible that pain arising from a joint is not restricted to the inflamed joint.

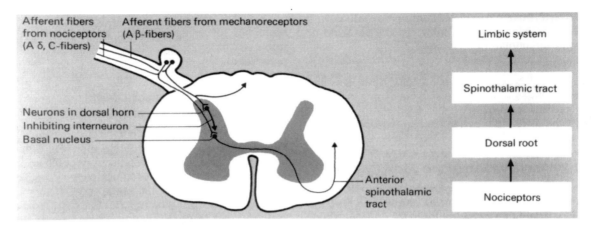

Figure 2.20. Fibers of nociceptors and mechanoreceptors in the region of the posterior horns. (Reprinted with permission from J Dvorak, V Dvorak. Manual Medicine–Diagnostics [2nd ed]. New York: Thieme, 1990.)

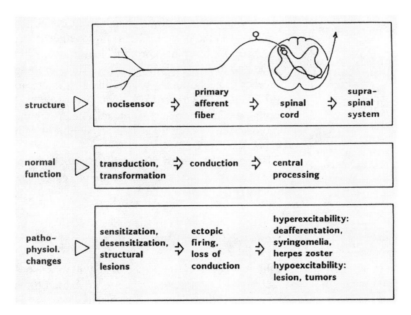

Figure 2.21. Transduction, transformation, and conduction of nociceptive information, including examples of pathophysiologic changes within the nociceptive system. At each level of the system, enhancement as well as diminution of the excitability may occur. Enhancement of excitability (sensitization) in the nociceptive system regularly leads to pathophysiologic pain sensations (e.g., allodynia, hyperalgesia, hyperpathia). (Reprinted with permission from RF Schmidt. Neurophysiological Mechanisms of Arthritic Pain. In MM Patterson, JN Howell [eds], The Central Connection: Somatovisceral/Viscerosomatic Interaction. Indianapolis: American Academy of Osteopathy, 1992.)

8. The mechanisms of the central sensitization have not yet been fully clarified.

Van Buskirk [54] presented an interesting model in which nociceptive reflexes are viewed as the source of the various changes that accompany somatic dysfunction (Figure 2.23).

In summary, information processing at both the spinal and supraspinal levels appears to be embedded in a background of far-reaching plasticity, more so than in isolated, one-on-one electrical pathway phenomena. This increased input from injured or inflamed areas has relevance at least on two levels: (1) the way and means by which the inputs are handled in the cord; and (2) the overall excitability of that area of the spinal cord [55].

From Palpation to the Facilitated Segment and Back

Palpatory examination findings have long been used by clinicians in identifying visceral reflex "reflections" onto the surface of the body. Early work was

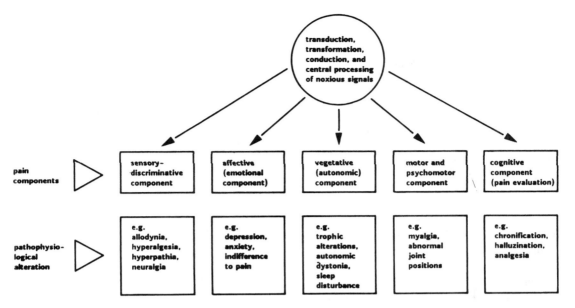

Figure 2.22. The various pain components activated by nociceptive signals and their potential pathophysiologic modifications. Note that pathophysiologic changes in the peripheral and central nociceptive systems may lead to pathophysiologic pain sensations; similarly, this may also happen in the central nervous structures dealing with emotion, and motivation and cognition can become disturbed. (Reprinted with permission from RF Schmidt. Neurophysiological Mechanisms of Arthritic Pain. In MM Patterson, JN Howell [eds], The Central Connection: Somatovisceral/Viscerosomatic Interaction. Indianapolis: American Academy of Osteopathy, 1992.)

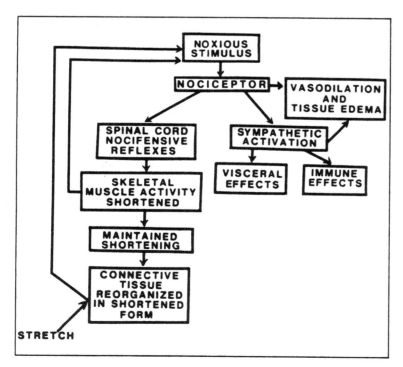

Figure 2.23. A model that underscores the nociceptive origin and maintenance of the somatic dysfunction. (Reprinted with permission from RL van Buskirk. Nociceptive reflexes and the somatic dysfunction: a model. J Am Osteopath Assoc 1990;90:792–809.)

done in this area by Denslow [56, 57]. He inferred from his observations of hyperirritability of tissues over the spinous process of a vertebra that there might be involved hyperactive autonomic reflexes in the associated segment. This led to the notion of the "facilitated" segment, a fundamental premise in the osteopathic profession. Korr [58] likened the facilitated segment to a neurologic lens that allows the *clinician* to focus on the activities in skeletal and visceral organs. We may now know more about many components of this entity called the "facilitated segment," yet the two central questions remain: (1) What are the factors that ultimately lower the threshold or that initiate the facilitation, and (2) what sustains it for prolonged periods of time? [59].

Palpatory evidence of somatic dysfunction has been related to segmental areas associated with that particular vertebra. Early palpatory findings include an increase in skin temperature and moisture of the skin, increased subcutaneous fluid, and increased muscle "contractility" or hypertonicity. These tissue changes can be localized at the anatomic reference site of the particular viscus involved [48]. Chronic changes have been correlated with thickening of skin and subcutaneous tissues, localized muscle hypertonicity, and hard and tense skin with hypersensitivity to palpation. I have noted a granular-grainy type of muscle texture when injecting into or "dryneedling" a muscle, for example, and this appears to be different than the "palpable taut band" usually associated with an active myofascial trigger point [60]. Previous studies [57, 61] have shown that an increase in somatic dysfunction in the thoracic spine may potentially be linked to some viscerosomatic reflex phenomenon. Beal demonstrated that a typical spinal somatic reflex pattern associated with cardiovascular disease involves the spinal segments of T1–T5, with the greatest incidence at T2–T3 on the left.

Thoracic Pain and Rib Pain

The above discussion attempts to set the stage and provide an insightful overview of the intricate interrelationships between the various mechanoreceptor, muscle receptor, and nociceptor pathways. Rib pain may be attributed to a joint dysfunction, either by inflammation or abnormal movement pattern (i.e., a "stuck rib" frequently observed by trained clinicians) or abnormal muscle balance surrounding a particular rib and its joint connections, including the neighboring vertebrae. The close proximity to the sympathetic nervous system may sometimes lead to reflex activity not encountered in the "healthy" state.

Some of the pain experienced in the chest wall is diffuse and difficult to localize. Foreman [62] believed this to be because central visceral terminals are sparse compared with somatic terminals (i.e., less than 10% of all afferent fibers in the thoracic and lumbar spine). Future studies within well-controlled designs will surely help shed light on some of the presently perplexing clinical situations, about which exist more hypotheses than explanations.

As pointed out by Schmidt [50] and Fig. 2.22, pain is a multifaceted entity, and the clinician knows that because of the reflex interactions, the patient's report of pain location is not necessarily congruent to the area where the pain generator is located.

Epilogue

Much of the information presented here shows how little is actually known about motor responses, both voluntary and involuntary; about the complexity of reflex patterns and their ability to be enhanced or diminished over time; and about possible interactions, direct or indirect, between nonneural tissues (fascia, bones, etc.) and neural networks (Fig. 2.24).

Exciting developments in the neuromusculoskeletal sciences over the past few decades are bound to lead to promising and relevant applications. Ultimately, new diagnostic and treatment modalities will be introduced and old ones will need to be modified or discarded altogether. As long as both clinicians and basic research scientists are willing to be engaged in a healthy dialogue, each others' queries will serve as starting points for new frontiers otherwise silent (or silenced!) for a long time.

Acknowledgments

Sincere thanks are extended to Ms. Sally Chu and Ms. Deborah Martin, at the Library of Mills-Peninsula Hospitals, Burlingame, California, for their expertise and impressive assistance. Thanks to Mr. Christian Fulmer for his assistance in manuscript preparation.

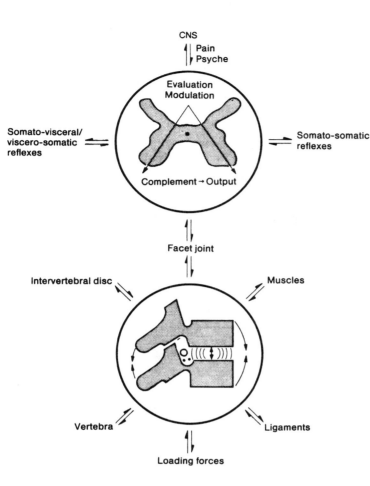

CNS

Pain
Psyche

Evaluation
Modulation

Somato-visceral/
viscero-somatic
reflexes

Somato-somatic
reflexes

Complement → Output

Facet joint

Intervertebral disc

Muscles

Vertebra

Ligaments

Loading forces

Figure 2.24. The facet (apophyseal) joint in its dual function (lower circle) as part of the spinal segment and all related mechanical structures, and (upper circle) as part of the reflexive neurologically mediated feedback mechanism. (CNS = central nervous system.) (Reprinted with permission from HD Neumann. Introduction to Manual Medicine. New York: Springer, 1989.)

References

1. Wheaton J. Introduction to Human Histology. New York: Harper & Row, 1984.
2. Despopolous A, Silbernagl S. Color Atlas of Physiology (4th ed). New York: Thieme, 1991.
3. Freeman MAR, Wyke BD. The innervation of the knee joint. An anatomical and histological study in the cat. J Anat 1967;101:505–512.
4. Wyke BD. Neurological mechanisms in the experience of pain. Acupunct Electrother Res 1979;4:27–35.
5. Wyke BD. Neurology of the cervical spinal joints. Physiotherapy 1979;65:72–79.
6. Wyke BD. The neurological basis of thoracic spinal pain. Rheum Phys Med 1967;10:356.
7. Dvorak J, Dvorak V. Manual Medicine—Diagnostics (2nd ed). New York: Thieme, 1990.
8. Auteroche P. Innervation of the zygapophyseal joints of the lumbar spine. Anat Clin 1983;5:17–18.
9. Jami L, Murthy KSK, Petit J. A quantitative study of skeletofusimotor innervation in the cat peroneus tertius muscle. J Physiol (Lond) 1982;325:125–144.
10. Laporte Y, Emmon-Denant F, Lami L. The skeletofusimotor or beta-innervation of mammalian muscle spindle receptors. J Physiol (Lond) 1962;161:357–373.
11. Janson JKS, Matthews PBC. The central control of the dynamic resonse of muscle spindle receptors. J Physiol (Lond) 1962;161:357–373.
12. Davidoff RA. Skeletal muscle tone and the misunderstood stretch reflex. Neurology 1992;42:951–963.
13. Houk JC, Singer JJ, Henneman E. The adequate stimulus for Golgi tendon organs with observations on the mechanics of the ankle joint. J Neurophysiol 1971;34:1051–1065.
14. Jankowska E, Roberts WJ. Synaptic actions of single interneurons mediating reciprocal Ia inhibition of motoneurons. J Physiol (Lond) 1972;222:623–645.
15. Ryall RW. Renshaw cell mediated inhibition of Renshaw cells: Patterns of excitation and inhibition from impulses in motor axon collaterals. J Neurophysiol 1970;33:257–270.

16. Eccles JC, Lundberg A. Integrative pattern of Ia synaptic actions on motoneurons of hip and knee muscles. J Physiol (Lond) 1958;144:271–298.

17. Fetz EE, Jankowska E, Johannisson T, et al. Autogenetic inhibition of motoneurons by impulses in group Ia muscle spindle afferents. J Physiol (Lond) 1979;293:173–195.

18. Harrison PJ, Jankowska E. Sources of input to interneurones mediating group I nonreciprocal inhibition of motoneurones in the cat. J Physiol (Lond) 1985;361:379–401.

19. Harrison PJ, Jankowska E. Organization of input to interneurons mediating group I nonreciprocal inhibition of motoneurones in the cat. J Physiol (Lond) 1985;361:403–418.

20. Jankowska E, McCrea D. Shared reflex pathways from Ib tendon organ afferents and muscle spindle afferents in the cat. J Physiol (Lond) 1983;338:99–111.

21. Jankowska E, Lundberg A. Interneurones in the spinal cord. Trends Neurosci 1981;4:230–233.

22. Lundberg A. Multisensory control of spinal reflex pathways. Prog Brain Res 1979;50:11–28.

23. Eccles JC. Presynaptic inhibition in the spinal cord. Prog Brain Res 1964;12:65–89.

24. Brink E, Jankowska E, Skoog B. Convergence onto interneurons subserving primary afferent depolarization of group I afferents. J Neurophysiol 1984;51:432–449.

25. Rudomin P, Solodkin M, Jimenez I. Synaptic potentials of primary afferent fibers and motoneurons evoked by single intermediate nucleus interneurons in the cat spinal cord. J Neurophysiol 1987;57:1288–1313.

26. Gottlieb GL, Agarwal GC. Response to sudden torques about ankle in man. II. Postmyotatic reactions. J Neurophysiol 1980;43:86–101.

27. Melville Jones G, Watt DGD. Observations on the control of stepping and hopping movements in man. J Physiol (Lond) 1971;219:709–727.

28. Lee R, Tatton WG. Long Loop Reflexes in Man. Clinical Applications. In JE Desmedt (ed), Progress in Clinical Neurophysiology. Basel: Karger, 1978;4:320–323.

29. Marsden CD, Merton PA, Morton HB. Is the human stretch reflex cortical rather than spinal? Lancet 1973;1:759–761.

30. Chan CWY, Melville Jones G, Catchlove RFH. The late electromyographic response to limb displacement in man II. Sensory origin. Electroencephalogr Clin Neurophysiol 1979;46:182–188.

31. Iles JF. Responses in human pretibial muscles to sudden stretch and to nerve stimulation. Exp Brain Res 1977;30:451–470.

32. Evarts EV, Tanji J. Gating of motor cortex reflexes by prior instruction. Brain Res 1974;71:479–494.

33. Tatton WG, North AGE, Bruce IC, et al. Electromyographic and motor cortical responses to imposed displacements of the cat elbow disparities and homologies with those of the primate wrist. J Neurosci 1983;3:1807–1817.

34. Marsden CD, Merton PA, Morton HB, et al. The effect of posterior column lesions on servo responses from the human long thumb flexor. Brain 1977;100:185–200.

35. Marsden CD, Merton PA, Morton HB. Servo action in the human thumb. J Physiol (Lond) 1976;257:1–44.

36. Adam J, Marsden CD, Merton PA, et al. The effect of lesions in the internal capsule and the sensorimotor cortex on servo action in the human hand. J Physiol (Lond) 1976;254:27–28P.

37. Diener HC, Ackermann H, Dichgans J, et al. Medium- and long-latency responses to displacements of the ankle joint in patients with spinal and central lesions. Electroencephalogr Clin Neurophysiol 1985;60:407–416.

38. Marsden CD, Merton PA, Morton HB. The sensory action of servo action in human muscle. J Physiol (Lond) 1977;265:521–535.

39. Matthews PBC. The human stretch reflex and the motor cortex. Trends Neurosci 1991;14:87–91.

40. Sherrington CS. Decerebrate rigidity and the reflex co-ordination movements. J Physiol (Lond) 1898;22:319–321.

41. Nolte J. The Human Brain—An Introduction to Its Functional Anatomy (3rd ed). St. Louis: Mosby, 1993.

42. Schwindt PC, Crill WE. Membrane Properties of Cat Spinal Motoneurons. In RA Davidoff (ed), Handbook of the Spinal Cord (Vols 2 and 3). New York: Marcel Dekker, 1984:199–242.

43. Baldissera F, Hultborn H, Iller M. Integration in Spinal Neuronal Systems. In VB Brooks (ed), Handbook of Physiology. Vol II. Bethesda: American Physiological Society, 1981;509–595.

44. Holmes O. Human Neurophysiology: A Student Text (2nd ed). London: Chapman and Hall, 1993.

45. Gilman S, Winans Newman S. Manter and Gatz's Essentials of Clinical Neuroanatomy and Neurophysiology (7th ed). Philadelphia: FA Davis, 1990.

46. Ader R, Cohen N, Felten D. Psychoneuroimmunology: Interactions between the nervous system and the immune system. Lancet 1995;345:99–103.

47. Cervero F. Visceral and Spinal Components of Viscero-Somatic Interactions. In MM Patterson, JN Howell (eds), The Central Connection: Somatovisceral/Viscerosomatic Interaction. Indianapolis: American Academy of Osteopathy, 1992; 77–85.

48. Beal MC. Viscerosomatic Reflexes. In MM Patterson, JN Howell (eds), The Central Connection: Somatovisceral/Viscerosomatic Interaction. American Academy of Osteopathy: Indianapolis, 1992;19–27.

49. Cervero F. Mechanisms of acute visceral pain. Br Med Bull 1991;47:549–560.

50. Schmidt RF. Fundamentals of Neurophysiology. New York: Springer, 1985.

51. Sato A. Reflex Modulation of Visceral Functions By Somatic Afferent Activity. In MM Patterson, JN Howell (eds), The Central Connection: Somatovisceral/Viscerosomatic Interaction. Indianapolis: American Academy of Osteopathy, 1992.

52. Schmidt RF. Neurophysiological Mechanisms of Arthritic Pain. In MM Patterson, JN Howell (eds), The Central Connection: Somatovisceral/Viscerosomatic Interaction. Indianapolis: American Academy of Osteopathy, 1992.

53. Melzack R, Wall RP. Pain mechanisms: A new theory. Science 1965;150:971–984.

54. van Buskirk RL. Nociceptive reflexes and the somatic dysfunction: A model. J Am Osteopath Assoc 1990;90: 792–809.

55. Patterson MM, Howell JH. The Central Connection: Somatovisceral/Viscerosomatic Interaction. Indianapolis: American Academy of Osteopathy, 1992.

56. Denslow JS. An analysis of the variability of spinal reflex thresholds. J Neurophysiol 1944;7:207–215.

57. Denslow JS. Neural basis of the somatic component in health and disease and its clinical management. J Am Osteopath Assoc 1972;72:149–156.

58. Korr IM. Proprioceptors and somatic dysfunction. J Am Osteopath Assoc 1975;75:638–650.

59. Korr IM. In MM Patterson, JN Howell (eds), The Central Connection: Somatovisceral/Viscerosomatic Interaction. Indianapolis: American Academy of Osteopathy, 1992;287.

60. Travell J, Simons D. Myofascial Pain and Dysfunction, Vol 1. Baltimore: Williams & Wilkins, 1983.

61. Beal MC. Palpatory testing for somatic dysfunction in patients with cardiovascular disease. J Am Osteopath Assoc 1983;82:822–831.

62. Foreman RD. The Functional Organization of Visceral and Somatic Input to the Spinothalamic System. In MM Patterson, JN Howell (eds), The Central Connection: Somatovisceral/Viscerosomatic Interaction. Indianapolis: American Academy of Osteopathy, 1992;178–202.

Selected Reading

Beal MC. Viscerosomatic reflexes: A review. J Am Osteopath Assoc 1985;85:786–801.

Carpenter MB. Core Text of Neuroanatomy (2nd ed). Baltimore: Williams & Wilkins, 1978.

Davidoff RA. Skeletal muscle tone and the misunderstood stretch reflex. Neurology 1992;42:951–963.

Dvorak J, Dvorak V. Manual Medicine—Diagnostics (2nd ed). New York: Thieme, 1990.

Glenn MB, Whyte J. The Practical Management of Spasticity in Children and Adults. Philadelphia: Lea & Febiger, 1990.

Greenman, PE. Principles of Manual Medicine. Baltimore: Williams & Wilkins, 1989.

Mitchell FL Jr. The Muscle Energy Manual. E. Lansing, MI: MET Press, 1995.

Neumann HD. Introduction to Manual Medicine. New York: Springer, 1989.

Nolte J. The Human Brain—An Introduction to Its Functional Anatomy (3rd ed). St. Louis: Mosby, 1993

PART II

Examination and Differential Diagnostic Procedures

Chapter 3

Imaging of the Thoracic Spine

Brian Demby

This chapter should actually be entitled, "When should I order anything other than an MRI." For a number of reasons magnetic resonance imaging (MRI) is fast becoming the "gold standard" for spinal imaging. The most important include the availability of multiplanar imaging (Figs. 3.1 through 3.3), high soft-tissue contrast, and noninvasiveness. These factors allow MRI to provide the best images of the thoracic spine available, short of cutting the patient open and looking. So why order anything else? Although MRI provides the best images, it is not always the best study. Magnetic resonance imaging is expensive (about $1,500 per examination), not always available or possible with all patients, and it images cortical bone poorly.

What imaging study should be ordered? This depends on the suspected pathologic condition. Each imaging modality has various strengths and weaknesses that can be exploited only after the clinician has completely reviewed the patient's history, physical examination results, and laboratory work. Ideally, the imaging study is ordered to confirm the suspected diagnosis. To make sure clinicians are thinking before ordering a study (and not just ordering every test possible), the "third-party payers"— i.e., insurance companies—are starting to look over our shoulders. In the future, reimbursement may be denied for imaging studies they consider unnecessary. The cost could come out of your pocket (Table 3.1). Now that I have your attention, in this chapter I develop a rationale and table for determining which

examination to order and why (Table 3.2). If you are still unsure, ask your radiologist. You can be sure that if he or she had to clinically work up patients, he or she would be asking you lots of questions.

Conventional Radiology

Advantages: Inexpensive, readily available, excellent view of cortical bone.
Disadvantages: Nonvisualization of soft-tissue structures.
Use: Rule out fracture, degenerative joint disease, or arthritic processes.

The thoracic spine series is the familiar x-ray examination of the thoracic spine. It is commonly performed in only two imaging planes, anteroposterior (AP) and lateral, although oblique views can be ordered. Subject contrast in x-ray imaging depends mostly on differences in density between the adjacent tissues. The five densities that can be adequately visualized as separate structures are metal, bone, soft tissue, fat, and air. Metal, bone, and air have high contrast because of their large differences in density. The soft tissues, however, have poor subject contrast because their densities are very similar. The soft-tissue structures include the muscles, tendons, ligaments, intervertebral discs, spinal cord, roots, and cerebrospinal fluid (CSF). The soft-tissue structures are the same density on plain films and cannot be individually distinguished.

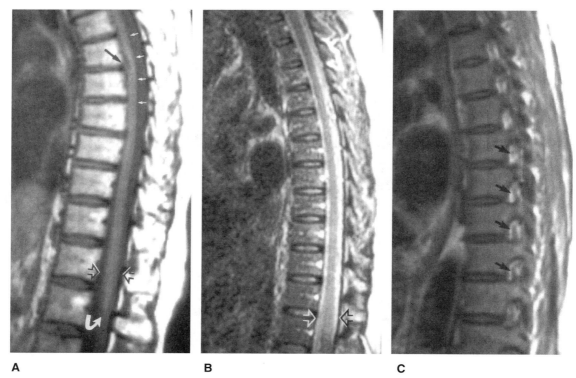

A   B   C

Figure 3.1. Sagittal and parasagittal images of the thoracic spine. A. Midline sagittal T1-weighted image (SE 600/20) shows a normal thoracic spinal cord. Note that the spinal cord in the upper and middle thoracic region lies anterior in position (small white arrows) as it follows the inner curvature of the normal thoracic kyphosis. More inferiorly, the thoracic cord lies within the middle portion of the spinal canal. The expansile portion of the distal thoracic spinal cord at the lumbar eminence (open arrows) is also well demonstrated, as is the tapering of the normal conus to its termination at approximately L1 (curved arrow). Note the incidental finding of a small thoracic disc herniation (black arrow) that was asymptomatic in this patient. B. Mid-sagittal T2- weighted image (SE 2000/80) demonstrates a normal thoracic spinal cord and conus outlined by high signal intensity from cerebrospinal fluid. This sequence produces a myelographic-like appearance of the image. Again, note the normal appearance of the expansile lumbar eminence (open arrows) at the distal thoracic spinal cord. Also note the anterior position of the thoracic spinal cord along the inner curvature of the normal thoracic kyphosis. C. Parasagittal T1-weighted image demonstrates the normal thoracic neuroforamina, which have a smooth, oval shape. Exiting nerve roots (small arrows) can be seen surrounded by perineural fat. (Reprinted with permission from KR Maravilla, WA Cohen. MRI Atlas of the Spine. New York: Raven, 1991.)

What does this brief review of "Physics 101" mean in practical terms? You cannot see a herniated disc compressing the spinal cord with plain films. A torn muscle or ligament is invisible. A tumor or infection that has not replaced or destroyed a large amount of bone or has no internal calcifications will not be visible. On the other hand, most bony pathologic conditions, especially those involving the cortical bone such as fractures (Fig. 3.4), can be easily and inexpensively identified. Plain films are also excellent for evaluating the bony alignment of the vertebral bodies (spondylolisthesis), fractures of the pars interarticularis (spondylolysis), degenerative changes (spondylosis or degenerative joint disease), and location of metallic foreign bodies. An estimate of the bone density and various spondyloarthritic processes can also be made. Some important notes about fractures: Bony overlap by ribs may prevent identification of fractures of the spinous processes in the thoracic spine and nondisplaced fractures may be inapparent on AP and lateral views. Oblique films, a nuclear medicine bone scan, or a computed tomographic (CT) scan may be needed to identify them.

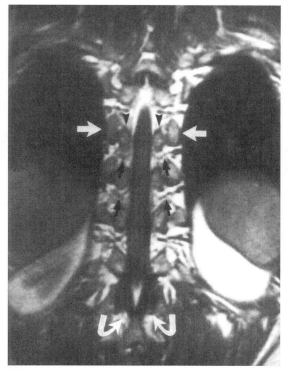

A

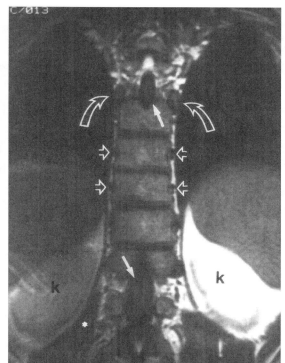

B

Figure 3.2. A. Coronal T1-weighted image through the mid-plane of the spinal canal shows the spinal cord surrounded by the low-signal cerebrospinal fluid space. Immediately lateral to the spinal cord are the pedicles (arrowheads). The osseous structures lateral to the pedicles are the heads of the ribs (horizontal white arrows). In the thoracic and lumbar spine, nerve roots exit within the neuroforamina inferior to their respective pedicles. The thoracic nerve roots within the neural foramina are surrounded by epidural fat and are oriented more horizontally (small black arrows) than the exiting cervical or lumbar nerve roots. Because there is normal kyphosis in the thoracic spine, lamina and facets (curved arrows) are visible in the lower thoracic region. B. Coronal T1-weighted image at a level anterior to that in Figure 3.2A. Because of the normal kyphosis, vertebral bodies are visible in the middle portion of the spine but spinal cord is seen superiorly and inferiorly (solid white arrows). The articulation of the heads of the ribs with the vertebral body can be seen at approximately T8 (curved open arrows). The intercostal vessels (straight open arrows) are seen on either side of the vertebral bodies outlined by retropleural fat. The kidneys (k) surrounded by retroperitoneal fat are visible bilaterally. On the right the superior portion of the psoas muscle can be seen (asterisk). (Reprinted with permission from KR Maravilla, WA Cohen. MRI Atlas of the Spine. New York: Raven, 1991.)

Myelography

Advantages: Indirect imaging of the disc, spinal cord, and roots.
Disadvantages: Invasive, nondirect imaging; CT scanning or MRI is better.
Use: When CT scanning or MRI are contraindicated or not available. Usually performed as a CT myelogram.

As radiology developed, the need to image the spinal cord led to the myelogram. First and foremost, a myelogram is very invasive. The procedure is basically a spinal tap with radiologic contrast material injected into the subarachnoid space surrounding the spinal cord. Complications are rare but include trauma to the nerve roots, infection (including within the subarachnoid space), headache, and allergic reactions to the contrast material. If given the option, both the patient and the radiologist would prefer a noninvasive study. The contrast material currently in use is water soluble, mixes with the CSF, and does not have to be withdrawn at the completion of the study. After the contrast is administered, multiple x-ray films of the spine are

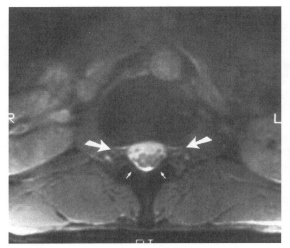

A

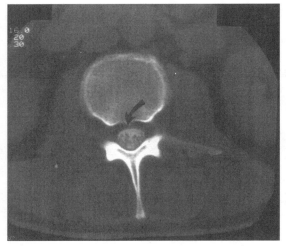

B

Figure 3.3. A. Axial GRE T2* image immediately inferior to the conus at L2. The "spider-like" configuration of nerve roots exiting from the tip of the conus is again seen, together with several roots that appear as individual punctate areas within the high-signal cerebrospinal fluid space. This section, which is obtained at the level of the neural foramina, shows nerve root sleeves (oblique arrows) surrounded by higher-signal epidural tissue lying within the neural canals. Ligamentum flavum is faintly visible as bands of intermediate signal deep to the posterior lamina (small arrows). B. Axial CT myelogram shows nerve roots as filling defects within the high-attenuation cerebrospinal fluid in the subarachnoid space (curved arrow) similar in appearance to the T2*-weighted MR image in Figure 3.3A. Unlike an MR image, the osseous structures are of high attenuation and thus clearly discernible from surrounding soft tissues on this CT myelogram. Note, however, that the exiting nerve roots within the neuroforamina are poorly shown when compared with the corresponding MR image. (Reprinted with permission from KR Maravilla, WA Cohen. MRI Atlas of the Spine, New York: Raven, 1991.)

Table 3.1. Imaging Options of the Thoracic Spine and Approximate Cost

Thoracic spine series	$35.00
Myelogram	$150.00
Bone scan	$100.00
CT scan	$500.00
CT myelogram	$800.00
MRI	$1,500.00

taken in AP, lateral, and oblique views to demonstrate the outline of the spinal cord and the filling of the nerve root sleeves. Although the intervertebral discs, spinal cord, and nerve roots are not directly visualized, their impressions on the contrast material within the CSF can be inferred. This allows the examiner to suggest the diagnosis of herniated nucleus pulposus (HNP), spinal stenosis, and tumors. Within the spinal canal, tumors are further subdivided by their location: intramedullary, intradural-extramedullary, or extradural. The disad-

Table 3.2 What to Order

Condition/Disease	Modality (in Order of Preference)
Fracture	1. T-spine series
	2. CT
	3. MRI
Herniated nucleus pulposis (HNP)	1. MRI
	2. CT
	3. CT myelogram
Infection	1. MRI
	2. Nuclear medicine bone scan
	3. CT
Neoplasm (involving the cord)	1. MRI
	2. CT
Bony metastasis	1. Nuclear medicine bone scan
	2. MRI
Arthritis	1. T-spine series
	2. CT
Cord abnormality	1. MRI
Congenital abnormality	1. MRI

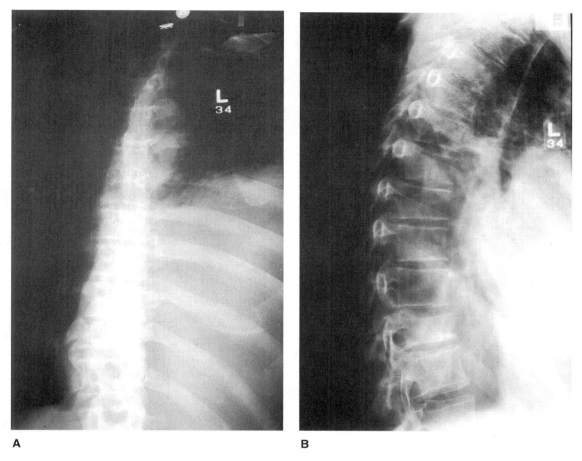

A   **B**

Figure 3.4. Anteroposterior (A) and lateral (B) plain films of the thoracic spine demonstrating an anterior compression fracture of a midthoracic vertebral body. Note that the soft-tissue structures such as the spinal cord, cerebrospinal fluid, and intervertebral discs cannot be visualized as distinct structures.

vantages are the invasiveness of the procedure, the lack of multiplanar imaging, and nondirect visualization. HNP is not directly seen; rather, an extrinsic impression of the opacified subarachnoid space at a disc level is visible. The differential diagnosis is most consistent with HNP, however, it could be another soft-tissue mass such as a hematoma, infection, or tumor. Remember, with plain films all soft-tissue structures look alike.

In the 1990s it is unusual to perform a myelogram without obtaining CT sections (see Fig. 3.3B) through the area of interest (a CT myelogram). The discogram (injecting contrast into a disc to tell if the annulus fibrosus is intact) is generally considered a dinosaur and should be left extinct.

Bone Scan

Advantages: Inexpensive study, images activity of the bone.
Disadvantages: Expensive equipment, poor anatomic image, nonspecific.
Use: Rule out bony metastasis, malingering patient, solitary versus multiple lesions, and infection workup.

The nuclear medicine bone scan is performed by intravenously injecting the patient with 99^mtechnetium MDP, a bone-seeking radiopharmaceutical. The ^{99m}Tc-MDP is thought to bind to the bone in relation to bone osteoid amount, mineralization of the osteoid, bone blood flow, and sympathetic nerve supply. A gamma camera obtains the image, which is then recorded on x-ray film. Nuclear imaging requires different, specialized equipment. There are many more personnel and government regulations than required for "regular" x-ray imaging. The image obtained is also different. It is a physiologic image of bone "activity" rather than an image of anatomic detail. The images are composed of dots of various intensity reflecting the bone "activity." The more "active" the bone, the darker and more numerous the dots over that area. An area of abnormality is often imaged as a "hot spot" or, conversely, a "cold spot." Various causes of altered "activity" include fractures, benign and malignant neoplasms, arthritis, osteomyelitis, and other bone disorders such as Paget's disease. Bone scans are the proverbial two-edged sword. They are very sensitive to areas of abnormality, but unfortunately very nonspecific. A "hot spot" in the spine may be secondary to an underlying fracture, neoplasm, osteomyelitis, or arthritic change. If the examination results are completely normal, it is very doubtful there is a significant bony abnormality. If positive, the clinician often must order another imaging test to determine the cause. Considering the cost of the equipment, the time required, and the computers used, the anatomic image produced is terrible. Often it is difficult to identify a specific vertebral body. The advantages are that this is the only imaging modality that displays the "activity" of the bone, and the entire skeleton can be rapidly and inexpensively visualized. The bone scan has some unique uses. It is the most cost-effective method to evaluate for bony metastases (the important exception is multiple myeloma). It can help distinguish between solitary and multiple lesions and determine anatomic distribution. Infectious etiologies such as cellulitis or osteomyelitis can be suggested on the bone scan. However, MRI is more sensitive and specific. If the bone scan results are perfectly normal, most bony disease processes can be excluded. This can be useful with a "malingering" patient to make sure you are not missing something.

Computed Tomography

Advantages: Excellent imaging of fractures and tumors involving the cortical bone, and spinal stenosis. **Disadvantages:** May require myelographic contrast (invasive procedure) to diagnose small HNPs. Not as good as MRI for imaging the cord, diagnosing infections, or detecting tumors not based in cortical bone.

Use: Rule out subtle fractures, lesion in cortical bone, HNP, and spinal stenosis.

An interesting story I heard, which may or may not be true, has to do with the development of the CT scanner. During the 1960s, the musical recording group the Beatles was such a success that their record company EMI. had money to invest. One project that the "Fab Four" money sponsored was the development of the CT scanner. The original scanner was in fact built by EMI.

The CT scanner revolutionized radiology in the 1970s in the same way that MRI is revolutionizing it now. CT imaging uses ionizing radiation, similar to plain x-rays, to produce an image. The major differences are vast improvements in spatial resolution, subject contrast, and imaging plane. The images are displayed as multiple sequential transaxial images (see Fig. 3.3B). This is analogous to viewing a loaf of bread by looking at each individual bread slice. The modern scanner can acquire images as thin as 1 mm, but for routine use 10-mm cuts are performed. The gantry of the machine can be angled slightly to provide oblique images (perpendicular to an angled disc space) if needed. Newer machines use the computer to reconstruct sagittal and coronal images from the axial data. Unfortunately, the reconstructed images are not as good as directly acquired images. Intravenous (IV) contrast agents such as iohexol (Omnipaque) can also be used to make lesions such as tumors and infections more conspicuous (enhanced). The distinction between recurrent postsurgical HNP and scar material can largely be resolved because disc material will enhance with IV contrast and scar will not.

The important point is that the improved spatial and contrast resolution of the CT scan finally allows direct visualization of the soft tissue structures individually. Finally, the intervertebral disc and the spinal cord can be viewed as separate distinct structures directly without the need for subarachnoid contrast in most cases. Rarely, myelographic contrast is still needed for the diagnosis of small HNPs. A CT scan is particularly useful for the diagnosis of HNPs, cortical bone lesions, spinal infections, spinal stenosis, and tumors involving both the soft tissue and the cortical structures. Although the images of computed tomography are light years better than those previously discussed, MRIs are better. The improved soft tissue contrast with MRI over CT scanning and the true multiplanar capability of

MRI are the reasons it is the preferred study for lesions not based in cortical bone such as disk or epidural infections, soft tissue and bone marrow neoplasms, and HNPs.

Magnetic Resonance Imaging

Advantages: Best imaging of the spine, especially the neurologic structures, noninvasive.
Disadvantages: Cost, nonavailability, multiple patient contraindications, poor visualization of cortical bone.
Use: Rule out tumors, infections, HNPs, congenital abnormalities.

As mentioned earlier, MRI is usually the best imaging study if a thoracic spine series does not provide all the necessary information. Unfortunately, MRI does not work for every patient. The contraindications to MRI include ferrometallic objects within the eyes and brain (aneurysm clips), a large number of computer-operated devices (such as drug infusion pumps, cardiac pacers, neurostimulators, and bone-growth stimulators), cochlear implants, and some prosthetic heart valves (Starr-Edwards pre-6000 models). Some relative contraindications include being unable to monitor and see the patient, inability of the patient to remain motionless for the required time, and claustrophobia.

MRI uses magnetic fields rather than ionizing radiation to create the image. At the current time MRI is believed to cause no adverse side effects (if the patient survives the shock of the cost, that is). Several types of images are available; T1 and some type of T2 images are the basic images acquired. The T1 and T2 images are generated distinctly different from each other and give us different types of information. T1 images are anatomy loving, because they are generated fast, causing less patient motion artifact than the more lengthy T2 images, which require the patient to remain motionless for several minutes. T1 images display fat as bright areas, muscle and water as gray, and tendons, ligaments, and cortical bone as black. T2 type images are pathology-loving. Water is displayed as bright areas on T2 images. Tissue that is infected, traumatized, neoplastic, or otherwise abnormal (demyelinating process of the cord) tends to accumulate more water than normal tissue and is displayed as bright areas on T2 images. True T2 image sequences are long, degraded by motion artifact, and costly to the radiologist in terms of patient input. Fast-spin echo (FSE) and gradient-echo images (see Fig. 3.3A) are new sequences designed to produce T2-weighted images faster. Gadolinium, an IV contrast agent for MRI that is analogous to the IV contrast agents used for CT scanning, can also be used. Gadolinium (Gd) accumulation in a tissue causes it to be displayed as a very bright area on T1 images. Our institution is constantly changing our imaging sequences as new advances develop. Currently our standard thoracic spine series includes T1 and FSE sagittal and T1 and FSE axial images. If gadolinium is administered we add T1 sagittal and coronal images and $100—the cost of the 5 ml of gadolinium used.

As a general rule, T1 data display the best anatomy and T2 data the best pathology. Look at the T2 images for the pathologic "bright spot" and correlate it with the sharper anatomy seen on the T1 images.

MRI is currently the preferred imaging study for the spine, particularly for tumors (Figs. 3.5 and 3.6), infections (Fig. 3.7), and congenital abnormalities such as tethered cord, meningocele, syringohydromyelia of the cord (Fig. 3.8), vertebral discs, and surrounding soft-tissue structures. Cord lesions such as transverse myelitis and multiple sclerosis (Fig. 3.9) are also imaged. HNP can be imaged both by CT scanning and MRI (Fig. 3.10), although most radiologists prefer MRI.

The imaging of neoplasms requires some extra comments. Plain films may be the most useful study for the radiologist to determine the type of tumor. To determine if there is widespread bony metastasis, a nuclear medicine bone scan is preferred. The diagnostic dilemmas of distinguishing between a compression-type fracture in a patient with known neoplasm versus neoplastic involvement versus osteomyelitis is best solved using MRI or, rarely, CT. Often a combination of plain films, bone scans, CT scanning, and MRI is needed for a complete evaluation.

MRI is currently undergoing rapid changes in imaging sequences, hardware, and software. Each new advance increases the image quality and utility of MRI (unfortunately, also the price).

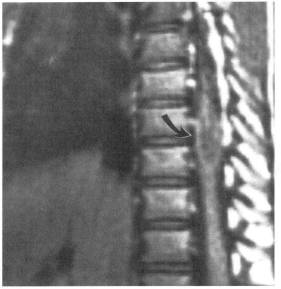

A

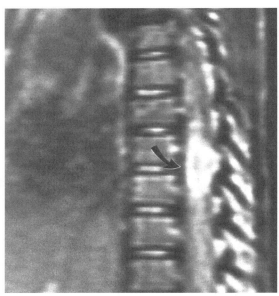

B

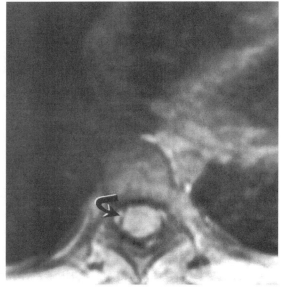

C

Figure 3.5. A 4-year-old child with an ependymoma of the thoracic spinal cord. A. Sagittal T1-weighted image (SE 600/20) shows a well-defined expansile mass within the midthoracic spinal cord (curved arrow). B. Spin-density image (SE 1800/40) shows increased signal intensity within the mass (curved arrow). At times, as in this case, intramedullary spinal cord lesions may be best seen on spindensity images because they may be partially obscured by high-signal cerebrospinal fluid on more heavily T2-weighted images. C. Axial T2* image (GRE 60/113, q = 20 degrees) shows poor definition of an expanded spinal cord with an inhomogeneous increased signal that is nearly isointense with the cerebrospinal fluid. A small area of diminished signal intensity along the right side of the cord (curved arrow) probably represents a small area of hemosiderin along the tumor margin. (Reprinted with permission from KR Maravilla, WA Cohen. MRI Atlas of the Spine. New York: Raven, 1991.)

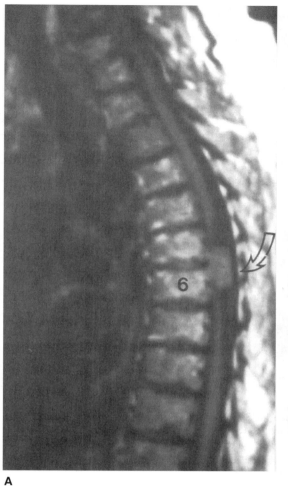

A

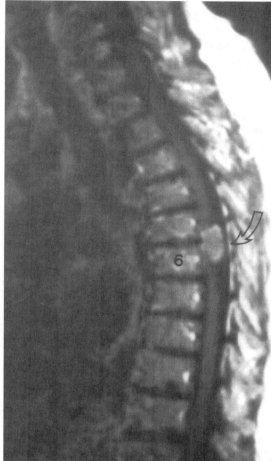

B

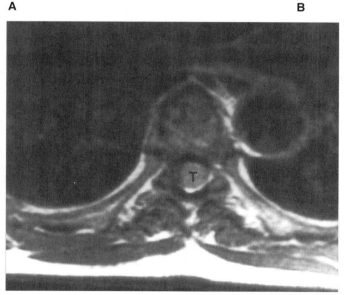

C

Figure 3.6. Spinal meningioma at the level of T5-6. A. Precontrast sagittal T1-weighted image (SE 600/20) demonstrates an intradural extra-axial mass that is minimally hyperintense to the deformed and displaced thoracic spinal cord (curved open arrow). B. Sagittal T1-weighted image after administration of gadolinium shows moderate contrast enhancement within the meningioma (curved open arrow). C. Axial postcontrast T1-weighted image (SE 600/20) shows the enhancing meningioma (T) located laterally and posteriorly within the spinal canal. (Reprinted with permission from KR Maravilla, WA Cohen. MRI Atlas of the Spine. New York: Raven, 1991.)

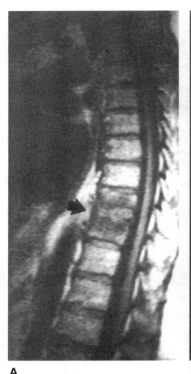
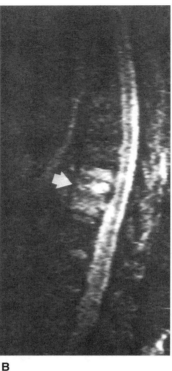

A   **B**

Figure 3.7. Pyogenic osteomyelitis and discitis. A. The classic findings of discitis with osteomyelitis—decreased disc space height, loss of the normal disc signal, and poor definition of the cortical end plates (arrow)—are present on this T1-weighted sagittal image (SE 600/20). Decreased signal in the vertebral bodies on either side of the disc space suggests cellular infiltration of the marrow space. The absence of a significant epidural soft tissue mass or cord displacement, clearly seen with MRI, is not appreciable with other noninvasive imaging studies. B. Sagittal STIR image (IR1500/43/160) of the same region confirms increased cellularity within both the disc space and vertebral bodies. The STIR sequences, which "suppress" signal from fat, are highly sensitive to the presence of cellular infiltration (increased water). The increased lesion conspicuity, however, is accompanied by loss of anatomic detail secondary to a decrease in the signal-to-noise ratio. Anatomic and morphologic detail are better evaluated using T1-weighted sequences. (Reprinted with permission from KR Maravilla, WA Cohen. MRI Atlas of the Spine. New York: Raven, 1991.)

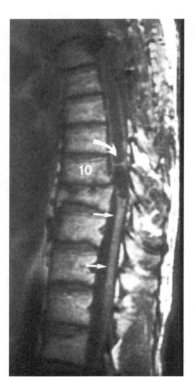

Figure 3.8. Posttraumatic syrinx in a 24-year-old paraplegic man 1 year after a T10–T11 fracture-subluxation. The syrinx on this T1-weighted sagittal image (SE 600/20) starts at T11 and extends upward, widening the spinal cord. Below T11 the cord is somewhat atrophic (small arrows). A septation is seen within this syrinx (curved arrow). These are commonly seen with benign syrinxes and represent incomplete, nonobstructive septae. There is residual deformity from the fractures including loss of height of the T10 and T11 vertebral bodies and posterior displacement of T11. Posttraumatic syrinxes may occur from one to several years after the initial spinal cord injury. Early diagnosis and treatment of these lesions are important, because a syrinx extending superior to the level of initial spinal cord injury may cause progressive loss of critical function in an individual who has already sustained a significant neurologic injury. (Reprinted with permission from KR Maravilla, WA Cohen. MRI Atlas of the Spine. New York: Raven, 1991.)

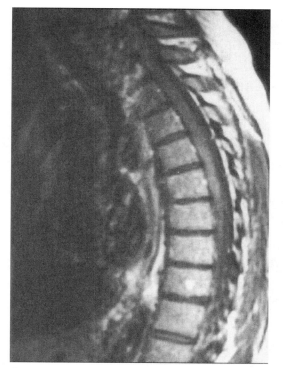

A

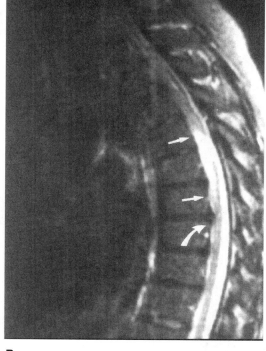

B

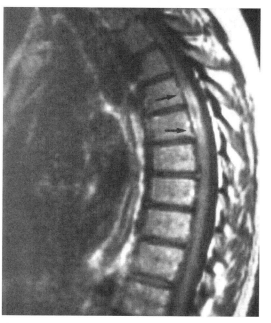

C

Figure 3.9. Spinal demyelination in a 42-year-old woman whose symptoms developed over 1 month. She was clinically felt to have a thoracic herniated disc. A. The spinal cord is of normal caliber on this T1-weighted image (SE 600/20). B. A T2-weighted image (SE 1800/80) shows increased signal with ill-defined borders extending over several midthoracic spinal cord segments (small arrows). Although a small thoracic disc herniation is present (curved arrow), it did not correlate with the patient's symptoms. C. A T1-weighted image after gadolinium enhancement shows an area of rim enhancement within the spinal cord (arrows) that corresponds to the area of high signal seen on the T2-weighted image in Figure 3.9B. Enhancement can be seen in patients with inflammatory or demyelinating disease of the central nervous system. In multiple sclerosis it correlates with an acutely demyelinating plaque rather than with the chronic, sclerotic plaques most commonly seen in demyelinating disease. Such enhancement may be, as in this case, very intense or very subtle. (Reprinted with permission from KR Maravilla, WA Cohen. MRI Atlas of the Spine. New York: Raven, 1991.)

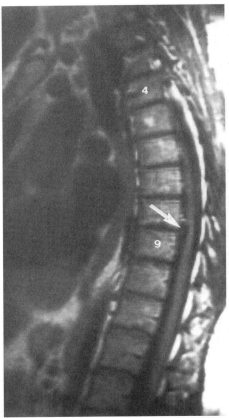 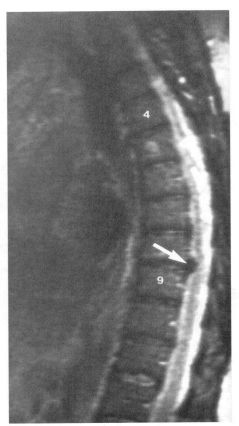

A   **B**

Figure 3.10. Thoracic disc herniation in a patient with long-standing back pain. Sagittal T1-weighted (SE 600/20) (A) and T2-weighted (SE 1800/80) (B) images show a T8–T9 disc herniation (arrows), which is of low signal intensity on all imaging sequences. Because it is almost isointense with cerebrospinal fluid on the T1-weighted image, the presence of the disc is more easily inferred from the flattening of the spinal cord at this level rather than from direct visualization.

On the T2-weighted image, the extremely low signal intensity of the posterior protrusion at the disc space suggests the presence of calcium within the disc. Incidentally noted at T5 is a rounded focus of high signal intensity, especially on the T1-weighted image. This represents a focal fat deposit. (Reprinted with permission from KR Maravilla, WA Cohen. MRI Atlas of the Spine, New York: Raven, 1991.)

Selected Reading

Curry TS, Dowdey JE, Murry RC Jr. Christensen's Introduction to the Physics of Diagnostic Radiology (3rd ed). Philadelphia: Lea & Febiger, 1984.

Helms CA. Fundamentals of Skeletal Radiology. Philadelphia: Saunders, 1989.

Lufkin RB. The MRI Manual. Chicago: Year Book, 1990.

Maravilla KR, Cohen WA. MRI Atlas of the Spine. New York: Raven, 1991.

Mettler FA, Guiberteau MJ. Essentials of Nuclear Medicine Imaging (3rd ed). Philadelphia: Saunders, 1991.

Runge V. Clinical Magnetic Resonance Imaging. Philadelphia: Lippincott, 1990.

Stark DD, Bradley WG Jr. Magnetic Resonance Imaging (2nd ed). St. Louis: Mosby-Year Book, 1992.

Webb WR, Brant WE, Helms CA. Fundamentals of Body CT. Philadelphia: Saunders, 1991.

Chapter 4
Clinical Electrophysiologic Testing

Frank B. Underwood

Clinical electrophysiologic testing consists of recording the electrical activity of the neuromuscular system. It includes nerve conduction studies, needle electromyography, and electronic reflex testing, but does not include surface electromyography. Surface electromyography is useful for kinesiologic studies but does not permit evaluation of individual motor units or individual muscle fibers. Despite the more common use of electrophysiologic testing in the evaluation of the cervical and lumbar spine, there are instances when this testing is indicated in the evaluation of patients who experience pain in the thorax. Therefore, practitioners should be familiar with the basic principles, testing procedures, and interpretation of electrophysiologic testing.

Historically, terms that have been used to describe clinical electrophysiologic testing have included "EMG/NCV," "electroneuromyography (ENMG)," and "electrodiagnosis." Although ENMG, EMG/NCV, and clinical electrophysiologic testing are descriptive of the techniques, they are somewhat awkward terms. Electrodiagnosis is not an appropriate term because the use of these techniques does not lead to a diagnosis [1]. For the purposes of this chapter, the term "EMG" will be used to refer to all components of clinical electrophysiologic testing.

The EMG examination is useful in the assessment of neuromuscular disorders but is not a sufficient nor requisite test to make a diagnosis. There are no abnormal findings that are pathognomonic of any particular disorder, with very few exceptions [1].

This examination is helpful to differentiate disorders of myelin, axons, and muscle. In addition, the specific site of a lesion can often be identified, and some information relative to the severity of the lesion can be obtained [2]. It may also be possible to provide some prognostic information based on the results of the examination [3]. It is crucial to understand that even if the EMG reveals that there is an axonopathy of a particular cervical nerve root, the EMG cannot be used to determine the cause of the axonopathy. The same concept applies to any other disorder identified with these procedures.

As with the neuromusculoskeletal screening examination described in Chapter 7, obtaining a comprehensive and accurate history is vital to conducting a meaningful EMG examination. The history will guide the physical examination that follows. In turn, the physical examination will guide the conduct of the EMG. Although the focus of the EMG should be on those muscles that demonstrate weakness and on the nerve roots or peripheral nerves that innervate the areas of the skin with diminished sensibility, the examination should not be limited to those areas. For example, if a patient has paresthesia in the lateral palmar aspect of the hand, with increased symptoms at night that are relieved by shaking the hand, the physical examination will likely focus on the wrist and hand. If the examination reveals decreased sensation in the tips of the lateral three and a half digits of the hand, along with weakness in palmar abduction of the thumb, the EMG will focus on the median nerve.

If there is slowing of the conduction of the median nerve across the carpal tunnel and evidence of denervation in the abductor pollicis brevis, the examiner may report that there is evidence of a combined myelinopathy and axonopathy of the median nerve at the wrist. However, unless the examination also includes other motor and sensory nerves and muscles that are proximal to the site of symptoms, associated pathologic conditions may be overlooked. It is known that many metabolic diseases (e.g., diabetes mellitus) make peripheral nerves more susceptible to entrapment [4, 5], and a proximal entrapment may make a distal site more vulnerable (the "double-crush" syndrome) [6, 7].

Principles

Electrophysiologic testing relies on the ability of the instrumentation to amplify bioelectric signals originating at the membrane of the nerve or muscle cell. Details of instrumentation will not be covered in this text; Kimura [2] and the chapter by Reiner and Rogoff [8] provide descriptions of the apparatus used. The genesis of bioelectricity will not be addressed either; any standard physiology or neuroscience text will provide adequate explanation (e.g., references 9–13).

The bioelectric potential changes that are recorded may either be initiated by the patient or elicited by an external stimulus. If the activity is elicited, the response is referred to as an evoked response [1]. Evoked responses may be recorded centrally (i.e., the response of the central nervous system) or peripherally. If the activity is initiated by the patient, the response is referred to as a volitional potential. Volitional potential recording is essentially synonymous with electromyography, whereas evoked potentials recorded peripherally are synonymous with nerve conduction studies. The term *evoked potential* is often used to refer to only those evoked potentials that are recorded centrally.

Evoked Responses

Recorded Centrally

Somatosensory evoked potentials (SSEPs) are recorded using surface electrodes placed on the scalp overlying the somatosensory cortex [14]. Surface stimulation of a peripheral nerve on the side contralateral to the recording electrodes is conducted with a stimulus amplitude just greater than motor threshold. The motor response is of no interest other than to monitor and standardize the amplitude of the stimulation. The action potentials that are initiated in the sensory fibers of the peripheral nerve are conducted proximally, and the time between the stimulus onset and the cortical response is measured. SSEP studies may also be conducted with surface recording electrodes over the ipsilateral spinal cord or a plexus [15, 16]. These studies are most useful in the early detection of sensory neuropathies, spinal cord injuries, and multiple sclerosis [14]. One advantage of SSEP recording is that segments of the afferent pathway not accessible to other evoked potential studies can be assessed. There is a recent report regarding SSEP recording of intercostal nerves in response to stimulation lateral to the sternum [17]. This technique may prove beneficial in the assessment of thoracic radiculopathies.

Brain stem auditory evoked potentials (BAEPs) and visual evoked potentials (VEPs) are useful for assessing the ability of the nervous system to receive and transmit auditory and visual information. Although useful in the detection of demyelinating diseases and multiple sclerosis [14], they are of little benefit in the evaluation of the thoracic spine.

Recorded Peripherally

Motor Nerve Conduction. Motor nerve conduction studies are obtained by placing electrodes on a muscle, then stimulating the nerve that supplies that muscle [18]. Most commonly, surface stimulation and recording are used, but a needle electrode may be required to isolate the response. For example, it is difficult to stimulate the suprascapular nerve to assess the motor nerve conduction to the supraspinatus muscle without also activating other shoulder girdle musculature. This could result in reporting a motor response when in fact the supraspinatus muscle is completely denervated. Therefore, a needle recording electrode in the supraspinatus muscle may be required. In some cases, such as the femoral nerve, needle stimulation may be more comfortable than surface stimulation.

The best muscle to study is the most distal superficial muscle in the nerve distribution. Figure 4.1 illustrates the method for assessing the motor nerve

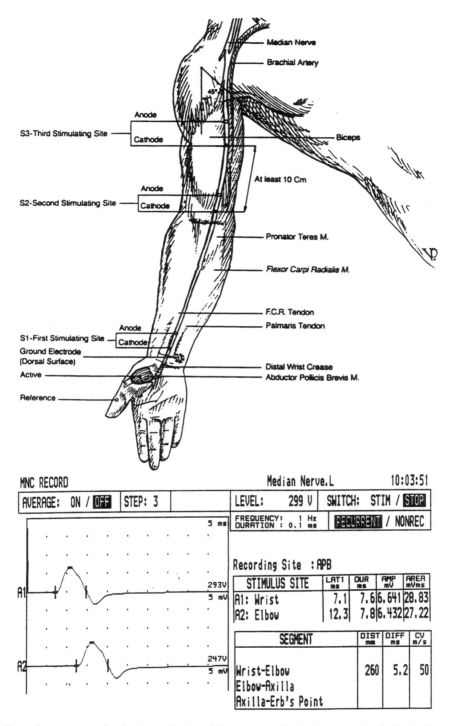

Figure 4.1. Electrode placement sites for determination of the motor conduction latency and velocity for the median nerve, and a typical response to stimulation at the wrist and elbow. (Top illustration reprinted from DE Nestor, RM Nelson. Performing Motor and Sensory Neuronal Conduction Studies in Adult Humans. Washington, DC: US Department of Health and Human Services, 1990.)

conduction of the median nerve as well as a typical recording. Essentially all nerves of the brachial plexus can be studied, but the ulnar, median, and radial nerves are the most common ones examined.

The distal motor latency is the time required for the action potential to travel from the point of stimulation to the neuromuscular junction (NMJ), across the NMJ, and down the sarcolemma. The response is a summation of all ionic currents produced in the muscle. The nerve is then stimulated at one or more proximal sites, and the nerve conduction velocity over various segments of the nerve can be calculated.

Motor nerve conduction studies provide information about the status of the myelination of the mixed peripheral nerve and the ability of the neuromuscular junction to transmit information. In addition, an indication of the status of the motor axons and the skeletal muscle fibers themselves can be obtained. A special type of motor nerve conduction study that involves repetitive stimulation of the peripheral nerve is sometimes used in assessing the status of the neuromuscular junction. Disorders such as myasthenia gravis and the myasthenic syndrome of Eaton-Lambert may be detected with repetitive stimulation techniques [2].

Sensory Nerve Conduction.   Conduction along the sensory fibers of a peripheral nerve may be assessed in an orthodromic or antidromic manner [18]. With orthodromic techniques, the receptors and terminal nerve fibers are stimulated distally, and the response is recorded from the nerve trunk proximal to the stimulation site. With antidromic stimulation, the nerve trunk is stimulated proximally, and the response is recorded distally from the terminal nerve fibers. Because there are differences in the values obtained with the two techniques, it should be noted in the report which technique was used. Figure 4.2 shows the technique for orthodromic recording of the median sensory nerve action potential and a typical recording of the response. The first tracing is with stimulation in the palm, and the second tracing is with stimulation in the web space between digits II and III.

As with motor nerve conduction, surface stimulation and recording is used most often, but needle electrodes may be helpful in certain cases. With many compression and metabolic neuropathies, sensory changes can be detected sooner than motor changes [2]. Whether this is because of an increased vulnerability of the sensory fibers or a more precise ability to detect sensory nerve changes is not clear.

Sensory nerve conduction studies are most helpful in the detection of demyelination disorders. However, if there is a loss of sensory fibers in the nerve trunk, the sensory response may be reduced in amplitude or absent. In addition, if there is a true loss of sensation in a particular nerve field, but the result of the sensory nerve conduction study is normal, a preganglionic lesion (i.e., a root lesion) is likely [2].

Electronic Reflex Studies

H-Reflex.   The H-reflex is the electrophysiologic equivalent of the monosynaptic stretch reflex (muscle stretch reflex [MSR]). When a mixed peripheral nerve is stimulated, an action potential is generated in the fibers innervating the muscle spindle. This action potential is conducted orthodromically through the posterior root ganglion to the lower motor neuron innervating the same muscle. The response of the muscle is the same as if the tendon had been stretched rapidly with a reflex hammer, except that the muscle spindle is bypassed [19, 20]. When recording from a muscle while stimulating the nerve innervating the muscle, two electrical responses can be recorded. The first is the result of the evoked action potential being conducted from the stimulation site to the muscle along the lower motor neurons. The second response is the result of the action potential conducted along the afferent limb of the reflex arc, then back to the muscle. Figure 4.3 illustrates the path taken by the action potential and a typical response.

The H-reflex is probably present in nearly all muscles of an infant but is suppressed as the central nervous system matures. In an adult, the H-reflex can be elicited consistently in the gastrocnemius-soleus and flexor carpi radialis [21] muscles, and occasionally in the hamstrings and quadriceps femoris [19]. Following an upper motor neuron lesion, the H-reflex often will return in the muscles that were innervated by the damaged neurons.

The H-reflex is helpful in assessing the status of the motor and sensory components of the reflex arc. A significant advantage of the H-reflex is that it provides a means of evaluating the component of the arc that is not easily accessible to direct stimulation—i.e., the far proximal or central part of the arc.

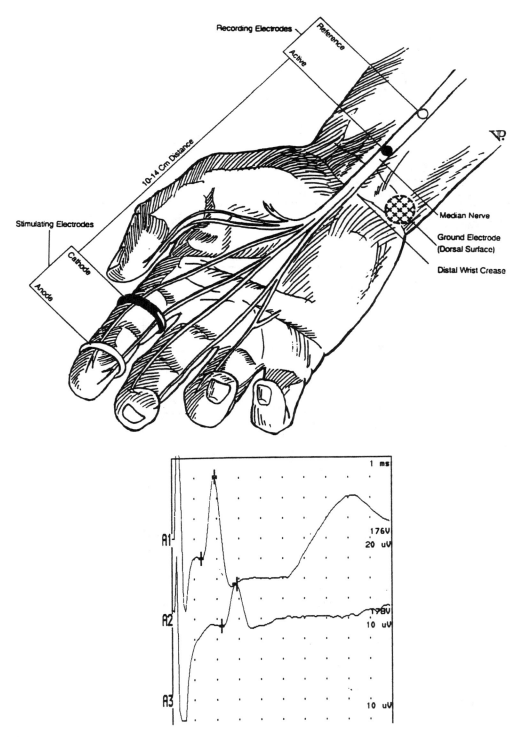

Figure 4.2. Electrode placement sites for determination of the orthodromic sensory latency for the median nerve, and a typical response to stimulation at the palm and wrist. (Top illustration reprinted from DE Nestor, RM Nelson. Performing Motor and Sensory Neuronal Conduction Studies in Adult Humans. Washington, DC: US Department of Health and Human Services, 1990.)

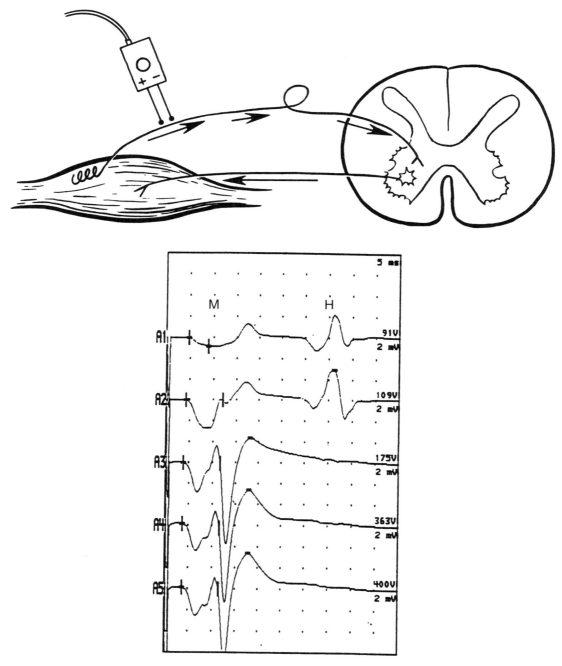

Figure 4.3. Anatomic pathway for the H-reflex and a typical response. Note the disappearance of the H-reflex with higher amplitude stimulation because of the anterior horn cell body being refractory.

F-Wave.   Although referred to as a reflex study, the F-wave is not a reflex. The only synapse involved in the F-wave is the neuromuscular junction, and there is no sensory component [19, 20].

The F-wave can be elicited from essentially any muscle that is accessible to conventional motor nerve conduction techniques. When the lower motor neurons in a mixed peripheral nerve are stimulated, the action potential is conducted both orthodromically to the skeletal muscle and proximally to the cell body in the anterior horn of the spinal cord. When the potential arrives at the NMJ, a response is elicited from the muscle. The potential that is conducted antidromically stops when it arrives at the cell body; however, approximately 10% of the motor neurons that were stimulated exhibit a rebound of the action potential. This rebounded action potential travels in an orthodromic fashion to the NMJ and causes a second, smaller response in the muscle [16, 19, 20]. Figure 4.4 shows the technique of eliciting the F-wave as well as a typical response.

The F-wave is useful for assessing the far proximal component of the motor neuron but does not include a sensory component. Because only 10% or so of the motor neurons rebound, the stimulation amplitude must be supramaximal and must be repeated at least 10 times [16]. For this reason, it can be quite uncomfortable for the patient.

Volitional Potentials

Volitional potentials can be recorded from any skeletal muscle using needle electrodes. Various types of needle electrodes are available; the distinctions among them and the rationale for the use of one type or another is beyond the scope of this chapter. It should be noted that the type of needle electrode used should be included in the report of electrophysiologic testing, because different electrodes result in some variance of the recorded potential.

The primary purpose of recording volitional potentials is to assess single motor unit activity, the sum of the activity of all motor units that can be recruited, and spontaneous activity in single muscle fibers or motor units. It is not possible to assess single motor units with any degree of accuracy using surface electrodes, and single muscle fiber activity cannot be detected. Therefore, information gleaned from surface electromyography is not useful in assessing neuropathies or myopathies.

Muscles must be observed while at rest, during minimal volitional effort, during maximal volitional effort, and during needle movement. It is desirable to examine a muscle in different locations to maximize the probability of detecting abnormal activity. The ability of the patient to relax a muscle is crucial

to a credible examination, but this is sometimes difficult to achieve. It is very painful to examine some muscles (e.g., abductor pollicis brevis), and volitional control of some postural muscles is not well developed (e.g., cervical paraspinals). Nevertheless, with patience on the part of the examiner and cooperation on the part of the patient, most muscles can be sampled adequately.

A normal muscle at rest is electrically silent. With minimal effort on the part of the patient, the repetitive discharge of a single motor unit can be recorded. The motor unit is typically biphasic or triphasic, has a firing rate of 3–15 per second, a duration of 3–16 msec, and an amplitude of 300–5,000 μV [1, 3]. As the patient increases effort and muscle tension, both temporal and spatial summation occur, resulting in more motor units firing and an increased rate of firing. At maximal effort, the motor unit activity fills the display screen with electrical activity in what is called a full interference pattern, or screen fill [2]. The isoelectric baseline is obliterated, because so many motor units are being recorded that there is never a period of electrical inactivity. As the needle is moved through a resting muscle, there are brief bursts of electrical activity, which stop almost immediately after the needle stops moving.

Spontaneous Activity

Fibrillations and Positive Sharp Waves

If the normal neural input to a muscle fiber is lost because of trauma or disease, the sarcolemma becomes hyperexcitable [2]. Normally, the acetylcholine receptors on the sarcolemma are confined to the region of the NMJ. When the neural input is lost, the receptors are thought to disperse throughout the sarcolemma and are thus capable of binding acetylcholine that leaks from adjacent healthy neurons. Activation of these receptors may create an action potential in the sarcolemma, thus causing the single muscle fiber to contract. Remember, it is not possible to volitionally recruit a single muscle fiber, unless the motor unit innervation ratio is one (one muscle fiber per neuron), which has not been observed [22]. The spontaneous firing of a single muscle fiber is called a fibrillation if it has a particular morphology, and a positive sharp wave if it has a different morphology. Although fibrillations and posi-

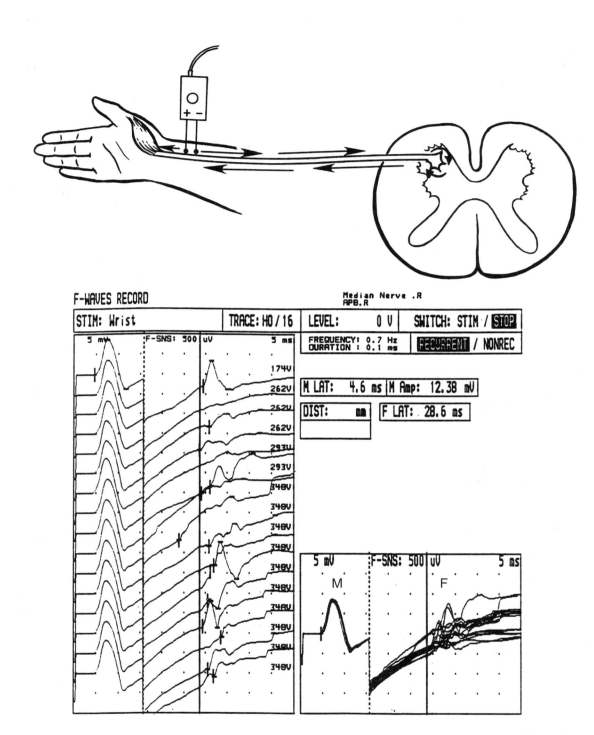

Figure 4.4. Anatomic pathway for the F-wave and a typical response. Note the variability in latency and morphology of the F-wave and the consistent M-wave. The smaller chart shows all 16 responses superimposed on each other.

tive sharp waves do occur in normal muscle on occasion, if they are abundant and widespread, they may represent an axonopathy. Fibrillations and positive sharp waves are not visible grossly, and the patient is unaware of them.

Fasciculations

A third type of spontaneous potential that may be noted during rest is the fasciculation. A fasciculation is the spontaneous discharge of a lower motor neuron, causing the firing of the entire motor unit. Fasciculations are often visible grossly, and the patient may be aware of the twitches. Although often thought to be associated with motor neuron disease (e.g., amyotrophic lateral sclerosis), fasciculations do occur in normal muscle, as well as in denervation and some myopathies.

Complex Repetitive Discharges

A fourth type of spontaneous activity is the complex repetitive discharge (CRD; formerly called *bizarre high-frequency discharges*). The CRD is more common in myopathy than neuropathy and does not occur in normal muscle. These discharges are characterized by bursts of electrical activity of various frequencies, amplitudes, and shapes. Within a burst, the morphology and frequency are generally constant (so, there may be a 5-second burst of triphasic potentials at a frequency of 15 per second, with an amplitude of 500 mV, followed by a 7-second burst of biphasic potentials at a frequency of 12 per second, with an amplitude of 700 mV).

Myotonic Potentials

Myotonic potentials are the last type of spontaneous activity that may be noted in a muscle at rest. Myotonic potentials do not occur in normal muscle and are essentially pathognomonic of one of the myotonias. However, they may also occur in hyperkalemic periodic paralysis, polymyositis, and in patients with disorders of carbohydrate metabolism [2]. Myotonic potentials are very high frequency bursts (up to 150 per second) of electrical activity that wax and wane in amplitude. The sound of myotonic potentials has been described in the past as "divebomber" potentials; however, their sound may be better described as a chainsaw accelerating and decelerating [2]. Myotonic

potentials are apparently related to a decreased chloride conductance of the sarcolemma; the loss of chloride conductance decreases the outward current carried by chloride, which destabilizes the sarcolemma.

Abnormalities

Large Polyphasic Motor Units

After the loss of lower motor neurons (neuropathies), a phenomenon called *collateral sprouting* may occur. In collateral sprouting the neurons that remain healthy further arborize and innervate muscle fibers that have lost innervation. As a result, the motor unit becomes larger, so that during minimal volitional effort, motor units of increased size are noted. In addition, the motor units may become polyphasic because of the increased distance the action potential must travel through the terminal arborization. As a result of the loss of motor units, the ability of the muscle to recruit spatially is decreased. Therefore, there is a greater reliance on temporal summation as the amount of force produced increases. This causes a rapid firing of the motor units when low and moderate amounts of tension are required.

Small Polyphasic Motor Units

In contrast to the increased motor unit size that may be noted in neuropathies, there is a decreased motor unit size in myopathies. Therefore, the motor units will be of smaller amplitude but will also fire rapidly. These small "myopathic" motor units may also be polyphasic.

With maximal volitional effort, fewer motor units will be noted with a neuropathy. This is described as an incomplete interference pattern; although the motor units that remain fire rapidly, they are unable to obliterate the baseline. A myopathy will generally cause an obliteration of the baseline with low to moderate effort, but the motor units will be of smaller amplitude. This is referred to as early screen fill of reduced amplitude.

Prolonged Insertional Activity

Movement of the needle through denervated muscle will cause an extended period of electrical activity after the needle stops moving. This is called pro-

Table 4.1. Classification Schemes for Peripheral Nerve Injuries

Classification Scheme			
Seddon	Sunderland	Tissue at Fault	Cause
Neurapraxia	Grade 1	Myelin	Ischemia, compression
Axonotmesis	Grade 2	Axon	Ischemia, compression, stretch
Neurotmesis	Grade 3	Axon and endoneurium	Stretch, crush
Neurotmesis	Grade 4	Axon, endoneurium, and perineurium	Stretch, crush, penetrating wound
Neurotmesis	Grade 5	Axon, endoneurium, perineurium, and epineurium	Penetrating or transecting wound

longed insertional activity and is a somewhat subjective estimate of membrane instability. In addition, needle movement may provoke a train of positive sharp waves, fibrillations, fasciculations, complex repetitive discharges, or myotonic potentials.

Interpretation of Findings

Clinical electrophysiologic testing can be used to determine whether a disorder is primarily of the muscle itself (myopathy) or of the nerve (neuropathy). If a neuropathy is detected, it can be determined whether the myelin is involved (myelinopathy) or the axon (axonopathy). Two classification schemes are commonly used for neuropathies—one developed by Seddon [23], the other by Sunderland [24]. Table 4.1 lists both classification schemes, along with the tissue involved and possible causes.

A discussion of "typical" findings in neuromuscular disease on electrophysiologic testing must be either very long or overly simplified. Because it is not the intent of this chapter to teach proficiency in the conduct of these examinations, the second option will be exercised.

Myopathy

Myopathies result in abnormal findings during needle electromyography, with a decrease in the motor evoked response, but without a slowing of nerve conduction velocity [1]. Typically, myopathies produce proximal weakness that progresses distally.

Myelinopathy and Axonopathy

In general, myelinopathies produce slowing of nerve conduction velocity without a change in amplitude of the evoked response, and without changes during needle electromyography [3]. Axonopathies usually result in a diminished amplitude of the evoked response with evidence of denervation during needle electromyography, but with no slowing of nerve conduction velocity. However, if severe, an axonopathy may eventually result in myelin damage, and a severe myelinopathy may eventually result in axonal damage [2]. Neuropathies usually begin distally and proceed proximally. However, Guillain-Barré is a neuropathy that begins with proximal weakness [2].

Radiculopathy

Compression or other damage to a single nerve root (radiculopathy) will result in EMG changes limited to a single myotome. Because most nerve roots contribute to the formation of more than one peripheral nerve, a radiculopathy will produce abnormal EMG activity in muscles supplied by more than one peripheral nerve. Generally, a radiculopathy will not produce alterations in the values obtained during nerve conduction testing because of the multiple roots forming that peripheral nerve [16].

Peripheral Neuropathy

Entrapment or compression of a single peripheral nerve will usually produce a slowing of the nerve conduction velocity across the segment that is compressed. Conduction velocity both distal and proximal to the site of the compression will remain normal. If the damage is confined to the myelin, the amplitude of the evoked response will remain normal. If an axonopathy is present, there will be changes noted on needle EMG in the muscles supplied by that nerve distal to the compression, and the amplitude of evoked responses may be diminished.

Table 4.2. Typical EMG Patterns Noted in Normal Muscle and in the Presence of Myelinopathy, Axonopathy, or Myogenic Lesions

Observation Condition	Normal	Myelinopathy	Axonopathy	Myogenic
Minimal contraction	Motor units of normal shape, amplitude, duration, and frequency	Motor units of normal shape, amplitude, duration, and frequency	Large (chronic) or small (acute) motor units with increased phases and duration	Small amplitude, short duration, possibly polyphasic motor units
Maximal contraction	Full interference pattern	Slightly reduced interference pattern of normal amplitude	Reduced interference pattern of increased or normal amplitude	Full interference pattern of reduced amplitude with minimal to moderate effort
Rest	Silence	Silence	Fibrillations, positive sharp waves, fasciculations	Silence; possibly fibrillations, positive sharp waves, complex repetitive discharges, myotonic potentials
Needle insertion	Short burst of activity	Short burst of activity	Prolonged	Abbreviated, normal, or prolonged

Polyneuropathies are rarely caused by mechanical trauma but are more often metabolic, toxic, or infectious in nature. These disorders (e.g., diabetes mellitus, ethanol abuse, Guillian-Barré, etc.) produce changes in multiple peripheral nerves. Polyneuropathies may be primarily sensory or motor, axonopathy or myelinopathy, or mixed.

In addition to the pattern of findings (i.e., proximal versus distal, single root versus single nerve versus multiple nerves, myelin versus axonal), the timing of the disease process is relevant to determining the cause. Table 4.2 shows typical EMG findings for myopathies, axonopathies, myelinopathies, and for normal muscle. Tables 4.3 and 4.4 show nerve conduction study findings for partial versus complete and myelin versus axonal involvement according to the time since the onset of the injury.

Specific Disorders

Myopathies

A patient with a myopathy will usually have symmetrical weakness; rarely is there unilateral involvement. The weakness is characteristically more pronounced in the proximal musculature. Although pain is not typically an initial complaint, weakness may alter the biomechanics of the shoulder girdle

sufficiently to cause musculoskeletal pain. Myopathies that may be encountered when evaluating the thoracic spine include the muscular dystrophies (e.g., Duchenne-type, limb-girdle, etc.), myopathies associated with disorders of lipid or glycogen metabolism (e.g., McArdle's disease), and others [2].

Radiculopathies

The most common cause of a radiculopathy is a herniation of the intervertebral disc. Because the discs in the thoracic spine do not herniate often, compression of thoracic nerve roots is not common, but it does occur [25]. Some researchers are challenging the idea that herniated discs in the thoracic spine are rare; see Chapter 1 for further discussion of this topic. Compression of any of the cervical nerve roots may cause pain in the shoulder girdle area.

Compression of a nerve root will generally not produce any alterations in the nerve conduction variables. Although there may be some EMG changes as soon as 7 days after the compression, the early changes are extremely subtle. At 3 weeks after onset, EMG changes will be confined to the myotome of the compressed root; Chapter 7 of this book lists the myotomes of the upper member.

Table 4.3. Nerve Conduction Findings After a Partial or Complete Loss of Myelin in a Nerve in the Forearm*

	Injury	Day of Injury	One Week After Injury
Stimulate at wrist			
Amplitude	Partial	Normal	Normal
	Complete	Normal	Normal
Latency	Partial	Normal	Normal
	Complete	Normal	Normal
Stimulate at elbow			
Amplitude	Partial	Diminished	Diminished
	Complete	No response	No response
Latency	Partial	Increased	Increased
	Complete	No response	No response
Velocity	Partial	Reduced	Reduced
(in forearm)	Complete	No response	No response
Stimulate at axilla			
Amplitude	Partial	Diminished	Diminished
	Complete	No response	No response
Latency	Partial	Increased	Increased
	Complete	No response	No response
Velocity	Partial	Normal	Normal
(in upper arm)	Complete	Because of no response, cannot calculate (unless a muscle proximal to the lesion is used)	

*A hand muscle is used as the recording site.
Source: Adapted from R Kellogg. Electrophysiologic evaluation. Clin Management 1991;11:34–42.

Peripheral Neuropathies

Disorders of peripheral nerves may occur in isolation (mononeuropathy) or may involve multiple nerves (polyneuropathy). Mononeuropathies are most commonly caused by direct trauma or compression in a tunnel, whereas polyneuropathies are usually associated with a systemic process. It is important to recall that many systemic processes increase the vulnerability of peripheral nerves to compression in a tunnel. For example, an individual may develop carpal tunnel syndrome with less compression of the median nerve if they consume excess ethanol than the compression that is required if they abstain. In addition, compression of a nerve or nerve root that is subclinical may make the nerve more susceptible to compression distally (the double-crush syndrome). If an individual has a C8 radiculopathy, the ulnar nerve can tolerate less trauma at the elbow than if the radiculopathy were absent. Additionally, surgical decompression at the elbow without also addressing the radiculopathy may be only partially successful at relieving the symptoms.

Sites of compression neuropathies involving the upper member have been addressed in several recent reviews (e.g., references 26–29). For this chapter, it is sufficient to state that all elements of the brachial plexus, from the roots to the peripheral nerves, are subject to compression or entrapment by normal tunnels, anatomically anomalous tunnels, normal movements, and abnormal biomechanics.

Thoracic Outlet Syndrome

That a constellation of symptoms constituting *thoracic outlet syndrome* (TOS) exists is generally well accepted. What are the subjects of sometimes acrimonious debate are whether TOS is common or rare and what the proper treatment of it should be if it is present [30, 31]. This debate is not addressed in this chapter, but the electrophysiologic findings that are generally interpreted as being consistent with a clinical diagnosis of TOS are presented.

TOS appears to occur as four distinct entities: arterial vascular, venous vascular, neurogenic, and disputed [31]. The results of the electrophysiologic examination are normal in the two forms of vascular TOS and in the disputed form [15, 32]. If there is true

Table 4.4. Nerve Conduction Findings After a Partial or Complete Axotomy in a Nerve in the Forearm*

	Injury	Day of Injury	One Week After Injury
Stimulate at wrist			
Amplitude	Partial	Normal	Diminished
	Complete	Normal	No response
Latency	Partial	Normal	Normal
	Complete	Normal	No response
Stimulate at elbow			
Amplitude	Partial	Diminished	Diminished
	Complete	No response	No response
Latency	Partial	Normal or increased	Normal or increased
	Complete	No response	No response
Velocity (in forearm)	Partial	Normal or reduced	Normal or reduced
	Complete	No response	No response
Stimulate at axilla			
Amplitude	Partial	Normal or increased	Normal or increased
	Complete	No response	No response
Latency	Partial	Normal or increased	Normal or increased
	Complete	No response	No response
Velocity (in upper arm)	Partial	Normal	Normal
	Complete	Because of no response, cannot calculate (unless a muscle proximal to the lesion is used)	

*A hand muscle is used as the recording site.
Source: Adapted from R Kellogg. Electrophysiologic evaluation. Clin Management 1991;11:34–42.)

compression of neural tissue in the thoracic outlet, the changes noted on EMG are the same as for any compression neuropathy. In the early stages, when the disorder is a primary myelinopathy, there will be a slowing of the nerve conduction velocity across the site of entrapment. Because the plexus is far proximal, and at least some of the potential sites of entrapment are proximal to the most distal site accessible to surface stimulation, the results of routine peripheral nerve conduction studies are often normal. The H-reflex and F-wave may be helpful, but because of the distance over which the potential must be conducted, minor delays in conduction may be missed. The axillary F central latency [2] or needle stimulation of the nerve roots [2] are sometimes helpful.

If the compression is severe, an axonopathy may develop. In this case, EMG changes (e.g., signs of membrane instability) may be noted in muscles innervated by peripheral nerves formed by the compressed structure. For example, if the lower trunk is compressed against the first rib, alterations in the motor units of the ulnar innervated muscles will be detected [15]. As with any other peripheral nerve injury, the double-crush syndrome must be considered.

This syndrome has been reported to accompany TOS [33]; whether the paraspinal muscles are involved is very helpful in distinguishing root involvement from purely peripheral nerve involvement.

Summary

Clinical electrophysiologic testing is an extremely useful tool when used appropriately. Even though diagnostic imaging (e.g., magnetic resonance imaging, computed tomography scans) provides a tremendous amount of information, the information is anatomic, not physiologic, in nature. Merely identifying an anatomic lesion does not mean that there is a loss of function as a result of the change in the anatomy. Furthermore, normal anatomy does not guarantee normal function.

The EMG examination can provide information relative to the severity, location, and chronicity of a lesion of the neuromuscular system. These examinations do not substitute for a thorough history and physical examination, and rarely provide enough information for a definitive diagnosis. Because of the delay between the onset of a lesion and the presence of detectable abnormalities, the timing of the examination in relation to the onset of symptoms must be considered.

References

1. Nelson RM, Nestor DE. Electrophysiological Evaluation: An Overview. In RM Nelson, DP Currier (eds), Clinical Electrotherapy. Norwalk, CT: Appleton & Lange, 1991;2:331–360.
2. Kimura J. Electrodiagnosis in Diseases of Nerve and Muscle: Principles and Practice. Philadelphia: FA Davis, 1988;2.
3. Kellogg R. Electrophysiologic evaluation. Clin Management 1991;11:34–42.
4. Dahlin LB, Archer DR, McLean WG. Treatment with an aldose reductase inhibitor can reduce the susceptibility of fast axonal transport following nerve compression in the streptozotocin-diabetic rat. Diabetologia 1987;30:414–418.
5. Dahlin LB, Meiri RF, McLean WG et al. Effects of nerve compression on fast axonal transport in streptozotocin-induced diabetes mellitus: an experimental study in the sciatic nerve of rats. Diabetologia 1986;29:181–185.
6. Dahlin LB, Rydevik B, McLean WG et al. Changes in fast axonal transport during experimental nerve compression at low pressures. Exp Neurol 1984;84:29–36.
7. Upton RM, McComas AJ. The double-crush in nerve entrapment syndromes. Lancet 1973;2:359–362.
8. Reiner S, Rogoff JB. Instrumentation. In EW Johnson (ed), Practical Electromyography. Baltimore: Williams & Wilkins, 1988;2:498–560.
9. Hille B. Membranes and Ions; Excitable Cells. In HD Patton, AF Fuchs, B Hille, AM Scher, R Steiner (eds), Textbook of Physiology. Philadelphia: Saunders, 1989;21:1–97.
10. Siegel GJ. Excitation, Conduction, and Transmission of the Nerve Impulse. In JB West (ed), Best and Taylor's Physiological Basis of Medical Practice. Baltimore: Williams & Wilkins, 1990;12:31–61.
11. Kutchai HC. Cellular Physiology. In RM Berne, MN Levy (eds), Physiology. St. Louis: Mosby, 1993;3:3–89.
12. Byrne JH. Resting Potentials and Action Potentials in Excitable Cells. In LR Johnson (ed), Essential Medical Physiology. New York: Raven, 1992;43–68.
13. Koester J. Membrane Potential; Passive Membrane Properties of the Neuron; Voltage-Gated Ion Channels and the Generation of the Action Potential. In ER Kandel, JH Schwartz, TM Jessell (eds), Principles of Neural Science. New York: Elsevier, 1991;3:81–118.
14. Liveson JA, Ma DM. Laboratory Reference for Clinical Neurophysiology. Philadelphia: FA Davis, 1992.
15. Aminoff MJ, Olney RK, Parry GJ et al. Relative utility of different electrophysiologic techniques in the evaluation of brachial plexopathies. Neurology 1988;38:546–550.
16. Herdmann J, Dvořák J. Electrophysiology of the normal and diseased spine. In Y Floman, J-PC Farcy, C Argenson (eds), Thoracolumbar Spine Fractures. New York: Raven, 1993;99–121.
17. Dreyfuss P, Dumitru D, Prewitt-Buchanan L. Intercostal somatosensory-evoked potentials: a new technique. Am J Phys Med Rehabil 1993;72:144–150.
18. Nestor DE, Nelson RM. Performing Motor and Sensory Neuronal Conduction Studies in Adult Humans. Washington, DC: US Department of Health and Human Services, 1990.
19. Cassvan A, Pease WS, MacLean IC et al. Late responses. Arch Phys Med Rehabil 1987;68(Suppl):19–22.
20. Jusic A, Tomic M, Fronjek N. Secondary potential of triceps surae muscles (F, FH, and H potentials) in healthy subjects. Electromyogr Clin Neurophysiol 1986;26:33–39.
21. Schimsheimer RJ, Ongerboer de Visser BW, Kemp B et al. The flexor carpi radialis H-reflex in polyneuropathy: Relations to conduction velocities of the median nerve and the soleus H-reflex latency. J Neurol Neurosurg Psychiatry 1987;50:447–452.
22. Christensen E. Topography of terminal motor innervation in striated muscles from stillborn infants. Am J Phys Med 1959;38:65–78.
23. Seddon HJ. Three types of nerve injury. Brain 1943;66:237–288.
24. Sunderland S. Nerve injuries and their repair: A critical appraisal. Edinburgh: Churchill Livingstone, 1991.
25. Hegde S, Staas WE Jr. Thoracic disc herniation and spinal cord injury. Am J Phys Med Rehabil 1988;68:228–229.
26. Toby EB, Koman LA. Thoracic Outlet Compression Syndrome. In RM Szabo (ed), Nerve Compression Syndromes: Diagnosis and Treatment. Thorofare, NJ: Slack, 1989:227–246.
27. Narakas A. Compression Syndromes about the Shoulder Including Brachial Plexus. In RM Szabo (ed), Nerve Compression Syndromes: Diagnosis and Treatment. Thorofare, NJ: Slack, 1989:227–246.
28. Torres-Ramos FM, Biundo JJ Jr. Suprascapular neuropathy during progressive resistive exercises in a cardiac rehabilitation program. Arch Phys Med Rehabil 1992;73:1107–1111.
29. Pecina MM, Krmpotic-Nemanic J, Markiewitz AD. Tunnel Syndromes. Boca Raton, FL: CRC Press, 1991.
30. Roos DB. The thoracic outlet syndrome is underrated. Arch Neurol 1990;47:327–328.
31. Wilbourn AJ. The thoracic outlet syndrome is overdiagnosed. Arch Neurol 1990;47:328–330.
32. Baumgartner F, Nelson RJ, Robertson JM. The rudimentary first rib: a cause of thoracic outlet syndrome with arterial compromise. Arch Surg 1989;124:1090–1092.
33. Askin SR, Hadler NM. Double-crush nerve compression in thoracic outlet syndrome. J Bone Joint Surg [Am] 1991;73:629–630.

Chapter 5

Bone Trauma and Disease of the Thoracic Spine and Ribs

Mary E. Reid

The thoracic spine is attached by the ribs to the sternum and has a high degree of inherent stability and rigidity. Anatomically, the thoracic spine is from T1 to T12. The thoracolumbar junction is defined as T12–L1. Functionally, there is a transition in anatomy from the lower thoracic spine into the upper lumbar spine. This is reflected in the fracture patterns associated with this area. The thoracic spine therefore has two segments with their own distinct fracture patterns. The two distinct injury patterns are related to the change in anatomy (Fig. 5.1). The facet joints in the upper and middle thoracic spine are generally in the frontal plane and allow a high degree of rotation, but the rotation decreases as the facet orientation transitions to that of the lumbar spine. The sagittally facing lumbar facets allow flexion and extension and almost no rotation. This change in stiffness between an upper segment that is flexible in rotation and a lower segment that is inflexible in rotation creates an area of high stress concentration, resulting in a high incidence of fractures in the thoracolumbar junction.

Thoracic Vertebral Fractures

There are over 160,000 spinal fractures each year and an average of 10,000 new spinal cord injuries each year in the United States. A high percentage of these involve the thoracic spine. The primary goal of treat- ment of these fractures is to preserve life, maintain neurologic function, and maintain or restore spine stability and alignment. Spinal fractures and spinal cord injuries (SCIs) should be highly suspected during the primary management of any trauma patient. Any unconscious victim of trauma should be assumed to have a spinal injury. In 3–5% of all spinal injuries, there is an additional injury within the spine at a separate noncontiguous segment. Spinal injuries are often missed on the initial evaluation of trauma patients. A delay in diagnosis of spinal injuries is associated with a low level of suspicion, failure to obtain x-ray studies, failure to recognize a fracture on x-ray films, altered mental status of the patient either because of intoxication or closed head injury, multiple levels of spinal fractures, and multiple trauma. Injuries that occur at levels from T1 to T10 are associated with damage to the spinal cord, whereas injuries of the thoracolumbar junction, T11–L2, may present as mixed spinal cord, conus medullaris, or nerve root injuries. Injuries at the level of L3 and below present as cauda equina injuries. Evaluation of trauma patients includes a history of the mechanism of injury. Facts from the injury scene help one understand the forces involved in spinal fractures. Any history of transient paralysis or previous spinal injury or surgery of the spine should be sought. Precautions must be taken to protect and immobilize the spine at all times during the patient evaluation via the use of a spine board and by log-rolling the patient. A rapid physical and neurologic examination is performed at the time the patient arrives at the hospital.

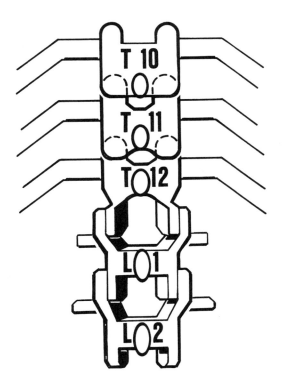

Figure 5.1. Differences in facet joint anatomy of the thoracic and lumbar spine.

This must be documented and recorded accurately. Follow-up examinations are repeated to document any changes. All clothing should be completely removed from the patient for the physical examination. The entire spine is examined. This includes palpation of the spinous processes and assessment for any step-off or gibbus, ecchymosis or tissue edema, and any wounds to the skin overlying the spine. The neurologic examination must include motor strength grading and determination of sensory levels and dermatomal distribution, with special attention to any perianal sensory sparing. The initial sensory level can be drawn on the patient's skin. Deep tendon reflexes (more accurately named muscle stretch reflexes; see Chapter 7), plantar reflex (Babinski), abdominal reflex, anal sphincter tone, and the bulbocavernosus reflex are all recorded. The bulbocavernosus reflex carries prognostic importance (Fig. 5.2). The absence of this reflex implies spinal shock or spinal cord injury.

In the case of neurologic injury, deleterious metabolic changes occur almost immediately to the spinal cord. Disruption of the vascular circulation to the spinal cord can be caused by mechanical defor-mity, blunt injury, edema, thrombosis, or vasoconstriction induced by local or systemic tissue necrosis. There is no proven therapy that will reverse ischemic damage to the spinal cord. There is recent evidence supporting the use of methylprednisolone in acute SCI patients. Treatment is begun with a loading dose of 30 mg/kg within the first 8 hours of injury. This is followed for the next 23 hours with 5.4 mg/kg per hour. There is evidence of improved neurologic recovery with this treatment [1].

Classification of Thoracic Spine Fractures

There are several classification systems of thoracic and thoracolumbar spine fractures. An earlier system described by Holdsworth [2] was based on a two-column model of the spine. The anterior column was described as the posterior longitudinal ligament and everything anterior to this. The posterior column involved the neural arch, pedicle, lamina, facets, and spinous process as well as the ligamentous structures attached to these. A newer modification of this system was proposed by Denis [3] and is easy to understand and often used to describe spinal fractures. The Denis classification system divides the spine into three segments (Fig. 5.3). The anterior column includes the anterior longitudinal ligament, the anterior vertebral body, and the associated annulus fibrosus. The middle column includes the posterior longitudinal ligament, the posterior aspect of the vertebral body, and the associated annulus fibrosus. The posterior column includes the pedicle, the facet joints, the lamina, the spinous process, and the interspinous ligaments. These columns are described as failing individually or in combination by either compression, distraction, rotation, or shear forces. Fractures are divided into categories depending on which columns are involved in the injury; with disruption of two or more columns the fracture is considered unstable.

Compression Fractures

Compression fractures result from axial loading combined with flexion or lateral bending. They are the most common type of thoracic fracture but have a predilection for the thoracolumbar junction. The fracture pattern is marked by a failure of the anterior column and can be subdivided into failure of both end plates or the inferior end plate only, but failure

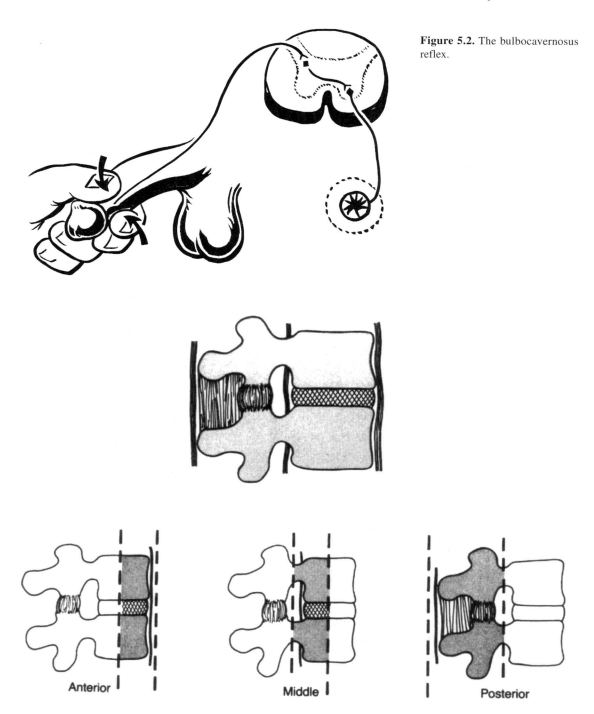

Figure 5.2. The bulbocavernosus reflex.

Anterior   Middle   Posterior

Figure 5.3. Denis's three-column model of the spine. The middle column is made up of the posterior annulus fibrosus and the posterior aspect of the vertebral body and disc. (Reprinted with permission from F Eismont, S Garfin, J-J Abitbol. Thoracic and Upper Lumbar Spine Injuries. In BD Browner, JB Jupiter, AM Levine et al. [eds], Skeletal Trauma. Vol. 1. Philadelphia: Saunders, 1992;744.)

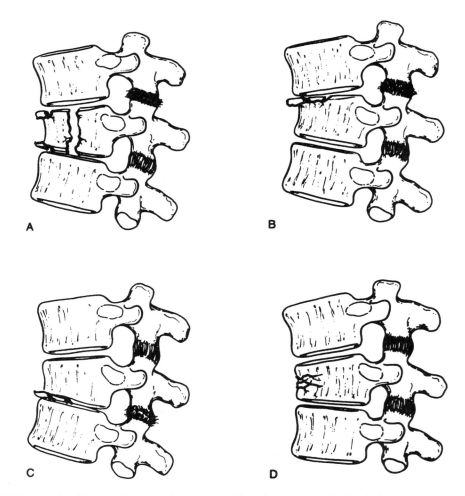

Figure 5.4. Denis's classification of compression fractures. These fractures may involve both end plates (type A), the superior end plate only (type B), the inferior end plate only (type C), or a buckling of the anterior cortex with both end plates intact (type D). (Reprinted with permission from F Eismont, S Garfin, J-J Abitbol. Thoracic and Upper Lumbar Spine Injuries. In BD Browner, JB Jupiter, AM Levine, et al. [eds], Skeletal Trauma. Vol. 1. Philadelphia: Saunders, 1992;744.)

of the superior end plate is a frequent pattern (Fig. 5.4). Compression of greater than 40% usually implies instability, but in some cases up to 50% is accepted as stable. When greater than 50% anterior wedging is present, progressive kyphosis may occur with time [4]. A kyphotic angulation of greater than 20 degrees is an indicator of instability. As the degree of angulation and compression increases, there is more need to assess the possibility of this being a burst fracture, and a computed tomographic (CT) scan is helpful. Compression fractures are usually not associated with neurologic deficit.

Burst Fractures

Burst fractures in the Denis classification are characterized by disruption of the middle column, usually with retropulsion of a bone fragment into the canal, decreasing the canal size (Fig. 5.5). There may be spreading of the posterior elements on an anteroposterior (AP) plain roentgenogram. A CT scan is very helpful in the evaluation of these fractures. Magnetic resonance imaging (MRI) has the advantage of visualizing the neural structures such as cord, cauda equina, or nerve roots. If the posterior column

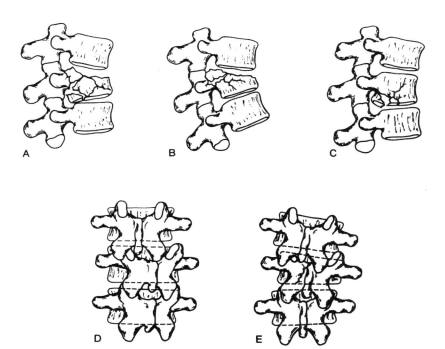

Figure 5.5. Denis's classification of burst fractures. Types A, B, and C represent fractures of both end plates, the superior end plate, and the inferior end plate, respectively. Type D is a combination of a type A burst fracture with rotation, which is best appreciated on the anteroposterior roentgenogram. The type E burst fracture is a result of a laterally directed force and hence appears asymmetric on the anteroposterior roentgeno- gram. The superior end plate, inferior end plate, or both may be involved with this fracture. (Reprinted with permission from F Eismont, S Garfin, J-J Abitbol. Thoracic and Upper Lumbar Spine Injuries. In BD Browner, JB Jupiter, AM Levine, et al. [eds], Skeletal Trauma. Vol. 1. Philadelphia: Saunders, 1992; 753.)

is involved, one-half of patients will have some neu- rologic injury. Most often these fractures occur at the thoracolumbar junction.

Fracture-Dislocation

Fracture-dislocations of the spine are considered to be very unstable injuries. These involve failure of all three columns of the spine. Spontaneous reduction can occur, thus not giving evidence of the degree of instability on plain roentgenograms. Fracture-dislo- cations are the result of considerable force. The forces can be a combination of rotation, flexion, dis- traction, compression, and shear. In the Denis clas- sification system, these injuries are subdivided into (1) flexion-rotation injuries, (2) shear-type fracture- dislocations, and (3) flexion-distraction injuries (Fig. 5.6). Neurologic deficit is present in 75% of cases. There is also a very high association with dural tears and additional intra-abdominal injury.

Flexion-Distraction Injuries

Flexion-distraction injuries were first described by Chance [5]. In this injury there may be failure of all three columns or just the posterior column. The spinal column is subject to large tensile force with the fulcrum being located anterior to the spine, as in a lap-belt injury. The injury through the spine is by avulsion and can be a pure bony injury, a pure soft- tissue injury, or a combination. These are potentially very unstable injuries, especially if the anterior lon- gitudinal ligament fails. These fractures are subdi- vided by Denis into four types depending on the involvement of bone or ligament (Fig. 5.7).

Extension Injuries

Extension injuries are considered a type of minor frac- ture pattern. These injuries occur when a compression force is applied over the posterior elements, and usu-

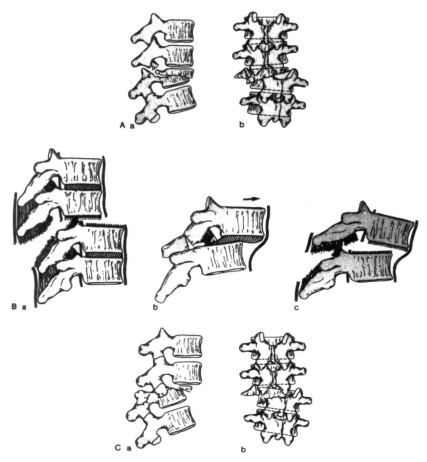

Figure 5.6. Denis's classification of fracture-dislocation of the spine. Type A is a flexion-rotation injury, either occurring through bone or through the disc. There is a complete disruption of all three columns of the spine, usually with the anterior longitudinal ligament remaining the only intact structure. Commonly this is stripped off the anterior portion of the vertebral body below. These injuries are usually associated with fractures of the superior facet of the more caudal vertebra. Type B is a shear injury. The type that produces anterior spondylolisthesis of the more cephalad vertebra usually fractures a facet, and that causing a posterior listhesis of the more cephalad vertebra normally does not cause a fracture of the facet joint. Type C is a bilateral facet dislocation. This is a flexion-distraction injury but with disruption of the anterior column in addition to the posterior and middle columns. This disruption through the anterior column may occur through either the anterior intervertebral disc or the anterior vertebral body. (Reprinted with permission from F Eismont, S Garfin, J-J Abitbol. Thoracic and Upper Lumbar Spine Injuries. In BD Browner, JB Jupiter, AM Levine, et al. [eds], Skeletal Trauma. Vol. 1. Philadelphia: Saunders, 1992;758.)

ally the strong anterior longitudinal ligament remains intact under a tensile force. This can result in laminar, spinous process, or pedicle fractures, as well as avulsion of the anterior portion of the vertebral body. These fractures are usually stable, but they may be unstable depending on the degree of injury. More severe hyperextension injuries occur in patients with ankylosing spondylitis, but they may rarely occur in patients with diffuse idiopathic skeletal hyperostosis (DISH) [6]. An ankylosed, osteopenic spine can be fractured with minimal trauma such as a fall [7]. Hyperextension injuries occur more often in the cervical spine than in the thoracic spine. These injuries may be difficult to diagnose because there may be spontaneous reduction, but they usually remain unstable. This injury pattern is not addressed by the Denis classification.

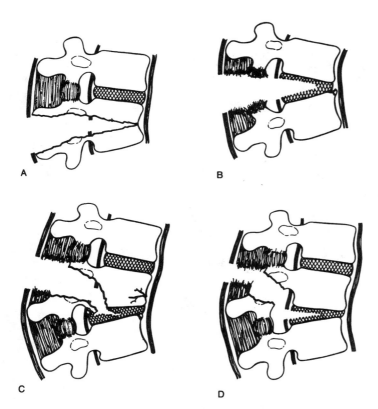

Figure 5.7. Denis's classification of flexion-distraction injuries. These may occur at one level through bone (A); at one level through the ligaments and disc (B); at two levels, with the middle column injured through bone (C); or at two levels with the middle column injury occurring through ligament and disc (D). (Reprinted with permission from F Eismont, S Garfin, J-J Abitbol. Thoracic and Upper Lumbar Spine Injuries. In BD Browner, JB Jupiter, AM Levine, et al. [eds], Skeletal Trauma. Vol. 1, Philadelphia: Saunders, 1992;754.)

Treatment

Treatment options for trauma to the spinal column are many and somewhat controversial. Nonoperative treatment has been used extensively in the past and still is applied to many fracture patterns. Assessment of stability does not dictate operative verses nonoperative treatment [8]. Fractures with canal compromise of more than 35% in the thoracic spine are considered to put the patient at risk for neurologic injury [9]. Treatment of stable injuries consists of bed rest, management of any associated ileus, and pain management. An external orthosis is usually applied, and ambulation is begun as pain decreases.

Surgical treatment is often used to restore the functional status of the spine. Goals of surgery include (1) decompression of the spinal canal, (2) restoration of normal alignment to the spine, and (3) provision of stability acutely and long term (Figs. 5.8, 5.9, 5.10, and 5.11). Surgical procedures may be through a posterior approach, an anterior approach, or a combined approach based on the fracture pattern and neurologic injury. Rapid reduction, decompression, and stabilization are indicated in incomplete neurologic lesions so that displacement and further impingement are prevented.

Posterior instrumentation remains the mainstay of treatment for unstable fractures. Decompression of the spinal canal can sometimes be achieved in acute injuries (less than 72 hours) by distraction to realign the spine [10]. In patients who are treated late after the injury, decompression may be done either through an anterior approach or through a posterior lateral or transpedicular approach. The timing of surgical treatment is still controversial. There is no conclusive evidence that immediate surgical treatment leads to better neurologic recovery. This is being evaluated by several centers. Emergency decompression is indicated in the presence of cauda equina syndrome or worsening neurologic status.

Rib Cage Fractures

Thoracic rib cage injuries can be minor, such as a simple rib fracture, or major, such as flail chest with

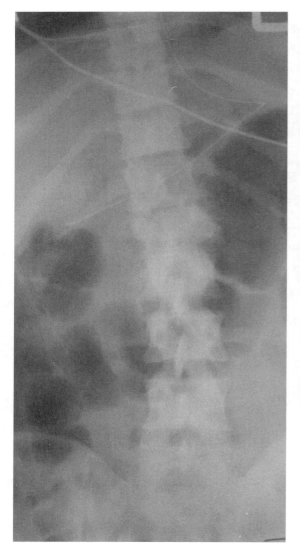

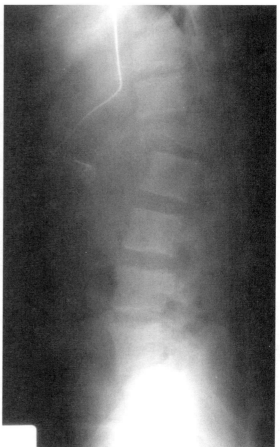

Figure 5.9. The lateral view of the L1 fracture-dislocation shows significant displacement of L1 causing significant injury within the spinal canal and profound neurologic deficit.

Figure 5.8. This anteroposterior radiograph shows the pattern of a fracture-dislocation of L1. There is displacement and abnormal alignment of the spine.

hemothorax or pneumothorax. If these injuries are treated with proper measures, most have an excellent prognosis.

Fracture of the ribs is a common injury, occurring more often in adults than in children. Usually rib fractures are the result of trauma, but pathologic fractures do occur in patients as a result of metastatic lesions or myeloma. The primary symptom of a rib fracture is pain on inspiration, resulting in hypoventilation. On physical examination there may be a palpable or visible defect, tenderness to palpa-

tion, crepitation from subcutaneous emphysema, or ecchymosis. A chest roentenogram is indicated primarily to exclude associated intrathoracic injuries such as pneumothorax, hemothorax, or pleural effusion. Fractures of the first or second rib can be the result of significant trauma, with associated injuries to the head, neck, or great vessels and a significant risk of death. In addition to rib fractures, costovertebral dislocations or costochondral and costosternal separation may occur.

Treatment

Treatment of simple rib fractures is symptomatic and supportive. Cough assistance or endotracheal

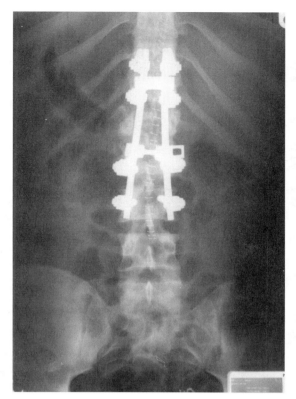

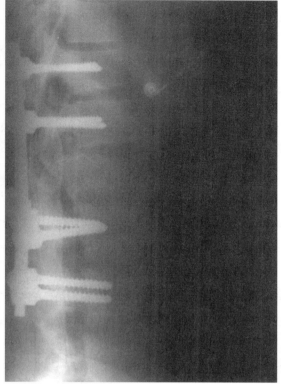

Figure 5.10. This anteroposterior film demonstrates re-alignment and fixation after open reduction and internal fixation with pedicle screws and rods.

Figure 5.11. The lateral film shows pedicle fixation with smaller diameter screws in the thoracic spine. Normal alignment was achieved but without complete reduction of L1.

suction may be necessary. Pain management allows for good cough effort and is achieved by narcotics in small amounts. Intracostal nerve blocks and muscle relaxants may also be used to alleviate pain (Fig. 5.12). However, intracostal nerve blocks may be associated with increased reflex bronchial secretions, which can lead to pneumonia, especially in elderly patients. Epidural or intrathecal morphine injection produces pain relief and improvement in pulmonary function in some patients during normal breathing. A combination of local anesthesia and continuous epidural analgesia is an effective way to treat pain and improve pulmonary function after chest trauma [11]. Adhesive taping or strapping should be avoided because it inhibits deep inspiration and may contribute to atelectasis. Simple rib fractures usually become stable in 1–2 weeks, with a firm healing by callus in approximately 6 weeks.

Flail Chest

A flail chest occurs when a segment of the chest wall does not have continuity with the remainder of the thoracic cage. Flail chest usually results from fractures in at least two sites in multiple adjacent ribs. The flail chest segment produces a paradoxical motion, moving in during inspiration and out during expiration. This in turn leads to splinting of the chest wall with inefficient ventilation and a decrease in vital capacity. Flail chest injuries may not be initially apparent because of splinting and may progress to respiratory distress. A chest x-ray film is indicated and arterial blood gas analysis may be helpful in making the diagnosis. The major difficulty in flail chest is the associated lung contusion, which can progress to the potentially lethal condition of adult respiratory distress syndrome (ARDS). Treatment of

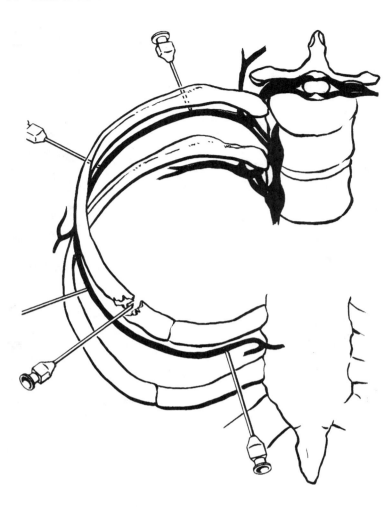

Figure 5.12. Intercostal nerve block to relieve pain of fractured ribs.

flail chest consists of expanding the lung and stabilizing the flail segment. Stabilization by open reduction and internal fixation is only very rarely indicated, such as when flail chest is associated with sternal fracture displacement or severe rib displacement. Endotracheal intubation with or without the use of positive end-expiratory pressure is the treatment used most often. Not all patients with flail chest injuries will need immediate endotracheal intubation, but all patients must be evaluated and monitored carefully [12].

Osteoporosis

Osteoporosis is an age-related disorder characterized by decreased bone mass and increased susceptibility to fracture in the absence of other recognized causes of bone loss. Generalized decreased bone density appears as excessive radiolucency on radiographic evaluation. This condition is referred to as osteopenia, which is the result of either the bone matrix not being calcified at a normal rate or, more commonly, a decrease in bone mass—that is, osteoporosis. A bone that has undergone osteoporosis will grossly have a normal appearance but will be much lighter with a thinner cortex, and the trabecular bone will appear much more porous than that of a normal bone. Bone loss is thought to be a consistent part of the aging process, but not all individuals will develop osteoporosis. This bone loss occurs more quickly in women. Women experience a period of rapid bone loss after menopause, which may approach 1–3% a year and is believed to occur as a consequence of the loss of estrogen. This rapid rate of bone loss may last up to 10 years. Peak bone

Table 5.1. Risk Factors for Osteoporosis

Biological	Disease States	Behavior	Drugs
Female sex	Scoliosis	Inactivity	Steroids
Northern European descent	Osteogenesis imperfecta	Malnutrition	Anticonvulsants
Low weight, small build	Diabetes	Poor nutrition	Methotrexate
Family history	Adrenal dysfunction	Exercise-induced amenorrhea	
Early menopause	Malabsorption syndromes	Smoking	
	Renal dysfunction	Alcohol abuse	
	Thyroid dysfunction		
	Parathyroid dysfunction		
	Liver disease		
	Hypogonadism		

mass or the maximal bone mass reached in life is achieved by the third decade of life and bone loss may begin as early as the fourth decade. Not reaching sufficient peak bone mass may contribute to the development of osteoporosis. There are two recognized forms of osteoporosis. Postmenopausal osteoporosis occurs in women within 10–20 years of menopause. The effect is seen most in the trabecular bone and results in vertebral crush and distal radius fractures. Senile osteoporosis occurs in both men and women over the age of 70 years. Women still predominate 2 to 1.

There are several known risk factors for the development of osteoporosis (Table 5.1). They encompass genetic and biological factors as well as behavioral and environmental factors. A major risk factor is early menopause; additional risk factors are caucasian race; small, thin body build; immobility; low calcium intake; and regular use of cigarettes, coffee, and alcohol.

Clinically, osteoporosis presents most commonly as acute back pain secondary to vertebral fracture. Radicular pain or neurologic disorders secondary to the fracture are uncommon. Occasionally, the condition is not associated with pain, and compression fracture of the spine will be diagnosed on routine lateral chest films or on spine films obtained for evaluation of progressive kyphosis or shortening. The investigation to diagnose osteoporosis usually begins with roentgenograms, but bone loss in the range of 30–50% must have occurred for osteoporosis to be visible on standard roentgenograms. Newer techniques such as single-photon absorption (SPA), dual-photon absorption (DPA), quantitative computer tomography (QCT), and, the most widely used, dual x-ray absorption (DEXA) allow measurement of bone density [13]. The sites of measurement are usually the vertebrae, forearm, or hip. These studies can be repeated at 6-month to 12-month intervals to evaluate progression or the effects of treatment in osteoporosis. Laboratory analysis of serum calcium, phosphate, and osteocalcin levels can be used to assess bone turnover, as can urinary hydroxyproline and pyridinium cross-links (Fig. 5.13) [14]. Patients with higher rates of bone turnover will profit most from treatment to decrease bone resorption. Complete blood counts and urine or serum protein electrophoresis can be used to evaluate patients for hematologic disease or for multiple myeloma. Thyroid function should be evaluated and the patient should be screened for renal and liver disease. If malabsorption is suspected, a serum carotene test is a quick screening method. A possible endocrine cause should be sought if the patient's history includes glucocorticoid use such as prednisone for the management of pulmonary or autoimmune diseases. Cortisol levels and a dexamethasone suppression test will help evaluate adrenal function. The combined direct and indirect effects of chronic glucocorticoid excess cause a profound decrease in bone mass (Cushing's syndrome). Urine collection for 24 hours can be used to evaluate calcium and phosphorus balance. The cause of low calcium secretion can be renal dysfunction, poor calcium absorption, or decreased dietary intake. If phosphorus secretion is high, it may indicate increased parathyroid activity. Serum parathyroid hormone levels as well as vitamin D levels can be used to further evaluate parathyroid function. High levels of osteocalcin, a bone glycoprotein, are associated with high bone turnover

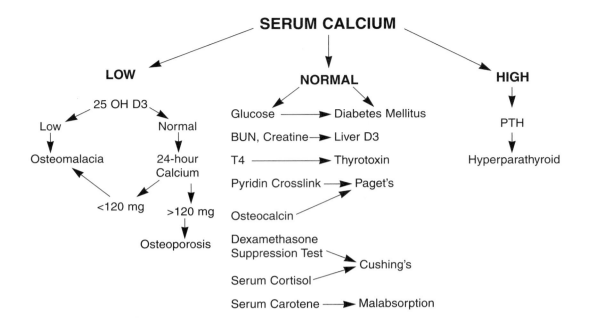

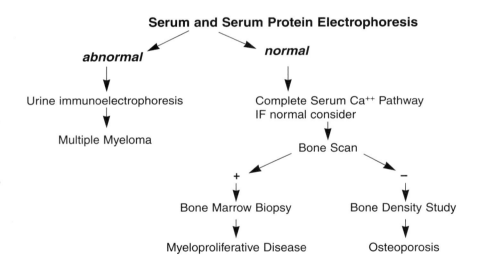

Figure 5.13. Algorithm for evaluation of compression fracture in the osteopenic spine.

such as Paget's disease, or renal osteodystrophy [15]. Further evaluation of an osteopenic patient may include transiliac bone biopsy, since it can be used to assess both the quality and quantity of bone. This procedure is minimally invasive and done routinely as an ambulatory procedure.

Treatment of Spinal Fractures in Osteoporosis

Compression fractures are usually seen in the thoracic or lumbar spine (Fig. 5.14). They are usually painful and can cause significant short-term morbidity, but they usually heal uneventfully, except when a

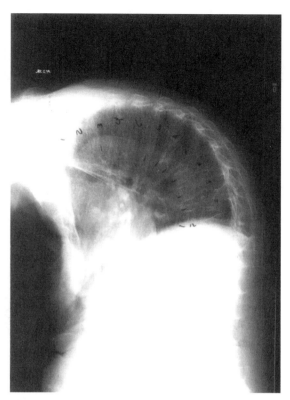

Figure 5.14. Compression fractures in a markedly osteo-porotic spine resulting in a severe kyphotic deformity.

residual kyphotic deformity develops. The goals of therapy are to alleviate pain and provide mechanical support to the spine. Indications for surgery include progressive deformity or instability of the spine with significant pain, or neurologic compromise. Because of the major surgical problems associated with the use of internal fixation on a mechanically weakened osteoporotic spine, most patients are treated nonoperatively. Initially, a brief period of bed rest will help reduce pain. A short-term oral narcotic pain medication may be necessary to control pain. An ileus may accompany a spinal fracture and must be suspected if enteral intake is not tolerated. As the initial episode of acute pain subsides, the patient may begin to increase mobility, usually with some form of orthosis. A molded, rigid thoracolumbar orthosis for lower thoracic fractures or a less restrictive three-point semirigid hyperextension orthosis will also be effective in discouraging kyphotic posture. Bracing

of the upper thoracic spine is difficult unless the neck is immobilized, which is usually not tolerated well by elderly patients. As pain relents, a rehabilitation program is begun. A cane may be helpful as ambulation is begun. A daily program of extension exercises and breathing exercises as well as strengthening of the pectoral muscles and trunk extensor muscles is begun. Strengthening the thoracic spinal musculature will help resist the flexion force of the developing kyphotic spinal deformity. A general conditioning program is also recommended, such as walking, since regular weight-bearing activity is essential to maintaining skeletal bone mass [16]. The patient should be taught to avoid unnecessary compression forces in lifting and bending. After 6–8 weeks, most patients have improved to normal activities, but if episodic pain persists, continued use of a brace is encouraged. The exercise program is recommended as a continued part of daily living for patients with osteoporosis. (See Chapter 12 for more details.)

The medical therapy for osteoporosis can take two approaches, to either increase bone formation or to decrease the rate of bone loss. Attempting to decrease bone resorption and then increase bone formation in a sequential manner is called coherence therapy [17]. Therapy begins with calcium supplements, vitamin D, and exercise as methods to decrease bone resorption. Estrogen, calcitonin, and bisphosphonates all work at producing a decrease in bone resorption. Bisphosphonates are an analog of pyrophosphatase and have a significant effect by blocking bone resorption and may become the most effective treatment of osteoporosis [18]. The therapies to stimulate bone formation include sodium fluoride, coherence therapy (phosphate/calcitonin or phosphate/bisphosphonate), and parathyroid hormone and 1,25 dihydroxyvitamin D_3. Estrogen replacement therapy is most effective for the prevention of progressive postmenopausal osteoporosis if begun in the perimenopausal period. Estrogen therapy can be used during any period where there is evidence that bone turnover is still active. Calcitonin is also effective in decreasing bone resorption but must be administered as a subcutaneous injection. Development of a nasal spray is ongoing. The use of sodium fluoride is experimental at this time; it does lead to increased bone mass but has not been proven to decrease fracture rates and has been associated with an increased rate of fracture in the appendicular skeleton [19]. Before treatment for osteoporosis is begun, a bone densitometry study is performed to establish a baseline for monitoring the response to treatment.

Ankylosing Spondylitis

Ankylosing spondylitis is a chronic inflammatory arthritis that leads to deformity and fusion of the spine. Additional names for the condition are rheumatoid spondylitis, pelvospondylitis ossificans, and Marie-Strümpell disease. It is not a variant of rheumatoid arthritis and is rheumatoid factor–negative. It is classified as one of the seronegative spondyloarthropathies along with Reiter's syndrome, psoriatic arthropathy, and colitic arthropathy. There are certain criteria that are associated with the diagnosis of ankylosing spondylitis. These include low back pain of at least 3 months' duration, limitation of spinal motion, decreased chest expansion, and sacroiliitis. Peripheral joint manifestations occur frequently in the larger joints, especially the hips and shoulders. Ankylosing spondylitis also involves the enthesis, where ligaments attach to bone, especially the Achilles tendon.

Clinical Features

Ankylosing spondylitis usually begins between the ages of 15 and 40 years and occurs more commonly in males at a ratio of 3 to 1. The onset is usually insidious, and complaints are most often related to spinal involvement or sacroiliitis. Patients usually have spinal pain and stiffness with normal neurologic findings. Low back pain and stiffness are worse in the morning or after resting and may improve with activity or mild exercise. Many patients will have associated complaints of peripheral joint involvement. As the disease progresses, strenuous activity such as heavy lifting may aggravate the pain. Physical findings usually include sacroiliac joint tenderness to palpation and a positive sacroiliac joint stress test (Gaenslen's sign and positive Patrick's or FABER maneuver). Gaenslen's test is performed with the patient supine with one buttock over the edge of the table. The leg is allowed to hyperextend over the edge of the table, stressing the sacroiliac joint. FABER stands for flexion, abduction, and external rotation of the hip and is also called the figure "4" test. It also stresses the hip and sacroiliac joint.

Usually a loss of lumbar lordosis is evident, as is a decrease in Schlinde's index (or Schober test), which measures the increase in the span of the lumbar spine. A mark is placed at the spinous process of L5 or at the midline at the level of the posterior superior iliac spine with the patient standing erect. A second mark is placed a measured distance of 10 cm above the first. This distance is measured when the patient is flexed forward without bending the knees. Less than 5 cm of change indicates decreased motion of the lumbar spine. Pain or tenderness on compression of the rib cage or decreased chest expansion indicates thoracic spine involvement. Rib expansion is measured at the nipple line and normally will exceed 2.5 cm. A progressive deformity of thoracic kyphosis may be assessed by the ability to place the back of the head against a wall while the patient's heels and back are against the wall. As the thoracic spine becomes kyphotic, the cervical spine may also lose motion and become kyphotic. This forward protrusion of the head results in a "chin on chest deformity." At this time the patient may have difficulty with ambulation because of limited forward vision.

Any patient with ankylosing spondylitis and a history of a recent fall should be presumed to have a spinal fracture until proven otherwise. Immediate immobilization and diagnosis are essential. Plain roentgenograms may fail to visualize a fracture and may need to be supplemented with a bone scan or tomograms. The most frequently fractured area is the cervical spine, but thoracic fractures may also be difficult to diagnose. The fracture usually originates through a disc space and continues through the posterior elements. Cauda equina syndrome with neurologic symptoms may be associated with these fractures when in the lumbar spine. This is best evaluated with an MRI scan [20].

Laboratory Evaluation

The erythrocyte sedimentation rate (ESR) is elevated in the majority of patients with ankylosing spondylitis, but it does not accurately reflect fluctuations in the disease actively. Rheumatoid factor is invariably negative, even in active peripheral joint disease. There is a strong association of the human leukocyte antigen B27 (HLA-B27) and ankylosing spondylitis; HLA-B27 is positive in 90% of patients with ankylosing spondylitis [21]. Only approximately

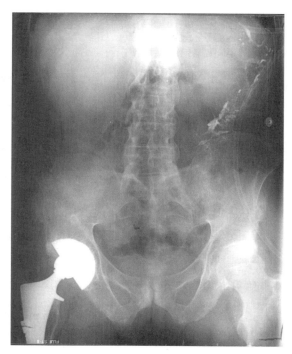

Figure 5.15. This anteroposterior roentgenogram shows the "bamboo spine" of ankylosing spondylitis, with a flowing osteophyte laterally and preservation of disc height. Also note complete ankylosis of both sacral iliac joints as well as bilateral hip involvement.

10–20% of HLA-B27–positive patients develop ankylosing spondylitis [22].

Radiography

Because roentgenograms may appear normal in early ankylosing spondylitis, scintigraphy is useful in evaluating patients who are suspected of having ankylosing spondylitis. The earliest changes seen on roentgenograms usually involve the spine and the sacroiliac joints. Sacroiliac joint involvement in ankylosing spondylitis may start unilaterally, but within years becomes bilateral. Radiographic changes in the spine include squaring of the anterior corners of the thoracic and lumbar vertebrae, formation of syndesmophytes, and, in some cases, advanced ankylotic bamboo spine (Figs. 5.15 and 5.16). Syndesmophytes are a manifestation of ossification of the paravertebral tissue, including the substance of the annulus fibrosus. Posterior spinal structures are involved including the zygapophyseal

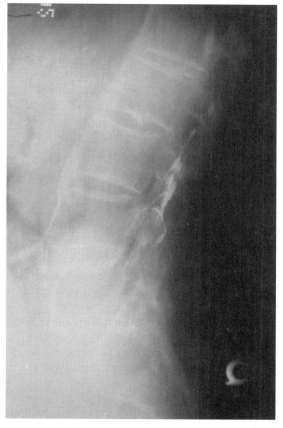

Figure 5.16. The lateral radiograph of a patient with ankylosing spondylitis shows the involvement of the anterior longitudinal ligament, preservation of the disc space, and involvement of the posterior elements.

joints, the interspinous and supraspinous ligaments, and the ligamentum flavum. Intervertebral disc height is usually maintained until late in the disease process. Atlantoaxial subluxation may be seen in ankylosing spondylitis or rheumatoid arthritis and is readily evaluated with flexion-extension lateral roentgenograms of the upper cervical spine.

Medical Management

The purpose of optimal management is to facilitate a normal, functional, and independent life. Patient education and a recommendation to not smoke should begin at the time of diagnosis. Physical therapy should be considered a lifelong commitment, initially begun with the supervision of a physiotherapist.

The goals of therapy are relief of pain and maintenance of mobility. Instruction should include maintenance of an erect posture, use of a firm flat mattress, and performance of a regular exercise program. Swimming is a highly recommended exercise. Nonsteroidal anti-inflammatory drugs (NSAIDs) work better than aspirin to suppress the inflammatory activity and may be a prerequisite to active physiotherapy because they may help diminish stiffness.

Surgical Treatment

Orthopedic reconstructive surgery is often used in the management of peripheral joint disease in ankylosing spondylitis. Total hip replacement has been shown to be efficacious in patients to decrease pain and increase function. Surgical indications for the correction of fixed flexion deformity are relative to the magnitude and functional limitations produced. A severe kyphotic deformity of the spine restricts the ability of the patient to look straight ahead and interferes with interpersonal communication, driving, and even walking. Initial evaluation is directed at determining the primary site of deformity, which may include fixed flexion deformity of the hips. Hip ankylosis should be treated before surgical realignment of any spinal deformity. The "chin-brow angle" is a means of quantifying the clinical deformity. The angle is measured from a vertical line to a line connecting the brow to the chin. The goals of surgery are to restore a horizontal gaze. The osteotomy may be directed at the area of worst deformity, but indirect correction by lumbar osteotomy at the L2–L3 level may be safer because this level is below the spinal cord. The operative technique was described by Smith-Peterson et al. [23] and involves a posterior midline approach to the spine and removal of a wedge of bone. The disc space fractures anteriorly as the osteotomy is closed. Some form of internal fixation is routinely used. A correction of from 40 to 55 degrees can be expected.

Diffuse Idiopathic Skeletal Hyperostosis

Diffuse idiopathic skeletal hyperostosis (DISH) is a relatively common disorder involving the spine and, to a lesser extent, the larger peripheral joints. It is also described under the terms of senile ankylosing hyperostosis, Forestier's disease, ankylosing vertebral hyperostosis, ankylosing hyperostosis of the spine, and spondylitis ossificans ligamentosa. The term *diffuse idiopathic skeletal hyperostosis* was suggested by Resnick et al. [24], and this has become the most widely used name because of its descriptive nature. It is a type of enthesopathy, or disease of the site of the attachment of ligaments or tendons to bone.

Clinical Features

DISH occurs most frequently in middle-aged and older men and is often associated with diabetes [24]. It may affect up to 10% of patients over 65 years of age. There is a 2-to-1 male predominance. The most frequent clinical complaint is back stiffness, which at times may be associated with thoracic and often lumbar pain. Because of the relative sparing of the posterior elements of the spine, there may be no limitation to spinal motion on physical examination. In addition, other skeletal manifestations, usually involving the shoulder, knees, or elbows, may be present. Chronic heel pain can be a frequent complaint. Cervical involvement may present as limited motion, dysphagia, or spinal stenosis with myelopathy. The etiology is not known. DISH is often an incidental finding because many patients may have minimal or no symptoms.

Diagnostic Evaluation

The major pathologic findings associated with DISH are seen on radiographic evaluation. The most characteristic radiographic abnormality of DISH is calcification and ossification of the anterior longitudinal ligament. The criteria for spinal involvement are flowing calcification along the anterolateral aspect of four contiguous vertebral bodies; preservation of intervertebral disc height; absence of apophyseal joint bony ankylosis; and sacroiliac joint sclerosis, erosion, or fusion [25]. The vertebral column develops anterior and lateral spurring in the early stages. The posterior portions are relatively spared. The lower thoracic spine is the most frequently affected area, but the entire spine may be involved. The flowing hyperostosis gives rise to a bumpy appearance of the spine that may resemble the "bamboo spine" in ankylosing spondylitis, but in DISH the bumps predominate on the lateral projection as the calcified anterior longitudinal ligament. Hyperostosis of the heads of the ribs may occasionally be noticed with spinal involvement. Diffuse idiopathic skeletal hyperostosis may also be associated with a rare syndrome, sternocostoclavicular hyperostosis, in which extensive ossification of the soft tissues between the anterior ribs, medial clavicle, and sternum is evident [26]. The diagnosis of DISH cannot be made in the presence of apophyseal joint erosions or radiographic sacroiliitis because these exclusions avoid confusing DISH with ankylosing spondylitis. Laboratory data are usually normal but may reveal a slightly elevated ESR. There is no strong evidence of association of HLA-B27 antigen with DISH, and it is therefore not classified with the seronegative spondyloarthropathies, ankylosing spondylitis, or Reiter's syndrome [27].

Treatment

The treatment of DISH is largely symptomatic and similar to that for osteoarthritis of the spine. Both prolonged rest or increased activity may aggravate the pain. NSAIDs may be helpful. Exercise is recommended to maintain mobility. The progression of the disease may continue with pain and stiffness and peripheral joint symptoms, but the significant limitations to movement seen in ankylosing spondylitis tend not to develop.

Scheuermann's Disease

Scheuermann, in 1920, first described the radiographic changes of anterior wedging and vertebral end-plate irregularity in the thoracic spine associated with kyphosis [28]. Scheuermann's disease is also known as juvenile kyphosis, vertebral osteochondritis, and osteochondritis deformans juvenilis dorsi. Scheuermann's disease of the thoracic spine is defined as an excessive thoracic kyphosis with wedging of 5 degrees or more in at least three adjacent apical vertebrae with vertebral end-plate irregularities. A thoracic kyphosis of greater than 45–50 degrees is usually considered abnormal, but there can be individuals with normal curvatures that exceed this [29]. Scheuermann's disease

has been reported to be transmitted in an autosomal dominant mode [30]. There is a slight predominance in females. The etiology is unknown, but pathologic specimens exhibit abnormal cartilage with deficient bone growth under the areas of abnormal growth plates. Disc material herniated into the vertebral bodies (Schmorl's nodes) is a common associated finding.

Diagnosis

The typical patient is an adolescent who presents because of spinal deformity. There may be associated pain at the apex of the deformity or in the low back. The kyphotic deformity is usually acute, helping to distinguish it from postural round back. The curve in postural round back is more flexible and can be seen to correct on physical examination or on roentgenograms taken with the patient supine over a bolster. Often there is associated increased lumbar lordosis and a 20–25% association with a scoliotic curve that usually does not progress. A thorough neurologic examination is important because cord compression can occur. Any hyperreflexia or ataxia needs further investigation. Hamstring tightness is often found on examination. The differential diagnosis includes tuberculosis (Pott's disease) or other infections, postural round back, congenital malformation, osteopenic conditions, inflammatory conditions including rheumatoid arthritis or ankylosing spondylitis, and tumor such as neurofibromatosis. Radiographic evaluation should include full-length standing AP and lateral views of the spine. Bending films may help assess flexibility and the ability of the curve to correct. The iliac crest should be included to judge skeletal maturity. The Cobb method is used to measure the curve. The degree of anterior wedging and the number of vertebrae involved are noted (Fig. 5.17). Decreased disc height, vertebral end-plate irregularity, Schmorl's nodes, or persistence of a separate fragment of bone anterosuperior to the front edge of a vertebral body (limbus vertebra) may also be present. Similar findings may be seen in the lumbar spine and associated with a form of lumbar Scheuermann's disease.

Treatment

Treatment is usually limited to those patients with a painful deformity, documented progression, and

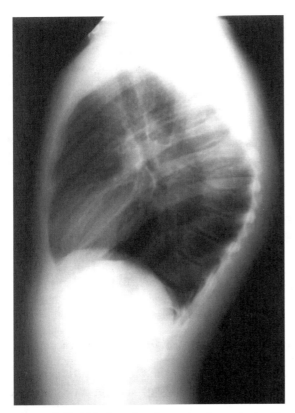

Figure 5.17. This lateral radiograph of a patient with Scheuermann's kyphosis demonstrates the wedging of the anterior portion of the vertebral bodies involved in the kyphosis.

at least 2 years of growth remaining. Younger children with a mild deformity can be initially treated by a program of exercise to strengthen the extensor muscles of the spine and stretch the hamstring and pectoral muscles and the anterior longitudinal ligament. In adolescents, Scheuermann's disease is effectively managed with bracing. An initial period of casting in hyperextension may be required for the more severe kyphosis. For the middle to upper thoracic curve a Milwaukee brace is used, and for thoracolumbar curves, T8 and below, an underarm molded brace may be used. Bracing is sometimes continued at least part time until signs of skeletal maturity are seen, but the length of bracing is controversial [31].

Contraindications to brace treatment include curves greater than 70 degrees, severe apical wedging, and a rigid curve. Surgery is considered in patients with severe deformity, disabling pain,

neurologic compromise, or continued progression despite conservative treatment. Spinal fusion is successful in decreasing deformity and relieving pain. The usual surgical management includes an anterior approach with discectomies and bone grafting followed by posterior instrumentation and fusion in a second, staged procedure.

References

1. Brackman MB, Shepard MJ, Collins WF et al. A randomized, controlled trial of methylprednisolone or naloxone in the treatment of acute spinal-cord injury. N Engl J Med 1990;322:1405–1411.
2. Holdsworth FW. Fractures, dislocations, and fracture-dislocations of the spine. J Bone Joint Surg 1963;45B:6–20.
3. Denis F. The three column spine and its significance in the classification of acute thoracolumbar spine injuries. Spine 1983;8:817–831.
4. White AA, Panjabi MM. Clinical Biomechanics of the Spine. Philadelphia: Lippincott, 1990.
5. Chance CQ. Note on a type of flexion fracture of the spine. Br J Radiol 1948;21:452.
6. McKenzie MK, Bartal EL, Pay NT. A hyperextension injury of the thoracic spine in association with diffuse idiopathic skeletal hyperostosis. Orthopaedics 1991;14:895–898.
7. Ferree BA, Wieser M, Clarke RP. Hyperextension spinal fracture. Orthop Rev 18;10:1061–1064.
8. Willen J. Unstable thoracolumbar injuries. Orthopaedics 1992;15:329–336.
9. Wood GE, Hanley EN. Thoracolumbar fractures: An overview with emphasis on the burst injury. Orthopaedics 1992;15:319–323.
10. McAfee PC, Yuan HA, Lasda NA. The unstable burst fracture. Spine 1982;7:365–373.
11. Dickson GR, Sutcliffe AJ. Intrathecal morphine and multiple fractured ribs. Br J Anaesth 1986;58:1342–1343.
12. Richardson JD, Adams L, Flint LM. Selective management of flail chest and pulmonary contusion. Ann Surg 1982;196:481–487.
13. Johnson CC, Slemenda CW, Melton LJ. Clinical use of bone densitometry. N Engl J Med 1991;324:1105–1109.
14. Einhorn TA. Bone Metabolism and Metabolic Bone Disease. In JW Frymoyer (ed), Orthopaedic Knowledge Update 4. Rosemont: American Academy of Orthopaedic Surgery, 1993.
15. Lian JB, Gundberg CM. Osteocalcin: Biochemical considerations and clinical applications. Clin Orthop 1988;226:267–291.
16. Dalsky GP, Stocke KS, Ehsami AA et al. Weight-bearing exercise training and lumbar bone mineral contents in post menopausal women. Ann Intern Med 1988;108:824–828.

17. Frost HM. Coherence treatment of osteoporosis. Orthop Clin North Am 1981;12:649–669.

18. Watts NB, Harris ST, Genant HK et al. Intermittent cyclical etidronate treatment of postmenopausal osteoporosis. N Engl J Med 1990;323:73–79.

19. Riggs BL, Hodgson SF, O'Fallon W, et al. Effect of fluoride treatment on the fracture rate in postmenopausal women with osteoporosis. N Engl J Med 1990;322:802–809.

20. Hunter T, Dubo HC. Spinal fractures complicating ankylosing spondylitis: A long term follow-up study. Arthritis Rheum 1983;26:751–758.

21. Khan MA, Vander Linden SM. Ankylosing spondylitis and other spondyloarthrapathies. Rheum Dis Clin North Am 1990;16:551–562.

22. Calan A, Fries JF. Striking prevalence of ankylosing spondylitis in "healthy" B27 positive males and females. N Engl J Med 1975;293:835–838.

23. Smith-Peterson MN, Larson CB, Aufranc OE. Osteotomy of the spine for correction of flexion deformity in rheumatoid arthritis. J Bone Joint Surg 1945;27:1–11.

24. Resnick D, Shaul SR, Robins JM. Diffuse idiopathic skeletal hyperostosis (DISH): Forestier's disease with extraspinal manifestations. Radiology 1975;115:513–521.

25. Resnick D, Niwayama G. Radiographic and pathologic features of spinal involvement in diffuse idiopathic skeletal hyperostosis (DISH). Radiology 1976;119:559–567.

26. Kohler H, Uehlinger E, Kutzner J et al. Sternocostoclavicular hyperostosis: Painful swelling of the sternum, clavicles, and upper ribs. Ann Intern Med 1977;87:192–194.

27. Spagnola AM, Bennet PH, Terasaki PI. Vertebral ankylosing hyperostosis (Forestier's disease) and HLA antigens in Pima Indians. Arthritis Rheum 1978;21:467–469.

28. Scheuermann HW. Kyfosis dorsalis juvenile. Ugeskr Laeger 1920;82:385–398.

29. Staganara P, de Mauroy JC, Dran G et al. Reciprocal angulation of vertebral bodies in the sagittal plane: Approach to references for the evaluation of kyphosis and lordosis. Spine 1982;7:335–342.

30. Halal F, Gledhill RB, Fraser FC. Dominant inheritance of Scheuermann's juvenile kyphosis. Am J Dis Child 1978;132:1105–1109.

31. Gutkowski W, Renshaw T. Orthotic results in adolescent kyphosis. Spine 1988;13:485–489.

Chapter 6

Medical Causes of Pain in the Thoracic Region

Wade A. Lillegard

Thoracic and chest wall pain that cannot be attributed to musculoskeletal pathologic entities may be referred pain from visceral pathologic conditions. Both visceral and somatic afferent nerves transmit pain messages from a peripheral stimulus and converge on the same projection neurons in the dorsal horn. When visceral afferents receive a strong stimulus, the brain may not recognize the source of the painful stimulus and interpret this visceral pain as somatic pain. The spinal segments that relay pain from the gallbladder, for example, also receive afferent fibers from the shoulder. Gallbladder disease, then, may be interpreted by the brain as shoulder pain. Furthermore, the visceral afferents' message of pain may ascend or descend a few levels before this confusion occurs, resulting in pain referred to proximal or distal somatic sites. This chapter will review common medical conditions that may manifest themselves as thoracic and chest wall pain and will describe the referral pattern of these conditions.

The approach to the diagnosis of referred thoracic pain is as follows:

1. Recognize that thoracic pain not readily attributable to a musculoskeletal cause may be referred from visceral pathologic conditions.
2. Realize the location of pain may or may not overlie the source of the pain.
3. Search for provocative and palliative factors in the pain. (a) Assess whether the pain varies with respiration (pleuritic pain) or not (nonpleuritic);

(b) determine whether the pain is acute or not acute; (c) follow the algorithm in Fig. 6.1 and search for historical or physical examination findings consistent with a diagnosis.

Thoracic Pain Referred from Thoracic Visceral Pathologic Conditions

Cardiac Pain

Pain arising from the myocardium results from a decrease in blood flow with a subsequent build-up of metabolites in the ischemic segment. Sudden, complete occlusion of the coronary artery causes an acute myocardial infarction. Angina pectoris is a symptom that represents an imbalance between myocardial perfusion and demand. Myocardial pain is characterized as a squeezing substernal sensation, tightness, or pressure.

History

Patients with acute myocardial infarction classically have an intolerable gripping or crushing substernal sensation with associated diaphoresis and shortness of breath. Pain from angina pectoris is generally more subtle and can be either exertional or variant. Exertional angina occurs when there is a fixed incomplete luminal occlusion that limits blood supply to the myocardium. When myocardial demand in-

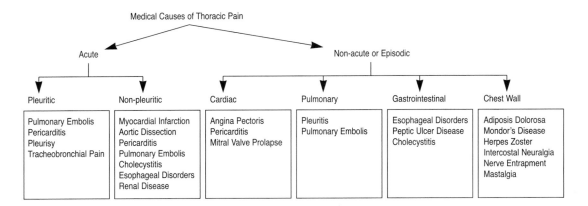

Figure 6.1. Algorithm for the classification of medical causes of thoracic pain.

creases (during exertion) pain results. This pain is quite variable in nature and may manifest as substernal or left-sided chest pressure, left shoulder pain (sometimes right), or neck and jaw pain. The significant feature of this pain, regardless of the location, is that it always worsens with exertion and is relieved with rest. Variant (nonexertional) angina is likely caused by coronary vasospasm over a fixed lesion. This pain has the characteristics of angina but is not always related to exertion.

Referral Pattern

Pain of myocardial origin frequently radiates over the left pectoral area to the left shoulder and along the left medial arm or neck and jaw. Pain occasionally radiates to the right shoulder and arm, or epigastrium (Fig. 6.2).

Treatment

Patients with any historical features consistent with acute myocardial infarction should be immediately transported via ambulance to an emergency room. Those with suspected angina should be evaluated expeditiously by their physician.

Aortic Dissection

Dissection of an aortic aneurysm causes marked distention of the aortic adventitial coat, which contains pain fibers.

History and Physical Examination Findings

Pain accompanying aortic dissection is of sudden onset and rapidly becomes severe. Pain is unrelenting and not changed by position. Patients appear in distress and may be pale or cyanotic. The blood pressure is often normal, but distal pulses are frequently decreased or absent.

Referral Pattern

Pain from an aortic aneurysm dissection is substernal and in the upper anterior chest when confined to the arch (see Fig. 6.2). It may radiate to the shoulder but rarely involves the arms. Once the dissection reaches the descending aorta, pain is felt in the back of the neck and the interscapular area.

Treatment

Patients with suspected aortic aneurysm dissections should be monitored and transported immediately to an emergency room via ambulance.

Pericarditis

Pericarditis is an inflammation of the pericardium. This can be secondary to infection (bacterial, viral, or fungal), systemic disease (rheumatoid arthritis, connective tissue diseases, or uremia), metastatic tumors, drugs (procainamide, hydralazine, phenytoin, anticoagulants), or it can be idiopathic.

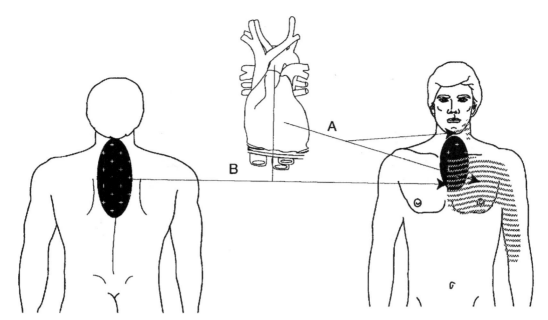

Figure 6.2. Common referral patterns for pain from my-ocardial ischemia and aneurysm dissection in the aortic arch. Myocardial ischemia (A) manifests as anterior and left an-terior chest pain or a "squeezing sensation," with radiation along the medial aspect of the left arm or to the jaw and neck. Dissection of an aneurysm in the aortic arch (B) causes severe anterior chest and neck pain when confined to the proximal arch, and upper back and interscapular pain as it dissects distal to the descending arch.

History and Physical Examination Findings

Patients with acute pericarditis have mild to severe chest pain that is aggravated by respiration, cough, and thoracic motion. The pain may be relieved with sitting and forward bending (ischemic heart pain generally is not related to position). Fever, chills, and weakness are common and tachypnea and cough are variable. When present, a systolic or di-astolic friction rub is diagnostic. Heart sounds may be muffled and there may be a narrowed pulse pres-sure and neck vein distention.

Referral Pattern

Both the visceral and parietal surfaces of the peri-cardium are generally devoid of pain fibers with the exception of the parietal surface opposite the fifth and sixth interspaces. Stimulation of these pain fibers from pericardial inflammation results in sharp referred pain felt at the superior border of the trapez-ius (similar to central diaphragmatic irritation). Fur-thermore, the inflamed (and largely insensitive) pericardium irritates the contiguous parietal surface of the mediastinal pleura. This may result in inflam-mation of mediastinal structures and referred pain to the epigastric and left parasternal area (Fig. 6.3).

Treatment

Patients with acute symptoms should be transferred immediately to an emergency room for evaluation. Others should be evaluated expeditiously by their primary care physician.

Mitral Valve Prolapse

Mitral valve prolapse results from thickened leaflets that are large and redundant. It affects approximately 4–7% of the population and is more common in women than men.

History and Physical Examination Findings

Chest pain is reported in 40–50% of affected patients and is characteristically sharp or sticking in nature. Some patients report a dull pain, and in 10–20% of

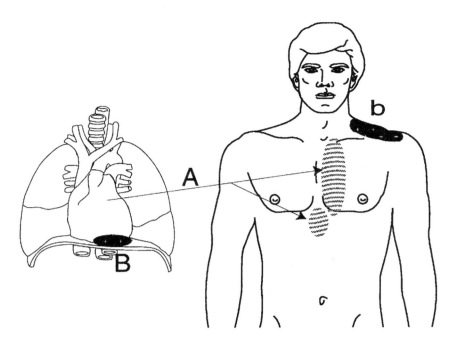

Figure 6.3. Referred pain from inflammation of the pericardial sac. Inflammation of the largely insensitive pericardial sac (A) causes irritation of the pain-sensitive contiguous mediastinal pleura, which causes pain in the epigastrium and left parasternal region. Irritation of the diaphragm (B) results in pain referred to the left trapezius (b).

patients it is angina-like. The pain is generally nonexertional and lasts momentarily but occasionally lingers minutes to hours. The pain episodes become more frequent during periods of emotional stress. The typical physical findings are a midsystolic nonejection click and a late holosystolic murmur.

Referral Pattern

Pain from mitral valve prolapse is typically retrosternal or left-sided chest pain and is not referred to distal sites.

Treatment

Patients with suspected mitral valve prolapse should be evaluated by their primary care physician for underlying causes and treatment.

Esophageal Disorders

Disorders of the esophagus include irritation from foreign bodies or tumors, erosion from acid reflux, and motility disorders.

History and Physical Examination Findings

Gastroesophageal reflux leads to a mild-to-severe burning sensation in the epigastric to retrosternal area. Pain is often worse at night because the supine position allows reflux of stomach acid into the esophagus. Patients may complain of a brackish taste and frequent belching. Patients with esophageal disorders have pain that may be sharp or constricting in nature and is related to swallowing (dysphasia). The maximal pain is at the level of the lesion and is generally retrosternal with occasional bandlike radiation. The physical examination findings are generally unremarkable.

Referral Pattern

Pain arising from a distended or eroded esophagus frequently is referred to somatic levels corresponding to the lesion. Lower level lesions therefore correspond to lower levels of sternal and back pain (Fig. 6.4).

Treatment

The patient should be referred to a primary care physician for evaluation and treatment.

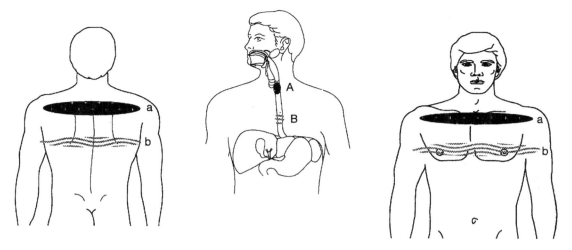

Figure 6.4. Thoracic manifestations of esophageal irritation. Esophageal irritation from erosion or distention causes a bandlike referred pain to the thorax at a level corresponding to the level of the lesion. Upper esophageal lesions (A) refer pain to the upper chest and back (a), and lesions closer to the gastroesophageal junction (B) refer pain to the middle chest and back (b).

Tracheobronchial Pain

Tracheobronchial irritation can occur from acute bacterial or viral tracheitis, sharp foreign bodies, carcinomas, and inflammatory lesions.

History

The pain from tracheobronchial irritation is generally a "burning" anterior chest and neck pain that is accentuated by coughing. Acute bacterial tracheitis occurs in both young and older children and is accompanied by acute onset of fever, dyspnea, and stridor. Bronchial inflammation from a foreign body or mass lesion is more subtle in presentation and may present with stridor, cough, vague retrosternal pain, shortness of breath, or a combination of symptoms.

Referral Pattern

Pain from inflammation of the tracheobronchial tree characteristically is referred to the upper portion of the sternum and lateral to the sternum at points corresponding to the major bronchi (Fig. 6.5).

Treatment

The underlying cause should be indentified and treated.

Pleurisy

The parietal pleura contains pain fibers that are conveyed through the chest wall through the intercostal nerves. Any irritation of the pleura thereby results in chest wall pain. Widening of the intercostal space during inspiration stretches the inflamed parietal pleura and accentuates the pain. Pleural inflammation has numerous causes: underlying lung insult from pneumonia or pulmonary infarction, direct entry of infection to the pleural space (empyema), hematologic or lymphatic spread (e.g., tuberculosis, uremia, cancer, collagen vascular disease), or pleural trauma (rib fracture).

History and Physical Examination Findings

Pain is generally over the site of pleurisy or the chest wall, of sudden onset, and characterized by a sharp stabbing pain that is aggravated by deep respirations and cough. Patients may guard the affected site and have shallow respirations. Auscultation of a pleural friction rub is pathognomonic but may be absent.

Referral Pattern

Irritation of the peripheral diaphragmatic rim refers pain to corresponding sites on the chest wall or ab-

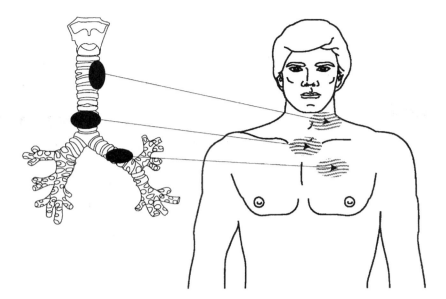

Figure 6.5. Chest pain referred from tracheobronchial lesions. Pain from irritation of the tracheobronchial tree is referred to sites on the neck and chest that correspond to the level of irritation.

domen. Irritation of the central diaphragm causes referred pain to the neck and shoulder (Fig. 6.6).

Treatment

The underlying cause must be identified and treated. Symptomatic treatment consists of heat, nonsteroidal anti-inflammatory drugs (NSAIDs), and codeine if needed. A 6-inch elastic wrap around the chest may offer additional relief.

Pulmonary Embolism

A pulmonary embolism is caused by a sudden lodging of a blood clot in the pulmonary vascular tree with resultant obstruction of blood flow. Complete obstruction leads to pulmonary infarction characterized by consolidation and necrosis of lung tissue. This is a medical emergency and should be diagnosed and treated immediately.

History and Physical Examination Findings

Thrombus formation generally occurs at a distant site such as the deep venous system of the leg or subclavian vein in the arm. Predisposing factors include recent surgery (within 1 month), trauma, im-

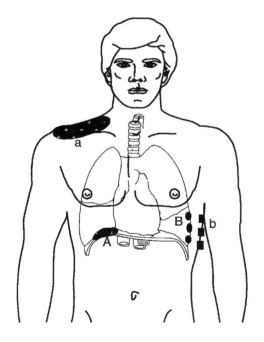

Figure 6.6. Thoracic pain patterns from irritation of the parietal pleura (pleurisy). Pleuritic irritation of the central diaphragm (A) results in pain referred to the ipsilateral shoulder (a). Inflammation of the peripheral pleura (B) directly stimulates the adjacent intercostal nerves, transmitting pain to areas on the thorax or abdomen directly overlying the inflammation (b). Pleuritic chest pain is aggravated by deep respirations.

mobilization, cancer, pregnancy, oral contraceptive use, obesity, and advanced age. Unilateral extremity swelling in such a patient is indicative of deep vein thrombosis and places the patient at high risk for a pulmonary embolism. Pleuritic chest pain will occur in those that have secondary pleuritis from a peripheral infarction. Severe pulmonary hypertension may cause dull substernal chest pain. Shortness of breath occurs in 80% of patients with a pulmonary embolism, and hemoptysis occurs in 20–30%. Patients are generally tachypneic with occasional rubs, crackles, and wheezing on auscultation. They may have a right ventricular heave, an increased P2 (pulmonic second heartsound), or a gallop. Patients without dyspnea, pleuritic chest pain, or tachypnea are unlikely to have acute pulmonary embolism. Those with unilateral extremity swelling and chest pain are at high risk.

Referral Pattern

Patients who have pleurisy secondary to a pulmonary infarction may have referred pain similar to that mentioned previously under pleurisy (see Fig. 6.6).

Treatment

Patients suspected of having a pulmonary embolism should be transferred immediately to an emergency room for further testing and anticoagulation therapy.

Thoracic Pain Referred from Pathologic Abdominal Conditions

Mechanism of Referral

Sensory impulses from visceral structures enter the posterior horn of the spinal cord and travel along with neurons of somatic origin. These visceral impulses then travel proximally or distally for several segments in the posterior horn before synapsing with neurons in the dorsal horn. While in the posterior horn, these impulses from visceral structures may interact with those of somatic origin and cause referred somatic pain. Pain in the abdomen is generally transmitted through T6–T12, and some structures in the chest are innervated as low as T9. Thoracic pain, then, can be referred from pathologic conditions of the abdominal viscera.

Cholecystitis

History and Physical Examination

Pain from cholecystitis (inflamed gallbladder) typically occurs 1–2 hours after ingestion of a heavy meal. There is sudden or gradual onset of severe pain, which peaks after 2–3 hours and resolves in approximately 10 hours. Passing gallstones (through the extrahepatic bile ducts) gives the sudden, intense paroxysmal pain of biliary colic. This pain is characteristically located in the right upper quadrant of the abdomen, the right subscapular area, or both. Patients with acute cholecystitis frequently have moderate fever from 100–103°F with occasional chills. Nausea and vomiting are common. Patients are generally in moderate to severe distress and unable to find a comfortable position. Tenderness is elicited in the right upper quadrant that worsens on deep inspiration (Murphy's sign).

Referral Pattern

Pain from gallbladder disease is generally transmitted along T8 and T9 nerve segments. Right upper quadrant pain or epigastric pain is characteristic. Gallbladder pain can, however, be located anywhere in the abdomen or thorax. Impacted stones in the cystic duct may cause pain only at the angle of the scapula or in association with pain in the right costal margin. Pain may also be transmitted to the right shoulder through stimulation of the phrenic nerve. Pain from either cholecystitis or biliary colic can be located in the anterior chest and confused with angina or myocardial infarction (Fig. 6.7).

Treatment

Patients with significant symptoms and fever should be evaluated immediately by a physician. Those with mild symptoms consistent with gallbladder disease should be evaluated by their primary care physician.

Peptic Ulcer Disease

Increased production of gastric acid or decreased cytoprotection of the stomach lining (e.g., from chronic NSAID use) leads to erosion of the gastric mucosa.

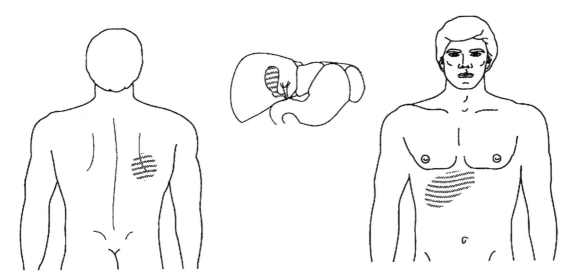

Figure 6.7. Referral pattern of gallbladder inflammation. Pain is generally felt in the right upper quadrant of the abdomen and epigastric area and commonly referred to the angle of the scapula on the right side.

Pain originating from the stomach is transmitted through the seventh to ninth thoracic dorsal roots.

History and Physical Examination Findings

Pain is generally burning and felt in the epigastrium below the xiphoid or left upper quadrant of the abdomen. Significant erosion may cause the patient to complain of a boring sensation through to the back. The burning pain of peptic ulcer disease typically begins 1–2 hours after a meal and is transiently relieved with the ingestion of antacids or food. The physical examination may reveal mild to moderate tenderness in the middle epigastric area.

Referral Pattern

Pain may "bore" straight through the epigastric area to the back. Perforation leads to free air accumulation under the diaphragm, causing referred pain to the shoulder (Fig. 6.8).

Treatment

Patients with suspected peptic ulcer disease should be evaluated and treated by their primary care physician. Urgent referral is indicated when the pain is moderate to severe to rule out a perforated ulcer.

Renal Disease

Pain originating from the genitourinary system involves the thorax only at the costovertebral angle. The pain is a result of either renal inflammation (from pyelonephritis) or distention (from sudden obstruction).

History and Physical Examination Findings

Patients with acute pyelonephritis generally have signs of urinary tract infection (polyuria and dysuria), which precede the development of flank pain. Patients have varying degrees of fever, chills, and sweats, and tenderness is elicited by percussing the costovertebral angle. Patients passing a kidney stone (renal colic) complain of a sudden onset of severe flank pain that radiates to the groin. No change in position relieves the pain and patients are in marked distress. They may or may not have ipsilateral flank tenderness.

Referral Pattern

Renal pain is transmitted through the lower two thoracic and first lumbar segments. Pain from acute pyelonephritis is localized over the ipsilateral costovertebral angle. Passing kidney stones causes di-

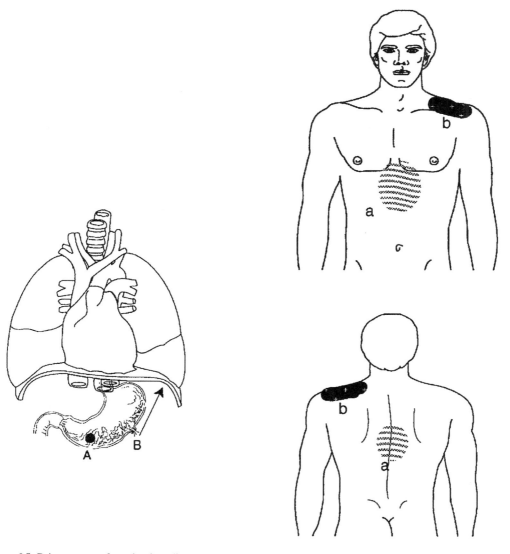

Figure 6.8. Pain patterns of peptic ulcer disease. Mucosal erosion (A) from an ulcer generally manifests as midepigastric pain, which can "bore" straight through to the back (a). Perforated ulcers (B) allow the release of stomach air, which collects under the diaphragm, causing pain referred to the shoulder (b).

lation of the ureter, which produces pain that radiates toward the groin.

Management

Patients with suspected pyelonephritis or renal colic should be evaluated immediately by a physician.

Thoracic Pain From Nonvisceral Medical Causes

Adiposis Dolorosa (Dercum's Disease)

Adiposis dolorosa is a disease characterized by painful subcutaneous fatty tumors and occurs primarily in postmenopausal women. Lethargy and emotional instability are common. The cause of pain in these fatty tumors is unclear but may be from a local neuritis of nerves stretched by the expanding tumor mass, or from fat necrosis.

History and Physical Examination Findings

Pain is often out of proportion to physical findings. Patients generally complain of fatigue, arthralgias, irritability, headaches, and nosebleeds. Fatty deposits typically occur over the medial aspects of the knees first, then on the back, neck, thighs, and arms. The face is uninvolved. Painful episodes are associated with emotional upset, tachypnea, paresthesias, and dyspnea. Patients with this disease are obese and other physical findings include cutaneous hyperesthesia over the tumors, weakness, hypotension, and facial flushing.

Referral Pattern

Pain is localized over and around the fatty tumor and is not referred to distal sites.

Treatment

Patients with this entity should be referred to a dermatologist or plastic surgeon. Oral prednisone, intravenous lidocaine given every other day, surgical excision, and liposuction have all been reported to be somewhat effective in relieving the pain.

Mondor's Disease

Mondor's disease is a thrombophlebitis of the subcutaneous veins of the chest region and occurs three times as often in men than women. It generally involves one or two segments of thoracoepigastric veins running obliquely from the epigastrium to the anterior axillary line over the lateral aspect of the breast. It less commonly involves the lateral thoracic veins along the lateral margin of the pectoralis. It is associated with traumatic events, breast surgery, infection, physical strain, rheumatoid arthritis, and breast cancer.

History and Physical Examination Findings

Patients develop insidious and progressive pain on the lateral chest wall. Physical examination will re-

veal one or more painful, superficial, palpable subcutaneous cords anywhere from the lateral aspect of the breasts to the epigastrium. There may be a protrusion or furrowing of the skin near the vein that is accentuated by tangential light or slight downward traction of the skin. There are minimal inflammatory changes in the skin and no associated fever or chills.

Referral Pattern

Pain is well localized over the thrombosed vein as described and it does not refer (Fig. 6.9).

Treatment

Symptoms usually resolve in 1–10 weeks without specific treatment. Patients with Mondor's disease should be referred to their primary care physician to rule out thrombophlebitis secondary to breast cancer, lymphangitis, arthritis, or mastitis.

Varicella-Zoster Virus (Shingles)

The herpes viruses have the ability to remain in the body after a primary chickenpox infection and are harbored in the nerve root ganglia. A competent immune system prevents further clinical manifestations during latent periods, but reactivation can occur with relative immunosuppression (from disease or stress). Herpes zoster is the clinical manifestation of the reactivated virus as it replicates and migrates to the skin along the involved dermatome, causing pain and a rash. The thoracic, lumbar, and ophthalmic sites are most frequently involved. Herpes is contagious and clinicians previously unexposed to chickenpox should avoid direct contact with the lesion.

History and Physical Examination Findings

Patients frequently have a prodromal phase of mild-to-severe burning pain in their chest over a dermatomal distribution. Within 2–3 days a characteristic rash will appear, starting as erythematous papules and progressing to vesicles. Vesicles cease to form after approximately 5 days and skin will return to normal color over the subsequent 2 weeks.

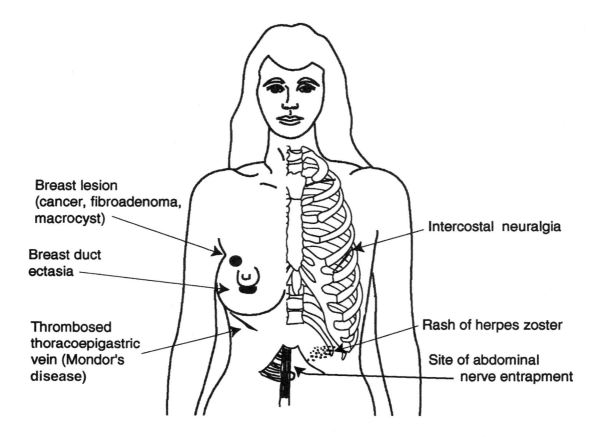

Breast lesion (cancer, fibroadenoma, macrocyst)

Breast duct ectasia

Intercostal neuralgia

Thrombosed thoracoepigastric vein (Mondor's disease)

Rash of herpes zoster

Site of abdominal nerve entrapment

Figure 6.9. Locations of pain from various chest wall lesions.

Referral Pattern

Pain is referred in a dermatomal distribution corresponding to the nerve root involved (see Fig. 6.9).

Treatment for Acute Herpes Zoster

Acyclovir, 800 mg five times a day for 7–10 days, has been shown to accelerate lesion healing but has little effect on pain and the development of postherpetic neuralgia. Symptomatic treatment consists of topical application of a soothing and drying agent such as Burrow's solution every 2 hours. Neuritis can be treated with oral amitriptyline, fluphenazine, acetaminophen, NSAIDs, or codeine. Oral steroids have been used but are of no documented benefit in preventing postherpetic neuralgia.

Postherpetic Neuralgia

Postherpetic neuralgia is pain that persists for greater than 1 month after the rash of acute herpes zoster resolves. This complication increases in frequency with age: from 4% between 30–50 years of age to 34% in those more than 80 years old. Pain resolves spontaneously in 50% of these cases within 3 months, 78% within 1 year, and 98% within 5 years.

History and Physical Examination Findings

The patient has a history of an episode of acute herpes zoster. The pain may be lancinating and paroxysmal or a steady burning pain or ache. The involved skin area on the thorax is often hyperesthetic to light touch and may show some scarring with hyper- or hypopigmentation from the antecedent rash. This area often has decreased sensation to pinprick.

Referral Pattern

The referral pattern is similar to that described for acute herpes zoster (see Fig. 6.9).

Treatment

No single therapy is uniformly effective. Ultrasound, transcutaneous electrical nerve stimulation (TENS) units, topical capsaicin cream, and low-dose amitriptyline have all been reported to be of some help.

Intercostal Neuralgia

Intercostal neuralgia is caused by an intercostal neuroma secondary to a prior thoracotomy, radical mastectomy, or fractured rib; it can also be idiopathic.

History and Physical Examination Findings

Patients may complain of paresthesias and burning thoracic pain in response to touch or thoracic movement. The pain generally subsides in weeks to months, but may last for years. Physical examination generally reveals a trigger point or tenderness at the site of the neuroma or scar. The patient may, however, have only a vague pain in the involved region of the thorax or abdomen that varies with position or respirations.

Referral Pattern

The pain is generally a burning pain in the thorax or abdomen that may radiate proximally to the spine (see Fig. 6.9).

Treatment

Intercostal or paravertebral nerve blocks with an anesthetic are useful primarily for diagnostic purposes. Destructive nerve blocks with alcohol or 10–15% phenol generally offer only transient relief. Ammonium sulfate selectively destroys unmyelinated c fibers, relieving pain without sensory or motor loss. One study reported excellent relief of pain in 60% of subjects treated with an intercostal nerve block using 10% ammonium sulfate. Surgical removal of the neuroma is sometimes necessary.

Nerve Entrapment

Lower anterior thoracic and upper abdominal pain may be secondary to nerve entrapment of any of the intercostal nerves (T9–T11) that traverse the rectus abdominus muscles.

History and Physical Examination Findings

Pain is generally felt along the outer border of the rectus sheath at the site of impingement. The pain is sharp, piercing, or burning and radiates horizontally. There is localized tenderness over the site of impingement that worsens as the patient lifts the legs or raises the head to tighten the rectus muscles. Nerve entrapment syndromes will be aggravated by this maneuver whereas pain from intra-abdominal pathologic conditions will lessen or be unchanged.

Referral Pattern

Pain manifested in the thoracic region is located medial to the subxiphoid costal margin and lateral to the proximal rectus sheath but may extend posteriorly along the course of the intercostal nerve toward the spine (see Fig. 6.9).

Treatment

Symptomatic treatment consists of trials of cold, heat, counterpressure massage, and abdominal binders. Local infiltration with an anesthetic agent will give transient relief and help to confirm the diagnosis. Good long-term results have been reported with lidocaine/steroid injections, and surgical treatment is rarely necessary.

Mastalgia (Breast Pain)

Breast pain is the most common breast symptom leading women to seek care. Most women, however, only have mild pain and need no more than reassurance that it is not caused by cancer.

The causes of breast pain can be conceptually divided into two categories: anatomic and physiologic. The anatomic factors include breast cancer, macrocysts, fibroadenomas, and duct ectasia. Proposed physiologic causes include caffeine stimulation of cyclic adenosine monophosphate (cAMP) and cyclic guanosine monophosphate (cGMP) in breast tissue, a hyperestrogenic state, decreased progesterone secretion, and increased prolactin. The anatomic causes are generally noncyclic in nature (pain does not vary with menses).

Physiologic breast pain is thought to be a result of an exaggerated response of the epithelium and stroma to chemical and hormonal stimulation, although unequivocal evidence of this is lacking. Caffeine has been purported to aggravate fibrocystic breast disease by inhibiting conversion of cAMP and cGMP, resulting in excess production of fibrous tissue and cystic fluid. There is no firm evidence that this is the case, and caffeine restriction has not been shown to be beneficial. Abnormal estrogen levels have not been well demonstrated in women with mastalgia. There is questionable evidence of a relative estrogen excess secondary to decreased luteal progesterone, and this has been the basis for treatment with progesterone or antiestrogens (danazol or tamoxifen). There is contradictory evidence of excess prolactin secretion in patients with mastalgia. This theory underlies the use of the prolactin inhibitor bromocriptine in treatment.

History and Physical Examination Findings

All patients with breast pain should be taken seriously. Their concern, as well as the clinician's, is to rule out cancer. Pain is the initial complaint in only 7% of patients with breast cancer, the pain is generally noncyclic, and the pain is well localized. Duct ectasia produces noncyclic subareolar pain with a nonbloody nipple discharge and dilated ducts. Macrocysts and fibroadenomas may produce pain and are readily identified on palpation (see Fig. 6.9). Patients should have a thorough breast examination, and mammography should be performed in all women over the age of 35 years. Any patient with suspicious lesions detected by either physical examination or mammography should be referred to a surgeon. Patients with severe cyclic mastalgia should keep a log of their symptoms and menstrual pattern for 2 months.

Treatment

Cyclic mastalgia can be considered an exaggerated physiologic response to hormonal stimulation, and approximately 80% of patients will respond to medication. Noncyclic pain, in the absence of anatomic abnormalities, is generally idiopathic and will not respond as well to hormonal therapy (around 40%). A trial of such is still warranted. The medications yielding the best results include danazol, bromocriptine, tamoxifen, and evening primrose oil.

Psychiatric

Anxiety disorder should be suspected in patients with atypical chest pain, multiple somatic complaints, and associated generalized anxiety or panic attacks.

Depression should be considered with a history of sleep disturbance, crying spells, loss of appetite, fatigue, and anhedonia (no interest in participating in normally pleasurable activities). A patient should be referred to his or her primary care physician if a psychiatric cause is suspected.

Selected Readings

Alpert MA, Mukerji V, Sabeti M, et al. Mitral valve prolapse, panic disorder, and chest pain. Med Clin North Am 1991;75:1119-1133.

Bauwens DB, Paine R. Thoracic Pain. In RS Blacklow (ed), MacBryde's Signs and Symptoms. Philadelphia: Lippincott, 1983;139–164.

Berkow R. The Merck Manual of Diagnosis and Therapy (16th ed). Rahway, NJ: Merck, 1992.

Carmichael JK. Treatment of herpes zoster and postherpetic neuralgia. Am Fam Physician 1991;44:203–210.

Catania S, Zurrida S, Veronese P et al. Mondor's disease and breast cancer. Cancer 1992;69:2267–2270.

DeFranzo AJ, Hall JH, Herring SM. Adiposis dolorosa (Dercum's disease): Liposuction as an effective form of treatment. Plast Reconstr Surg 1990;85:289–292.

DeGowin RL. DeGowin & DeGowin's Bedside Diagnostic Examination (5th ed). New York: Macmillan, 1987.

Gateley CA, Miers M, Mansel RE et al. Drug treatments for mastalgia: 17 years experience in the Cardiff mastalgia clinic. J Royal Soc Med 1992;85:12–15.

Goldhaber SZ, Morpurgo M. Diagnosis, treatment, and prevention of pulmonary embolism. Report of the WHO/International Society and Federation of Cardiology task force. JAMA 1992;268:1727–1733.

Gurevich I. Varicella zoster and herpes simplex virus infections. Heart Lung 1992;21:85–93.

Miller RD, Johnston RR, Hosobuchi Y. Treatment of intercostal neuralgia with 10 percent ammonium sulfate. J Thorac Cardiovasc Surg 1975;69:476–478.

Morrow M. Management of Common Breast Disorders. In JR Harris, S Hellman, CI Henderson, DW Kinne (eds), Breast Diseases (2nd ed). Philadelphia: Lippincott, 1991;63–73.

Reilly BM. Chest Pain. In BM Reilly (ed), Practical Strategies in Outpatient Medicine (2nd ed). Philadelphia: Saunders, 1991;440–524.

Whitley, RJ. Therapeutic approaches to varicella zoster infections. J Infect Dis 1992;166(suppl 1):S51–S57.

Wyngaarden JB, Smith L, Bennett JC. Cecil Textbook of Medicine (19th ed). Philadelphia: Saunders, 1992.

Chapter 7

Neuromusculoskeletal Scan Examination with Selected Related Topics

John S. Halle

Purpose and Philosophy of the Scan Examination

The patient will usually attempt to aid the examiner by identifying where the problem arises. Although this is an ideal starting point, the examination needs to be broad in scope and must consider dysfunction from adjacent regions to ensure that the patient's real problem is not overlooked. The examination should also consist of a nucleus of elements that are examined with virtually every patient to provide focus to the evaluation and to ensure that one or more important points are not missed. This includes consideration of potential "red flags" suggesting a serious pathologic condition. These elements of scope, consistency, and red flags are the basic purposes of the scan examination.

A focused regional examination often follows the scan examination and builds on the information elicited during the scan examination. Although categorized conceptually as two different procedures, the scan examination and the focused regional examination are not two separate entities; rather they are interrelated elements. This chapter deals with just the framework that makes up a scan examination; other sections of this text deal with specific focused examination procedures.

The philosophical perspective taken here includes several points. First, the focus of the examination is usually to identify somatic dysfunction rather than discrete pathologic entities or a disease process. So-

matic dysfunction has been defined as "impaired or altered function of related components of the somatic (body framework) system; skeletal, arthrodial, and myofascial structures; and related vascular, lymphatic, and neural elements" [1]. There are several advantages to this approach over relying solely on a pathologic state. This definition reminds the clinician to consider the whole individual, rather than thinking of the patient as simply a specific system that does not function optimally. It stresses that all of the related components of the somatic system need to function together for optimal health. Focusing on dysfunction also provides the clinician with objective elements that can be assessed and reassessed over time to quantify progress. For example, if a patient's range of motion is initially limited, it can be measured, described, and followed over time. This is helpful not only in assessing the response to treatment, but also when communicating with other health care professionals and may have more meaning in terms of understanding the problem than a specific diagnostic label. Also, the problem with diagnosis in areas such as the thoracic and lumbar spine is that the vast majority of cases are not amenable to a precise diagnosis [2].

A second point related to the scan examination is the issue of when is it needed. Some clinicians have recommended that a scan or neurologic examination is needed only when the presenting problem is an extremity problem or when the patient has symptoms such as radicular pain, weakness, numbness, or paresthesias [3, 4]. Whereas radicular problems and extremity pain are clear indications for a scan examination, the approach taken here is slightly more conservative than that advocated above. Because a scan examination can be accomplished in a matter of minutes, it should be performed as part of the initial neuromusculoskeletal evaluation of all patients except those who have a definite history of trauma to a specific joint [5]. For individuals who have sprained an ankle or injured a joint in athletic competition, proceeding to a focused examination may be appropriate. Few thoracic problems are that clear cut, however, and virtually all patients with a thoracic problem warrant a brief scan examination. Even when trauma has preceded the problem, it should be kept in mind that "trauma has been related to symptoms in 10% of patients with neoplasm, compared with 10% to 30% or more in patients with discogenic pain" [6]. Therefore, even in cases where trauma is related as the source of the problem, a brief scan examination is indicated. Certainly, if there is any doubt regarding whether an examination of this type should be done, it should be done.

A third point regarding the scan examination is how much should be done at one time. While the description presented here will encompass both upper and lower quadrant screens, it is both appropriate and customary to screen only the quadrant adjacent to the problematic region. For upper thoracic problems, an upper quadrant or cervical scan examination is indicated. For lower thoracic problems, a lower quadrant scan examination is indicated. In those thoracic spine cases where a direct quadrant association is not clear, both quadrants can be scanned, although this is the exception rather than the rule. A related point is that even a specific quadrant scan examination may not always be performed in its entirety because of patient limitations such as acute pain. In these cases, the clinician needs to use professional judgment, accomplish what can be done, and complete the evaluation at a later, more appropriate, time.

Two final points associated with the scan examination are the place of pain in the examination and the recording of the data obtained. Pain is the reason that the vast majority of patients seek care, and it is therefore a very important element in the patient/evaluator relationship. Having said that, the clinician should not be led by pain. Rather, an attempt should be made in the initial scan examination and all subsequent examinations to base treatment on the identified somatic dysfunction and objective data.

As will be discussed later, pain thresholds can change over time. Additionally, pain can be referred, and since it is largely subjective, it is not necessarily related to the severity of the underlying condition. A hypothetical illustration of this is the case of an individual who was seen for severe back pain but had normal neurologic findings. After a manipulative procedure, the patient reported a decrease in pain but left the clinic with a foot drop. Whereas the level of pain was decreased, the patient was clearly not improved. Thus, pain is an indirect measure that should not lead the clinician. Second, since memory is finite, even during a brief scan examination, take a few seconds and record what is found. The data will be more accurate if it is collected throughout the examination, rather than relying on memory.

The Scan Examination Components

The scan examination is a quick procedure that is usually completed in approximately 10 minutes. As a clinician becomes familiar with the procedure, he or she will usually tailor the examination to his or her particular style, but all of the essential elements listed below are typically included. The following is an outline of a scan examination model. Each of the components mentioned will be discussed in greater detail later in the chapter.

A. Subjective examination
B. Objective examination
  1. Observation
  2. Range of motion
  3. Motor assessment
  4. Sensory assessment
  5. Vascular status
  6. Reflexes
  7. Focused examination
    a. Clearing tests/special tests
    b. Palpation
    c. Laboratory studies
C. Assessment
D. Plan and goals

Subjective Examination

Listening to patients describe in their own words what has brought them to see you can provide great insight concerning the problem at hand. In most cases, a patient will tell the clinician what is wrong if the clinician has developed appropriate listening skills and is able to help direct the interview with appropriate questions. It is estimated that more than 80% of the information needed to clarify the presenting problem is provided by a thorough subjective examination [7, 8]. Therefore, the subjective examination or history not only provides a logical starting point for informational exchange with the patient, but it also provides a wealth of valuable clues concerning the patient's current problem.

The initial questions in the interview should be open ended, so that patients will describe in their own words and terms what is wrong with them. Initially, questions that can be answered with either "yes" or "no" should be minimized, so that patients are actively communicating information to the clinician. Also, the questions posed by the examiner should not lead the patient, but rather provide a framework from which appropriate informational exchange can occur. As the interview progresses, however, it may become necessary to be more directive, so that the patient does not take charge of the conversation and needlessly waste time. Therefore, the interview should be broad-based initially and become more focused with less open-ended questions and more closed-ended or follow-up questions over time. A more complete description of the techniques associated with the patient interview is provided by Goodman and Snyder [7].

Important questions that should be addressed during the interview are provided in Table 7.1. Additional questions should be added to this abridged list depending on the specific region evaluated and the response provided to the baseline list of questions. In addition to addressing the topics outlined in Table 7.1, be aware that how a question is asked can have an effect on the response obtained. A good example of this is the examiner's inquiry about the patient's age. Because certain pathologic conditions are more common in specific age groups, it is generally agreed that determining the patient's age is vitally important. The question "How old are you?" implies that age may be a problem and probably is not the best way to start off the interview. Instead, if the question is rephrased to "What is your age?", the tone of the question is more neutral and may be received more favorably. The consideration of how questions may sound to the patient can result in an improved quality of dialogue.

A second element of the subjective examination is to consider the possibility that the patient's problem may be caused by a systemic disease process or some other condition that is not amenable to manual therapy techniques. These questions are red flags that are suggestive of serious pathologic conditions or systemic involvement and should be considered for medical referral. One clear-cut example is a patient who has a fever. This individual should be referred to a primary care physician for evaluation for the fever. A more complete listing of potential red flag questions is provided by Goodman [9].

Whereas the subjective examination has the potential for providing a wealth of information, its dynamic and free-flowing nature also provides an environment where significant amounts of time are expended and important items can potentially be overlooked. One solution to this problem is to use a medical history screening card, which the patient fills out before the interview. Although use of a medical history screening card is not essential, it provides the examiner with a uniform base of questions, so that important information is not missed. Additionally, it serves as a useful screen for red flags from the onset of the evaluation. A sample medical history screening card is provided in Table 7.2.

Place of Pain in the Subjective Evaluation

As alluded to previously, pain is the symptom that brings the patient into the clinic in the majority of cases. Although a valuable symptom, the caution remains that the clinician does not want to be led by pain. Instead, it is often useful to both note the pattern and nature of the pain, and document the semiquantifiable quality known as pain to aid in the assessment of a patient's progress over time. The quantification of pain may also be useful by providing an index of appropriateness secondary to the assessed dysfunction. In other words, a value that was obviously rated too high for a given dysfunction may be an indication of symptom exaggeration.

Pain may be quantified in a variety of ways. One of the simplest methods is to use a 10-point scale where the patient is asked to rate the pain compared with a very severe problem. For example, the patient is asked to rate the average pain over the last 24 hours from 1 to 10, with 1 representing minimally perceived pain that they had to think about to notice,

Table 7.1. Subjective Examination Information

Question	Reason Information Sought	Example	Red Flag
What is your age?	Age specificity present with some diseases	Vertebral body epiphyseal aseptic necrosis (Scheuermann's disease)	—
Sex? (Typically observed and noted, not asked)	Sex specificity present with some diseases	Juvenile rheumatoid arthritis	—
Current occupation?	Occupation may relate to either the onset of symptoms or serve as a factor in treatment	Heavy industrial worker versus secretary	—
What problem has caused you to seek medical care?	Identifies the patient's perception and location of the current dysfunction	Trauma versus problem of insidious onset	—
Onset of problem?	Identifies length of time current dysfunction present	Acute versus chronic condition	—
Any past medical history of similar or related problem? (If so, how was the condition treated and what was the result?)	Provides insight into past history of dysfunction, rehabilitation status, and effectiveness of prior treatment	Recurring rib dysfunction	—
How is your general health? Have you experienced any unexplained weight losses?	Provides insight into other possible problems that may contribute to current problem	Rheumatoid arthritis, cancer, cardiac problems, etc.	*
Any recent infections, fever, or surgery?	Provides information regarding systemic disease that may be related to this problem	Recent history of bladder infection related to low thoracic or lumbar pain	*
What aggravates your symptoms?	The pathomechanics of provoked pain are identified by the patient	Flexion of the cervical spine reproducing upper thoracic pain	—
What relieves your symptoms?	Provides additional insight into pathomechanics and possible treatment approach	Lying on the affected side decreases pain (this is called autosplinting and may suggest pleuropulmonary involvement [9]). Also, beware of nothing relieving symptoms— suggests nonmechanical problem	*
Is there a specific pattern of pain over a 24-hour period?	Mechanical problems tend to become worse throughout the day and are relieved by rest	Muscle strain aggravated by repetitive use	—
Does the pain ever wake you from a sound sleep? If so, are you able to roll over and go back to sleep?	Provides information about the pattern of pain and alerts the examiner to the possibility of nonmechanical problem	Osteoid osteoma (Pattern of night pain, typically relieved by aspirin [6])	*
What hobbies or recreational pursuits do you engage in?	May relate to onset of symptoms or identify factors that will need to be considered in treatment	Serious rugby player versus avid reader	—
Are you aware of strength or sensory changes?	Provides insight into function of the neuromusculoskeletal system	C5 dermatome identified as area of decreased sensation	—
Any episodes of dizziness or vertigo?	Symptoms may be present with vestibular or vertebral artery problems	Vertebral artery problem	*
Current medications?	Relates potentially to both this problem and other medical problems	Steroids—long-term use may be associated with osteoporosis	—

Table 7.1. *(continued)*

Question	Reason Information Sought	Example	Red Flag
Have x-rays or other special tests been performed? If so, do you know the results?	Provides a more complete picture of what has already been done	X-rays, laboratory work obtained	—
On a scale of 1–10, with 10 representing excruciating pain and 1 representing minimal pain, where would you rate the pain over the last 24 hours?	Provides a pseudo-objective level of the patient's current perception of pain—this can be used to gauge progress later	Pain currently 4/10	—

*Potential red flags that suggest additional work-up required or referral to appropriate medical specialist.

and 10 representing a severe toothache that requires immediate attention. This method can be performed without any special charts, and the results are recorded as part of the subjective evaluation (see Table 7.1). To record this, the value reported by the patient is placed in the numerator, and 10 is placed in the denominator. This provides any other health care provider with an easily interpreted index of pain. The mean value over 24 hours is usually sought, which is more representative of the patient's condition than one moment in time, which may have been exceptionally good or bad. In addition to this technique, there are many other excellent ways of quantifying pain that use charts, questionnaires, and other mechanisms [10–13]. An example of a pain card is provided in Fig. 7.1.

In addition to attempting to quantify the subjective commodity of pain, it is also important to be aware of some of the general types of pain. The following section briefly outlines some aspects of pain that should be considered during the scan examination.

Pertinent Aspects of Pain

Referred Pain.   Convergence of afferent information is the most common explanation for the phenomenon of referred pain. The mechanism associated with referred pain is hypothesized to be a result of the convergence of both visceral and cutaneous nociceptive afferents at the dorsal horn of the spinal cord, where they synapse on projection neurons [14]. Convergence is a result of several factors. First, an organ and a given dermatome level

that were initially contiguous during embryonic development may end up in different anatomic locations in adulthood because of organ migration. Second, with both visceral and cutaneous nociceptive afferents synapsing on common projection neurons, a nondedicated signal is carried to the cortex. Because of this convergence of peripheral and visceral afferent information on projection neurons, higher centers cannot distinguish the exact source of the stimulation and often erroneously interpret the signal as arising from the peripheral cutaneous nociceptive afferents [14]. This type of somatic and visceral input convergence appears to be particularly prevalent in the thoracic region because of the association of sensory neurons for pain with the sympathetic nervous system [15]. The cell bodies for these sensory pain neurons are located in the dorsal root ganglia from approximately T1 to L2 [15]. As a consequence, when evaluating the thoracic region, the examiner should be very aware of the potential for referred pain. These referred pain patterns often tend to be very stereotypical (see Chapter 6).

Localized Pain.   An axiom that is often true is, the more superficial the pain, the more readily localized. This has been shown with a number of studies in which hypertonic saline was injected into structures and the area of pain mapped [16]. The precision of the mapping associated with superficial stimuli appears to be a result of the innervation density of a particular area [16]. In the face or hands, for example, with small receptor fields and a large innervation density, pain is accurately localized. This is in contrast to deep somatic or visceral structures,

Table 7.2. Medical History Screening Card

Date:
Patient's Name: DOB: Age:
Diagnosis: Date of Onset:
Physician: Therapist: Precautions:

Medical History

| | | *Do Not Complete. For the Therapist.* | | |
Have you or any immediate family member ever been told you have:	Circle one:	*Relation to Patient*	*Date of Onset*	*Current Status*
Cancer	Yes No			
Diabetes	Yes No			
Hypoglycemia	Yes No			
Hypertension or high blood pressure	Yes No			
Heart disease	Yes No			
Angina or chest pain	Yes No			
Shortness of breath	Yes No			
Stroke	Yes No			
Kidney disease/stones	Yes No			
Urinary tract infection	Yes No			
Allergies	Yes No			
Asthma, hay fever	Yes No			
Rheumatic/scarlet fever	Yes No			
Hepatitis/jaundice	Yes No			
Cirrhosis/liver disease	Yes No			
Polio	Yes No			
Chronic bronchitis	Yes No			
Pneumonia	Yes No			
Emphysema	Yes No			
Migraine headaches	Yes No			
Anemia	Yes No			
Ulcers/stomach problems	Yes No			
Arthritis/gout	Yes No			
Other	Yes No			

Medical Testing

1. Are you taking any prescription or over-the-counter medications?   Yes   No
   If yes, please list:
2. Have you had any x-rays, sonograms, computed tomography (CT) scans, or   Yes   No
   magnetic resonance imaging (MRI) done recently?
   If yes, when?   Where?   Results?
3. Have you had any laboratory work done recently (urinalysis or blood tests)?   Yes   No
   If yes, when?   Where?   Results?
4. Please list any operations that you have ever had and the date(s) of surgery:
   Surgery/Date:

General Health

1. Have you had any recent illnesses within the last 3 weeks (e.g., colds,   Yes   No
   influenza, bladder or kidney infection)?
2. Have you noticed any lumps or thickening of skin or muscle anywhere   Yes   No
   on your body?
3. Do you have any sores that have not healed or any changes in size, shape,   Yes   No
   or color of a wart or mole?
4. Have you had any unexplained weight loss in the last month?   Yes   No

Table 7.2. *(continued)*

5. Do you smoke or chew tobacco?	Yes	No
If yes, how many packs/day?		
For how many months or years?		
6. How much alcohol do you drink in the course of a week?		
7. How much caffeine do you consume daily (including soft drinks, coffee, tea, or chocolate)?		
8. Are you on any special diet prescribed by a physician?	Yes	No

Special Questions for Women

1. Last Pap smear:		
2. Last breast examination:		
3. Do you perform a monthly self-breast examination?	Yes	No
4. Do you take birth control pills or do you use an intrauterine device (IUD)?	Yes	No

Special Questions for Men

1. Do you ever have difficulty with urination (e.g., difficulty in starting or continuing flow or a very slow flow of urine?)	Yes	No
2. Do you ever have blood in your urine?	Yes	No
3. Do you ever have pain on urination?	Yes	No

Work Environment

1. Occupation:		
2. Does your job involve:		
prolonged sitting (e.g., desk, computer, driving)	Yes	No
prolonged standing (e.g., equipment operator, sales clerk)	Yes	No
prolonged walking (e.g., mill worker, delivery service)	Yes	No
use of large or small equipment (e.g., telephone, fork lift, typewriter, drill press, cash register)	Yes	No
lifting, bending, twisting, climbing, turning	Yes	No
exposure to chemicals or gases	Yes	No
other: please describe	Yes	No
3. Do you use any special supports:		
back cushion, neck cushion	Yes	No
back brace, corset	Yes	No
other kind of brace or support for any body part	Yes	No

For the physical therapist

Vital signs:
    Resting pulse rate:
    Oral temperature:
    Blood pressure: 1st reading: 2nd reading:
    Position: Extremity:

Source: Reprinted with permission from CC Goodman, TK Snyder. Differential Diagnosis in Physical Therapy. Philadelphia: Saunders, 1990.

which poorly localize pain. Additionally, the quality of the pain differs between superficial and deeply located structures. Superficial pain tends to be sharp, prickling, or burning, while that from deep structures often is a dull ache [16].

Somatic Pain: Localized and Referred.   Somatic pain is often categorized into either superficial or deep somatic pain [17]. Superficial somatic pain arises from stimulation of receptors in the skin and is generally well localized because of the innervation density described in the preceding paragraph. Deep somatic pain, on the other hand, arises from stimulation of receptors in skeletal muscle, joints, tendons, and fascia, and may be poorly localized or referred [16, 17]. With hypertonic saline injections in muscle, the perceived pain was often not present in the muscle of origin but was referred to other

PLEASE GIVE THIS FORM TO THE DOCTOR AT THE TIME OF
THE EXAMINATION

MARK THE AREAS ON YOUR BODY WHERE YOU FEEL THE DE-
SCRIBED SENSATIONS. USE THE APPROPRIATE SYMBOL. MARK
AREAS OF RADIATION. INCLUDE ALL AFFECTED AREAS. JUST TO
COMPLETE THE PICTURE, PLEASE DRAW IN YOUR FACE.

NUMBNESS	≡≡≡	PINS AND NEEDLES	ooo ooo ooo
BURNING	xxx xxx xxx	STABBING	/// ///

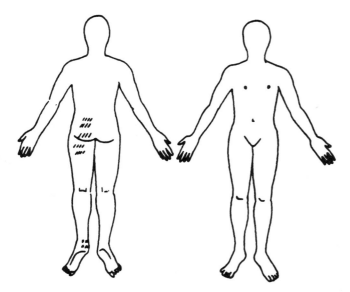

Figure 7.1. Pain card. (Reprinted with permission from V Mooney, D Cairnes, J Robertson. A system for evaluation and treatment of chronic back disability. West J Med 1976;124:373.)

muscles innervated by the same spinal nerve root [16]. Similar predictable referral patterns were also found when ligaments and periosteum were stimulated [16]. Thus, pain originating from a dermatome, myotome, or sclerotome may be referred and perceived at a site apart from the point of origin. A dermatome is that region of skin supplied by the afferent fibers projecting to a single dorsal (sensory) root of a spinal nerve. Myotomes and sclerotomes are similar, in that myotomes are the area of a muscle supplied by the afferent fibers projecting to a single dorsal root, and a sclerotome is the area of bone tissue supplied by the afferent fibers projecting to a single dorsal root. They are also similar in the sense that pain of both muscle and bone origin tends to be poorly localized [18]. Bone pain differs from muscle pain, however, in that it is usually more pronounced at night and is not affected by joint movement or resistance [18]. Whereas dermatomes, myotomes, and

sclerotomes for a given dorsal root all have a similar embryonic origin, the conscious perception of pain may differ slightly for each of these pathways because of migration during development. Additionally, whereas all three of these may refer pain, only dermatomal patterns are routinely used clinically. This is because of overlapping and discontinuous zones, which make attempts at mapping nonfunctional for distributions such as myotomes [19].

A functional key point associated with somatic pain is that it can usually be provoked during the physical examination when the somatic structure is stressed. Visceral pain often cannot be reproduced during the examination, which thus provides insight into the origin of the pain.

Radicular Pain.   Radiculalgia is defined as "neuralgia due to irritation of the sensory root of a spinal nerve" [20]. As this definition implies, it is usually caused by the irritation of a nerve root, most commonly the portion of the nerve root that lies between the spinal cord and the spinal canal. In the neuromusculoskeletal system, radicular pain is often associated with a peripheral nerve, with the pain perceived as migrating distally from the site of the dysfunction [4]. Radicular pain is one type of referred pain, referred along a given nerve distribution.

Because radicular pain is often demonstrated clinically, a common misconception is that all radiation of pain involves peripheral nerves. When dealing with referred pain, the clinician needs to consider all possible sources of the patient's pain and not fall into the trap of thinking only of the involvement of nerves. As has been mentioned previously, many soft tissues can also refer pain to other areas [19].

Visceral Pain.   Visceral pain arises from all organs and from blood vessels of the head, the body, and the extremities. Because of the extensive convergence in the thoracic region discussed previously, autonomic pain signals that are referred from other regions of the body may also be involved (see Chapters 2 and 6 for details).

Ischemic Pain.   Ischemic pain typically occurs during exercise and is caused by intramuscular pressure occluding the intramuscular blood vessel [18]. A characteristic associated with ischemic pain is that during a provoking exercise, the pain increases until the activity is stopped, then the pain disappears quickly. The mechanism of this type of pain appears to be related to both hypoxia and the accumulation of metabolites [18]. Whereas pain from intermittent claudication in the leg is commonly recognized, ischemic conditions can also affect the thoracic spine. When evaluating this region, be aware that narrowing of the axillary artery by a cervical rib can result in one of the presentations of thoracic outlet syndrome, with pain found in the upper extremity [18].

Efferent Activity Causing Pain.   Pain is usually related to afferent signals from the periphery projecting to higher levels. In cases of reflex sympathetic dystrophy (RSD), pain may have been the initial causative agent, but the syndrome is maintained at least in part by efferent activity. The mechanism is hypothesized to be a result of sympathetic efferent activity causing pain by direct activation of damaged nociceptive afferents or by nonsynaptic electrical cross-talk (ephaptic transmission) [14]. The concept that sympathetic efferent fibers participate in the sensitization of afferent fibers has not been widely recognized and has received relatively little attention [21]. Yet, this mechanism helps explain the relative success encountered in treating some of these patients with sympathetic blocks.

An important point associated with RSD and the evaluation of the thoracic spine is that conditions related to its development range from minor blunt trauma, osteoarthritis of the spine, and other degenerative diseases, to herpes zoster and peripheral nerve injury [21, 22]. Because all of these conditions are found in individuals with thoracic pain, they must be considered in the assessment. Additionally, the ultimate prognosis depends on early recognition and aggressive treatment. Individuals with persistent pain that remains out-of-proportion to their injury and that is not responding to treatment need to be referred for additional workup with a pain specialist or other appropriate professional.

Altered Pain Thresholds Secondary to Tissue Damage.   Another factor to keep in mind when assessing pain is that it is not necessarily linearly representative of the condition of the underlying tissue. Pain levels change over time, not only in response to factors such as mental state or fatigue, but also in response to tissue injury [14, 23]. With conditions such as inflammation, the sensation of pain in response to a given external stimulus is enhanced after the initial stimulus [23]. This can occur with thermal receptors, mechanoreceptors, and pain receptors [23]. Thus, something as innocuous as light touching of the skin induces pain once the area has been conditioned. This decrease in threshold of a painful response occurs not only at the site of the injury (primary hyperalgesia), but it can also occur in the surrounding undamaged tissue (secondary hyperalgesia) [14, 23]. Potential mechanisms associated with the phenomenon of enhanced response to a given painful stimulus include lowered pain thresholds, improved synaptic efficiency, sensitization of nociceptors with diffuse collateral branches, sensitization of central nociceptor neurons, and the release of a variety of chemical mediators [14, 23]. The bottom line associated with this research is that after injury, particularly one that has resulted in chronic pain, there is a leftward shift of the stimulus-response function [23]. Therefore, the subjective grading of pain has additionally a measure of physiologic plasticity associated with it.

Objective Examination

The subjective examination should have provided one or more working hypotheses that can be explored. The objective examination thus builds on the information obtained from the history by examining specific structures and systems to either confirm or rule out the working hypothesis. The objective elements of the scan examination are used to provide routine baseline information and to clear adjacent regions so that a focused regional examination can proceed with confidence. The scan examination will be presented here with subsequent chapters providing a detailed description of focused regional examination procedures for the thoracic spine.

Observation

Observation of the patient begins in the waiting room or the first time that the clinician comes in contact with the individual. The carriage (posture), facial expression, and general demeanor of the patient should be observed. While recognizing that most individuals are a little intimidated simply by virtue of being in a health care professional's office, the patient's affect can give valuable clues regarding how the individual is dealing with the present dysfunction. Depression or symptom exaggeration may be evident in the patient's manner, and it will be important to assess these elements as part of the evaluation of the whole individual.

It is probably ideal to initially meet the patient in a location that requires the individual to walk back to your office or evaluation area. This enables you to observe the patient walking without the individual being aware that he or she is being observed. Note the cadence, stride length, and associated movements such as arm swing. Also note the general posture and facial expressions as the patient walks to the evaluation area. Correlation of this impression with the formal evaluation is valuable in determining the consistency of the data collected.

Observation in the Examination Room

Ensure that the region of interest is adequately exposed on the patient. For evaluation of the thoracic spine, men should remove their shirts and women should be in a halter top. If shorts are needed for access to the low back or hips, ensure that this clothing is available. Patients should remove shoes and socks before inspection to guarantee that any limb length asymmetries noted are indeed real or not apparent because of an overlooked shoe lift or construction asymmetry. Observe at a minimum the following elements: gait, posture, and trunk and extremities for atrophy.

In terms of gait, have the patient ambulate again and reassess the general components of gait. This should correlate with what was observed as the patient walked to the examination room. Assess posture, looking specifically for asymmetries from the floor up and for normal spine contours. Planning increases the likelihood of noting a problem, so the examination should be efficient but systematic. One method is to examine the patient while he or she is standing with the feet approximately shoulder width apart. Perform a posterior-anterior inspection of the patient's feet, lateral malleoli, fibular heads, greater trochanters, posterior superior iliac spines, iliac crests, spine, inferior borders of the scapulae, shoulders, and the position of the head. As part of this inspection, be sure to note the space between each of the upper extremities and the trunk. Occasionally, a discrepancy in space between the arm and trunk will help the examiner focus in on a subtle asymmetry. Then, observe the patient from the side and note the alignment of the lower extremities, curves of the spine, position of the shoulders, and position of the head. Be aware that a normal variant is that most individuals carry their dominant shoulder slightly lower than the nondominant shoulder [5]. Also, while not a normal variant, a high percentage of individuals in our society have a forward head and protracted shoulders, which predisposes them to a variety of problems. As part of the inspection and performed simultaneously, inspect the patient for atrophy. All sides of the individual should be examined.

Range of Motion

The scan examination for range of motion will ideally be very brief. Generally, if an individual demonstrates complete, pain-free, active range of motion, then the joints away from the region being examined are clear. Therefore, for lower thoracic spine dysfunction where the lower quadrant is of interest, having the patient squat and return to standing is a very quick general gauge of the region's range of motion. For the trunk, have the individual flex, extend, and side-bend bilaterally and rotate the trunk bilaterally. For the upper quadrant, ask the patient to bilaterally reach as far down the back as possible, which causes the individual to flex, abduct, and externally rotate. Then, ask the patient to bilaterally reach up the back as far as possible, which requires extension, internal rotation, and some adduction. For the head and neck, have the patient perform the same general motions as for the trunk. If any asymmetry of movement is noted, then a more detailed investigation is required with goniometric measures used to quantify the extent of the difference. If a noticeable scoliosis is noted, particularly in an adolescent, the examiner needs to document the curve. Furthermore, determine if it is nonstructural—that is, if it is flexible and corrects with bending to the convex side—or structural—that is, it does not correct with bending to the convex side [24]. Additional information on scoliosis is available from articles by Lonstein [24] and Keim [25].

Whereas the scan examination is designed to quickly screen the joints, detection of a limitation in range of motion or the production of pain will require a more focused inspection. This will typically involve three components:

1. Active range of motion—motion that the individual performs under his or her own power. This assesses contractile elements as well as the capability of the joint.
2. Passive range of motion—examines more specifically the capability of the joint, with muscle function eliminated. In the case of weakness or pain associated with a contractile element, the passive range of motion will often be greater than the active range of motion.
3. Overpressure—provided at the end of range to assess the quality of the joint.

Motor Assessment

When assessing motor function, it is not necessary to check every muscle in a region. The scan exami-

nation for the shoulder and hip girdle and the extremities will typically involve at least one resisted test representative of each nerve root level within a given nerve plexus, and an examination of each major peripheral nerve. Often these are done simultaneously, which minimizes the number of muscle groups examined. For example, C7 is the primary nerve root level supplying the triceps, and the triceps is innervated by the radial nerve. Thus, testing the triceps looks at both possible C7 nerve root involvement and radial nerve involvement. As long as the strength is normal, no additional examination of either of these two elements is needed. In cases of observed weakness or patient complaints of specific muscle weakness, however, the motor examination must include detailed testing of all potentially involved muscles.

For the scan examination, it is usually enough to examine bilaterally just the quadrant of interest. If the patient has an upper thoracic problem, then the upper quadrant should be examined for motor function. For a lower thoracic problem, the lower quadrant should be inspected. See Tables 7.3 and 7.4 for the motor scan examination for the upper and lower quadrants.

Motor Examination Grading Scheme

Motor function should be graded according to a commonly used framework such as the National Medical Research Council Scale [26, 27]. Possible values on this scale range from 0 to 5. Motor function is recorded by placing the obtained grade in the numerator and recording the full scale value of 5 in the denominator. A summary of that scale is:

0 = no muscle contraction.
1 = trace contraction but no significant movement of the joint on which the muscle acts.
2 = movement of the joint through its full range by the muscle if gravity is neutralized.
3 = movement of the joint through its full range by the muscle against gravity.
4 = movement of the joint by the muscle against both gravity and active resistance.
5 = normal strength.

Grading Motor Function in the Presence of Pain.
If the individual experiences pain with a resisted contraction, resulting in yielding of the muscle with any

Table 7.3. Upper Quadrant Scan Motor Evaluation

Resisted Action	Muscle Tested	Root Level*	Peripheral Nerve
Shoulder abduction	Deltoid	C5–6, primarily C5	Axillary
Elbow flexion	Biceps brachii	C5–6	Musculocutaneous
Elbow extension	Triceps brachii	C5–7, primarily C7	Radial
Wrist extension	Extensor carpi radialis longus, brevis, and extensor carpi ulnaris	C5–8, primarily C6	Radial
Wrist flexion	Flexor carpi radialis and flexor carpi ulnaris	C6–T1 (radialis [C7] provides the majority of power for flexion (33))	Median for radialis and ulnar for ulnaris
Finger flexion	Flexor digitorum superficialis, flexor digitorum profundus, and lumbricales	C7–T1, primarily C8	Median for superficialis, both median and ulnar for profundus and lumbricales
Finger abduction	Dorsal interossei	C8–T1, primarily T1	Ulnar

*Range of root levels taken from Kendall et al. [60]. Primary root levels taken from Hoppenfeld [33].

Table 7.4. Lower Quadrant Scan Motor Evaluation

Resisted Action	Muscle Tested	Root Level*	Peripheral Nerve
Hip flexion	Iliopsoas	L1–L4	Femoral to iliacus and lumbar plexus to psoas
Knee extension	Quadriceps	L2–L4	Femoral
Hamstrings	Biceps femoris, semimembranosus, and semitendinosus	L4–S3	Sciatic (peroneal branch to lateral hamstrings, tibial branch to medial hamstrings)
Dorsiflexion with inversion	Tibialis anterior	L4–S1, primarily L4	Deep peroneal
Great toe extension	Extensor hallicus longus	L4–S1, primarily L5	Deep peroneal
Ankle eversion	Peroneus longus and brevis	L4–S1, primarily S1	Superficial peroneal nerve
Ankle plantarflexion	Gastrocnemius and soleus	L5–S2, primarily S1	Tibial
Hip extension	Gluteus maximus	L5–S2	Inferior gluteal nerve

*Range of root levels taken from Kendall et al. [61]. Primary root levels taken from Hoppenfeld [34].

strength value below normal (5/5), then the muscle test is invalid [28]. The test is invalid because it cannot be conclusively determined if the observed weakness was indeed secondary to the pain or the result of an underlying process such as a compressed nerve root. While true muscle function cannot be ascertained in this case, many clinicians will record what they were able to assess. For example, a yielding to pain with moderate resistance could be recorded as "4/5*", with the asterisk indicating pain limited.

Contractile Versus Inert Structures.   The concept of contractile versus inert structures was popularized by Cyriax [29] and is very useful when assessing

motor function. Simply stated, contractile elements consist of the muscle, tendon, and tendon-periosteal junction. During a muscle contraction, if any of these are involved, pain will be elicited. Inert structures are basically everything else—tissues that possess no inherent capacity to contract and relax. Categorization of structures into these two basic groups is essential when attempting to ascertain the cause of pain. If an active range of motion procedure elicits pain, for example, it is not clear if the pain is caused by the muscles moving the joint or the joint structures being moved. If, on the other hand, the joint is not moved and muscle function is tested isometrically and pain remains, it is presumed to be caused by involvement of the muscle, the tendon, or the tendon-periosteal junction. This type of categorization facilitates the identification of the cause of a given dysfunction.

Sensory Assessment

The sensory scan examination, like the motor scan examination, does not need to be very involved. Generally, a patient with a sensory deficit resulting from a peripheral nerve problem will identify the area of anesthesia when questioned [28]. Therefore, since the intent of the scan examination is to ensure that important information is not inadvertently overlooked, a brief assessment of sensory function will usually suffice. Like the motor examination, usually either the upper or the lower quadrant is assessed, depending on the patient's complaint. Be aware that questioning a patient regarding sensory function will often yield identification of areas of paresthesia rather than anesthesia [4], but these can easily be sorted out during the examination.

Light touch is a commonly assessed sensory modality. It is usually performed by gently brushing along the area of interest with either a wisp of cotton or the examiner's fingertips. If an area of decreased sensation is determined, then further investigation with other sensory modalities is indicated. Recall that light touch, two-point discrimination, vibration, and proprioception are carried by the dorsal column–medial lemniscal pathway. Pain, temperature, and crude touch, on the other hand, are carried by the anterolateral system (spinothalamic tract). Figure 7.2 diagrams both dermatomes and peripheral nerve cutaneous fields. Whereas the scan examination is typically restricted to light touch, other sensory modalities often assessed include pain, two-point discrimination, proprioception, vibration with a 128-Hz tuning fork [8], and double simultaneous stimulation [28].

Noteworthy Points Associated with the Sensory Scan Examination

There are a number of points of interest regarding the sensory scan. First, there is a great deal of overlap of dermatomes because of overlapping innervation of adjacent dorsal roots. This is especially true in the thoracic spine, where one dermatome may be completely absent with no loss of sensation [30]. Second,

the amount of dermatomal overlap depends on the modality. Pain dermatomes mapped with a sharp object have less overlap than light touch dermatomes mapped with a mechanical stimulus [31]. Therefore, a common recommendation is that when investigating areas of cutaneous sensory loss, begin in the area of anesthesia and work outward until the border region of normal sensation is identified [32]. A pin may be used to obtain this delineation. Third, while a pinprick has the advantage of making it easier to identify a single dorsal root injury through the use of the modality of pain, be extremely cautious with the use of sharp objects in routine sensory testing. Pinwheels are commonly used, yet if the skin were inadvertently compromised, the instrument would need to be autoclaved before it is used on another patient to ensure against the spread of diseases such as AIDS. While no one intends to break the skin on a sensory examination, the potential exists and it should be considered in the selection of assessment tools. A recommendation is to use a safety pin rather than a pinwheel for mapping out the area of anesthesia and discard the safety pin after use. Fourth, if an assessment of vibration or proprioception is done for conditions such as multiple sclerosis or pernicious anemia, the deficit is usually present in the lower extremities before it is present in the upper extremities [28]. Therefore, if the lower extremities are normal, testing of the upper extremities is probably not needed. Fifth, double simultaneous stimulation can be done with either light touch or pinprick when a general area deficit (such as the entire extremity) is encountered [28]. This rapid test examining for a possible cerebral lesion is done by having the patient close his or her eyes and applying light touch or pinprick bilaterally [28]. If the patient reports perception of the modality on one side only, this suggests a significant sensory deficit on the involved side [28]. If sensation is equal bilaterally at the start of the test, leave the stimulus in place for 10 seconds and then reassess the patient's sensory perception [28]. In some cases adaptation will have occurred, resulting in the patient reporting stimulation on only one side after this time delay. This is indicative of a subtle sensory deficit on the involved side [28]. Another clue to a central nervous system lesion that affects sensation is that it is typically not painful, unlike most peripheral nerve injuries, which have pain accompanying sensory loss [28]. Sixth, stocking glove paresthesias are suggestive of possible vascular insufficiency [4].

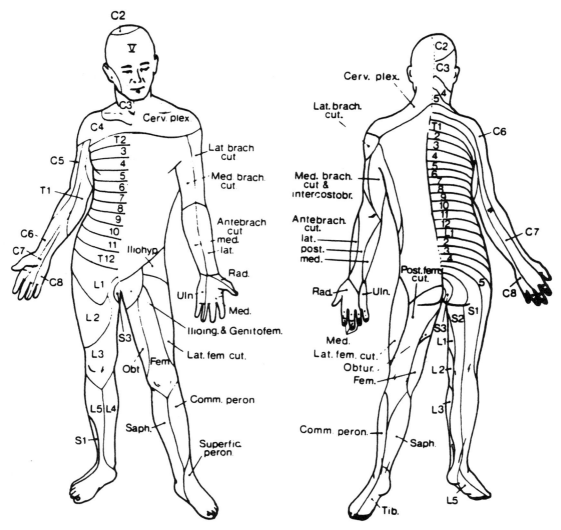

Figure 7.2. Dermatomes and peripheral nerve cutaneous distributions. (From J Gilroy. Basic Neurology [2nd ed]. Tarrytown, NY: Pergamon, 1990. With permission of McGraw-Hill, Inc.)

Vascular Status

Vascular status is often omitted during a scan examination, apart from some of the special tests that will be discussed later under thoracic outlet syndrome. If done, examination of the nail beds, capillary refill, and normal pulse are the only data that are usually obtained. The dorsalis pedis pulse may be taken in the lower extremities and the radial pulse elicited in the upper extremities. While part of a thorough evaluation, signs such as clubbing of the fingernails or chronic open wounds will often lead the evaluator to perform more detailed vascular evaluations when needed.

Reflexes

Reflex assessment is a vital component of the scan examination, especially on any patient suspected of having neurologic involvement. Reflexes allow the clinician to evaluate the status of both the afferent and efferent limb of the peripheral nerve, the sensory organ, and the effector organ, and often to obtain information about the status of the central nervous system. Since these are typically easy to elicit, are stereotypical, and do not decrease with repeated trials, the use of reflexes is an extremely valuable element of the evaluation. Additionally, since the strength of the stimulus determines the amplitude of the response, they are typically graded. Specific reflexes that will be discussed include muscle stretch reflexes, pathologic reflexes, and superficial skin reflexes.

Muscle Stretch Reflexes

A muscle stretch reflex (MSR), in its most basic form, is a simple reflex arc, with the muscle spindle as the sensory receptor. The MSR is typically assessed by tapping the mid-substance of a tendon and noting the reaction of the homonymous skeletal muscle. If any of the elements in the reflex arc are dysfunctional, then the reflex will be diminished or absent. A diminished reflex usually indicates a lower motor neuron problem, such as a compressed or lacerated peripheral nerve.

The MSR also provides information regarding the status of the upper motor neuron. Whereas the basic reflex path described in the preceding paragraph is monosynaptic and occurs at a given segmental level, the lower motor neuron is subject to descending influences from cortical and brain stem pathways such as the corticospinal tract, rubrospinal tract, and lateral vestibulospinal tract. The combined influence of these pathways onto Sherrington's "final common pathway," the lower motor neuron, is generally inhibitory. Thus, when the combined higher level influences are functioning properly, they tend to modulate down the segmental reflex response. On the other hand, if there is damage to a tract such as the corticospinal tract, a disinhibition occurs at the segmental level of the spinal cord, and the MSR response is typically enhanced. In this way, the status of the upper motor neuron is indirectly assessed with MSR testing.

Whereas diminished or absent responses are a sign of a lower motor neuron problem and enhanced responses are a sign of an upper motor neuron problem, the critical issue in interpreting MSRs is the symmetry of the reflexes between sides. If an individual has a symmetrical response bilaterally, generally he or she does not have either a lower or an upper motor neuron problem, regardless of the absolute activity of the MSR demonstrated. For example, normal individuals have bilaterally absent responses to tendon taps. On the other hand, it is the asymmetrical response that suggests a problem. If the side of the asymmetry is diminished, then a lower motor neuron problem would be suggested. Similarly, an enhanced response

on the involved side would suggest an upper motor neuron problem. The variable response provided by spinal level and descending influences makes MSRs valuable for clinical assessment.

The activity of MSRs is graded as follows: a grade of 0 indicates no response, a grade of 1+ indicates a diminished or hypoactive response, a grade of 2+ indicates a normal or expected response, a grade of 3+ indicates an enhanced or hyperactive response, and a grade of 4+ indicates hyperactivity with clonus [32]. Again, it is stressed that a grade other than 2+ is not by itself suggestive of a neurologic problem if both sides are symmetrical. The presence of clonus, however, even if it were bilateral, would warrant additional investigation.

Five MSRs are commonly assessed, three in the upper extremities and two in the lower extremities. Each muscle tested is considered to have a primary neurologic level, which assists with localization of an identified response. Whereas root level innervation of a particular muscle is not restricted to a single level, the response can be viewed as an assessment of the primary component of the peripheral nerve tested. The three upper extremity responses are (1) biceps, predominantly C5; (2) brachioradialis, predominantly C6; and (3) triceps, predominantly C7 [33]. The two MSRs assessed commonly in the lower extremity are (1) quadriceps, predominantly L4; and (2) soleus, predominantly S1 [34]. Additionally, the medial hamstrings are occasionally tested as an L5 predominant reflex, although this MSR is a little more difficult to elicit.

Noteworthy Points Associated with MSRs.   The name originally given to MSRs was "deep tendon reflexes" or DTRs. Because the tendon is the region tapped by the reflex hammer, this term was embraced and has been widely used by practitioners. A DTR is a misnomer, however, in that the sensory organ responsible for the reflex is the muscle spindle, not the Golgi tendon organ. Whereas muscle spindles facilitate the homonymous muscle, Golgi tendon organs actually cause an inhibition of the muscle of origin when activated. The currently accepted term of MSR correctly identifies the reflex as being caused by a stretch of the muscle, rather than a stretch of the tendon.

The Jendrassik maneuver is a technique commonly used to enhance an MSR that is difficult to elicit. To enhance the upper extremity response, the patient would be asked to cross the ankles so that the lateral aspects of each foot are in contact, then isometrically attempt to abduct the legs. The upper extremity MSR would be obtained while the patient was performing this procedure. To enhance the lower extremity response, the patient's fingers are interlocked while the patient isometrically attempts to pull the elbows apart while the lower extremity MSRs are simultaneously tested. It appears that this easily observed enhancement is a result of facilitation of synaptic transmission at the segmental level of the spinal cord rather than by altering muscle spindle sensitivity, although the exact mechanism has not been clearly elucidated [35]. Since this technique does alter the response, however, if it is used in the scan examination, the recorded note should reflect that the MSR was elicited while the patient was performing a Jendrassik maneuver.

The Jendrassik maneuver illustrates that for the most reproducible results, standardization should be used during reflex testing. Boissonnault [3] pointed out that a change in position, such as from sitting to supine, or a change in head or neck posture may cause inconsistent or false-negative findings. He speculated that these altered positions change the pressure exerted on the nerve resulting in variable results. Ideally, standard positioning should be used when assessing MSRs, with consideration of weight-bearing and the effects of posture on foraminal size.

One additional interesting point associated with MSRs is that it is possible that they are affected by referred pain. Mooney and Robertson [36] have shown experimentally in three patients with low back pain that MSRs were depressed before administration of an arthrogram and local anesthetic injection. After this procedure, the reflexes were normal. The authors attributed this change to the elimination of reflex inhibition, a neurophysiologic mechanism that has been clearly demonstrated with muscle activation secondary to pain or joint effusion [37, 38].

Pathologic Reflexes

Primitive reflexes are normally integrated by individuals as they develop. For example, Babinski's sign is a normal primitive reflex in humans at birth and is integrated by supraspinal levels within the first 5–7 months of life [39]. If an injury or disease process results in a loss of this normal suppression by the cerebrum on the segmental level of the brain stem or spinal cord, then the integrated primitive reflex is released. This released reflex is termed a pathologic reflex.

Babinski's sign is the most common pathologic reflex tested in the lower extremity, and its presence is pathognomonic of corticospinal tract damage [32]. Babinski's sign is elicited by stroking the outer border of the foot with a blunt object such as a key or the end of a reflex hammer [40]. The normal response is flexion of the great toe and the lateral four toes. An abnormal response is extension of the great toe with fanning of the lateral toes. The test result is recorded as present or not present, with a present Babinski's sign indicative of corticospinal tract damage. A common mistake is to apply too much pressure when stroking the foot, eliciting a mass flexion withdrawal response because of the noxious stimulation. Many other pathologic reflexes can be assessed in the lower extremity [32].

A pathologic reflex similar to Babinski's sign for the upper extremity is Hoffmann's sign. This is elicited by flicking the distal phalanx of either the patient's index or middle finger while the hand is relaxed [39, 40]. A "clawing motion" or flexion of the thumb and index finger is indicative of a present Hoffmann's sign [39, 40]. Unlike Babinski's sign, some normal individuals exhibit a present Hoffmann's sign [40]. The key to interpreting this test is asymmetry from one side to the other. See Chusid [39] for other upper extremity tests.

When scanning either the upper or lower quarter, a pathologic reflex test is essential for any patient with a suspected neurologic problem. Whereas other procedures such as the MSR indirectly examine for upper motor neuron problems, pathologic reflex testing is the only direct method used in the scan examination for this important category of lesions.

Clearing Tests

Clearing tests are designed to clear one area before a detailed examination of a second area, where pain may have been referred. Special tests, on the other hand, are usually those tests that allow an in-depth examination of the hypothesized area of dysfunction. For example, when the clinician suspects that the patient's problem is in the upper thoracic spine, the cervical spine and thoracic outlet must be cleared to ensure that the dysfunction is not really a dysfunction in one of those areas referring pain to the thoracic spine. Once the clearing tests have been done with no positive supporting evidence of an outside problem, then the special tests would be used to ex-

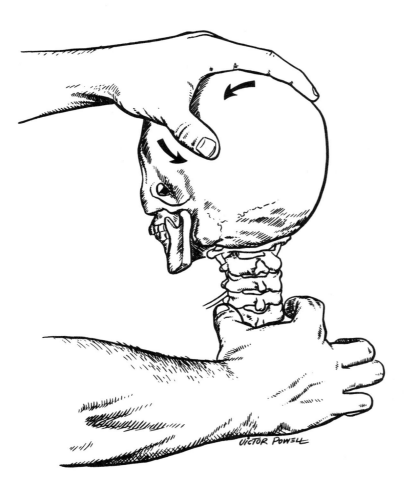

Figure 7.3. Enhancing the specificity of the foraminal encroachment test.

amine the thoracic spine in detail. This section will review several commonly used clearing tests. Specific special tests are discussed elsewhere in this text.

Upper Quadrant Clearing Tests

The abridged list of tests reviewed here can be used to quickly scan the cervical spine and thoracic outlet for potential problems before focusing on the thoracic region. See Bourdillon et al. [1], Boissonnault [3], Saunders and Saunders [4], Cyriax [29, 42], Magee [30], Greenman [41], and Aspinall [43, 44] for a more detailed listing of clearing tests.

Foraminal Encroachment Test. The purpose of the foraminal encroachment test is to examine the exiting cervical nerve roots as a possible source of the patient's pain. Often as a result of degeneration of the cervical spine with osteophyte formation, decreased disc space, chronic postural problems, or alterations in normal mo-

bility, the intervertebral foramina will be implicated as a source of peripheral symptoms. The test is performed with the patient in a sitting position and the head and neck abducted, rotated away from the midline, and extended. Slight overpressure is applied, and the patient is questioned about the effect of this position on the symptoms. The combined rotation, side-bending, and extension maximally closes the intervertebral foramina on the side to rotation, and a positive test is indicated by a reproduction of symptoms on the ipsilateral side [4]. This test can be made more specific by stabilizing a cervical segment with one hand and then using that hand as a fulcrum (Fig. 7.3) in an attempt to narrow one foramen. For example, stabilizing C6 with the hand and then extending, left side-bending, and left rotating the neck over your hand might produce pain or tingling in the left C6 dermatome, suggesting a left C6 root irritation or compression.

This test should be done after the cervical range of motion procedures outlined earlier, specifically cervical rotation to end of range. The rationale is that as little as 45 degrees of rotation ipsilaterally and 50 degrees of rotation contralaterally can possibly cause vertebral artery compression [30]. If the patient had experienced symptoms associated with possible vertebral artery involvement, such as vertigo, dizziness, or nystagmus, then a more detailed examination such as that described by Aspinall [44] should be performed. A careful examination up to this point, noting patient responses to the range of motion procedures and adequate questioning during the subjective examination, is usually adequate for a patient with probable thoracic spine dysfunction, and specific vertebral artery tests are normally not performed as part of the scan examination. The importance of the vertebral artery test as part of a routine examination remains controversial [4, 30, 41].

Compression Test. With the patient sitting, downward pressure is gently applied on the top of the head, causing a compression of the axial skeleton. If this downward pressure results in a reproduction of the patient's symptoms, it may implicate narrowing of the intervertebral foramina, facet joint pressure, or muscle spasm [33]. A slightly more specific variant of this same test is to have the patient bend the head to the involved side, then apply a compression force on the head [30]. This decreases the intervertebral foraminal space slightly before compression and may yield a clearer result. This combined side-bending and compression test is also sometimes referred to as Spurling's test [30]. Specific levels of involvement can often be hypothesized by observation of distribution of pain and altered sensation.

Distraction Test. The distraction test is the opposite of the compression test, with a distraction force applied to the chin and occiput in a rostral direction. The proposed mechanism of the procedure is to open the intervertebral foramina, joint capsules, or facet joint, thus decreasing or eliminating the patient's symptoms [33]. If the results of this test are positive, it gives an indication that cervical traction may be an effective form of treatment.

Upper Limb Tension Test. The upper limb tension test is the functional analog of the straight leg raising test in the lower quadrant scan examination, and a positive response implicates the peripheral nerve trunks or the cervical nerve roots [45, 46]. The purpose of the test is to exert a longitudinal traction force on the involved structures and reproduce the patient's symptoms. The test is most useful as a method of recognizing somatic pain referred from the cervical spine to the shoulder that is not identified by the foraminal encroachment test or compression test. The test is composed of three successive maneuvers that progressively add a greater stretch on the peripheral nerve trunks of the tested arm [45].

To perform the initial position of the test, the patient is positioned supine. The arm, which is moderately flexed at the elbow, is passively moved into shoulder abduction, extension, and external rotation. Shoulder abduction should be between 100 and 130 degrees, shoulder external rotation approximately 60 degrees, and shoulder extension approximately 10 degrees [45]. This places the shoulder joint in the middle of its available range of motion and should not stress the capsule or joint receptors (Fig. 7.4) [45]. The patient is questioned regarding symptoms, and if appropriate, movement into the second position is performed. The second maneuver builds on the first by extending the elbow and supinating the forearm [45]. Be sure to stabilize the shoulder before extending the elbow joint, so that excessive stress is not placed on the shoulder. This increases the stretch and the patient should be questioned again regarding the symptoms (Fig. 7.5). The third and final position is achieved by extending the wrist and fingers while the previous position is maintained. This produces a maximum stretch of the neural and dural tissue [45] (Fig. 7.6). Again, the patient should be questioned regarding symptoms.

The normal response for the initial position is perhaps a mild stretch, while positions two and three may produce a stretch sensation to a deep stretch or ache in the region of the cubital fossa [45]. Note that while there are symptoms associated with a normal response, these symptoms are not reproduced at the shoulder. The provocation of shoulder pain, other than a mild sensation of anterior shoulder stretch, should be considered abnormal and is indicative of a positive upper limb tension test (ULTT) [45]. Additional follow-up tests for further confirmation of the cause of the symptoms obtained are available in Kenneally et al. [45], Butler [46, 47], and Elvey [48].

While this test is not specific for a given nerve root or peripheral nerve, it should be recognized that the various positions will accentuate the stretch to upper extremity nerves. The median nerve is stretched by all positions of the ULTT and is the pe-

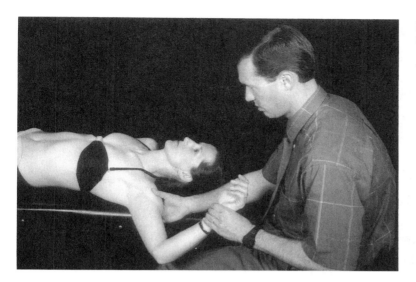

Figure 7.4. Upper limb tension test—initial position.

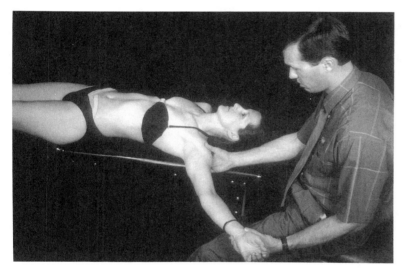

Figure 7.5. Upper limb tension test—second position.

ripheral nerve most affected [45]. The musculocutaneous and ulnar nerves are also exposed to stretch with this procedure, with the combined motion of shoulder abduction, extension, and external rotation stressing the musculocutaneous nerve (position two), and the addition of wrist and finger extension stressing the ulnar nerve (position three) [45]. In addition to implicating nerve root problems, the clinician should be aware that other cervical spine structures such as dural tissue attached to the zygapophyseal joints may also yield a positive result [45]. As with other procedures, collaborative findings need to be examined in context with the rest of the examination.

Thoracic Outlet Syndrome Tests.   As the neurovascular bundle made up of the subclavian artery, vein, and brachial plexus leaves the superior rim of the thoracic cage, there are several potential sites of impingement that can result in referred signs and symptoms to the thoracic cage and upper extremity [4, 49–52]. The typical sites of impingement are (1) the interscalene triangle, composed of the anterior and middle scalene and the first rib; (2) the costoclavicular space, created between the clavicle and the first rib; and (3) the axilla, specifically where the neurovascular bundles pass beneath the coracoid process and the tendon of the pectoralis minor. Because arterial, venous, and neural structures can be involved individually or

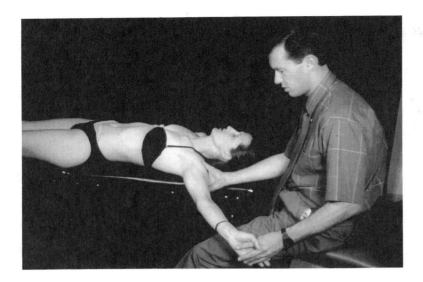

Figure 7.6. Upper limb tension test—third position.

collectively, the signs and symptoms of thoracic outlet syndrome (TOS) vary widely. Arterial compression can cause ischemic pain, vascular symptoms that are more severe in cold weather, fatigue during activity, and Raynaud-like symptoms [4, 50, 51]. Severe cases can progress to gangrene [50]. Venous signs and symptoms include edema, stiffness of the fingers, pain, and fatigue [4, 51]. Neurologic involvement is characterized by pain and paresthesias, commonly in the ulnar distribution but also reported in the median distribution [4]. Other common findings include atrophy of intrinsic muscles of the hand and symptoms that are worse at the end of the day or night [4, 49–51]. Many tests have been developed to aid in the differential diagnosis of TOS, since these impingements are often difficult to distinguish from thoracic or cervical problems. The following three tests are commonly used in the scan examination to clear these areas.

ADSON'S TEST. Adson's test is used to clear the interscalene triangle. The patient is either seated or standing, and the examiner locates the radial pulse at the wrist. The arm is extended and externally rotated passively, while the patient is asked to extend and rotate the head to the ipsilateral side, while taking and holding a deep breath (Fig. 7.7). This position is maintained for approximately 10 seconds, while the effects on the radial pulse and symptoms are assessed. If the pulse is diminished or abolished and the symptoms are reproduced, the result is positive [4, 49–51]. The test should also be repeated with the head turned to the opposite side, since some individuals exhibit the greatest response with a contralateral head turn [4, 50] (Fig. 7.8).

COSTOCLAVICULAR OR MILITARY BRACING TEST. The costoclavicular procedure tests the costoclavicular space. The patient is either seated or standing, and the radial pulse is palpated. The patient is asked to assume a pronounced shoulder retraction and depression posture, analogous to an exaggerated military attention position. Again, diminishment or obliteration of the pulse accompanied by reproduction of symptoms would indicate a positive result. This may be aided by providing longitudinal traction on the arm [51] (Fig. 7.9).

HYPERABDUCTION TEST. Hyperabduction of the arm stretches the neurovascular bundle around the coracoid process while it is held in place by the tendinous attachment of the pectoralis minor. Like the other two tests, the radial pulse is located, and information concerning the reproduction of symptoms is sought. A positive test diminishes or eliminates the pulse and reproduces the symptoms.

Noteworthy Points Associated with the Thoracic Outlet Syndrome Tests. Whereas these clearing tests are useful elements of the scan examination, it should be clearly understood that these are not pathognomonic for a specific dysfunction. All of the tests have a high percentage of false-positive results in normal individuals and they may be inconsistent [51]. As a result, both sides should be tested on all individuals and the results compared, and the findings must be viewed in the context of the entire examination. Second, the structure implicated in most patients with positive TOS test findings is neural. It has been reported

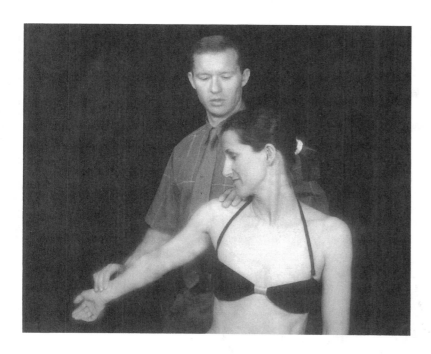

Figure 7.7. Adson's test with patient's head rotated to the ipsilateral side.

that 90–97% of all positive findings are the result of neurologic compression, with venous problems accounting for 2% and arterial compression accounting for approximately 1% of the identified incidence [4]. It is noteworthy, however, that while small in actual percentage, arterial compression problems can lead to the most serious complications. A third important point is that sensory signs and symptoms usually precede motor involvement in these cases [51]. Last, both postural and anatomic variants have been implicated as causing TOS signs and symptoms [50, 51].

Upper Quadrant Scan Considerations

The purpose of the upper quadrant scan examination is to clear the cervical spine so that the clinician can focus on the suspected region of dysfunction for a patient with a thoracic complaint. It also serves to force the clinician to consider the entire scope of causes that might produce the patient's current signs and symptoms. In addition to radicular pain, it is now clear that the anterior cervical disks and associated ligamentous structures can refer pain to the mid-thoracic area [53]. Autonomic pathways can be involved as a result of the relationship of the sympathetic nervous system with the thoracic spine, and conditions such as Horner's syndrome should be considered during the scan examination. Addition-

ally, with all thoracic problems, both systemic and visceral causes of signs and symptoms such as the cardiovascular, pulmonary, gastrointestinal, and urogenital systems may need to be ruled out.

Lower Quadrant Clearing Tests

Since pain is usually referred distal to the site of origin [4], most lower thoracic problems will not be the result of distal problems referring pain proximally. As a result, there is typically less involved in the lower quadrant screening than the upper quadrant examination. Two useful tests, however, are the straight leg raising test and the FABER test. The straight leg raising test is used to determine radicular involvement in the lower extremity and the FABER test is a quick screen for hip dysfunction on the involved side. Through the use of these two tests, lower lumbar and sacral radicular problems and potential hip dysfunction are quickly screened.

Straight Leg Raising Test. The straight leg raising test is done with the patient supine and relaxed. The leg is passively raised with the knee maintained in extension through the available range. Reproduction of unilateral hip, thigh, or leg pain when the leg is raised to approximately 35–70 degrees is suggestive of sciatic nerve involvement [54]. Con-

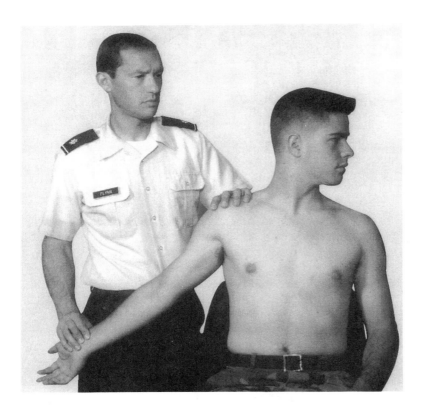

Figure 7.8. Adson's test with the patient's head rotated to the contralateral side.

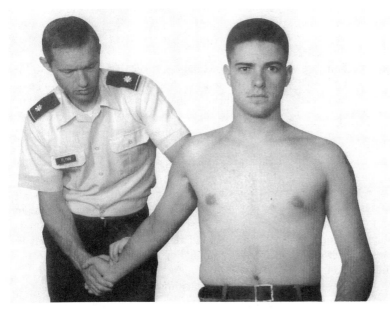

Figure 7.9. Costoclavicular or military bracing test.

tralateral hip, thigh, or leg pain is suggestive of a space-occupying lesion such as a herniated disk, and is sometimes called the cross-over straight leg raising test [54]. Further confirmation can be ob-

tained by taking the leg to the point of irritation, then lowering the leg slightly to ameliorate the symptoms, then passively dorsiflexing the ankle. Reproduction of the symptoms with this maneuver implicates sciatic nerve involvement. Neck flexion may also be used during this test to increase the stretch on the sciatic nerve, lumbosacral nerve roots, and the dura mater [54].

Sciatic nerve involvement is not likely if the patient's symptoms are reproduced with less than 30 degrees of hip flexion, since this is the range where slack in the nerve is taken up [55]. The nerve is maximally stretched from 35–70 degrees, and this is the range in which symptoms should be reproduced. Pain reproduction beyond 70 degrees suggests hamstring involvement or joint pain [54].

During the scan examination, this test can practically be performed during the motor function test of the lower extremities. Ask the patient to extend the leg fully while in the sitting position. If the patient is unable to do this without pain, then the straight leg raising test is not needed, since this stretches the sciatic nerve in a manner similar to the straight leg raising test. If this sitting straight leg test does reproduce symptoms, then the variants of the straight leg raising test described above can be used to examine the symptoms in more detail.

The FABER Test. The FABER test derives its name from the combined motions of flexion, abduction, and external rotation, and it is occasionally called Patrick's test. With the patient positioned supine, the knee is flexed and the hip is passively brought into flexion. The foot on the examined side is set on the patient's contralateral knee, and then the hip is gently lowered into abduction and external rotation. Limitation of motion or reproduction of pain suggests a problem of the hip joint, the iliopsoas muscle, or the sacroiliac joint [56].

Special Tests

If the upper or lower quadrant has been cleared, then special regional tests are employed to thoroughly investigate a given region. These tests are detailed in other sections of this text.

Palpation

Palpation is part of the focused regional examination and has intentionally been left until near the end of the examination for two reasons. First, it provides the clinician with an opportunity to collect a broad base of collaborative information before focusing on a specific structure or joint. Second, it enables the clinician to establish rapport with the patient before potentially inflicting discomfort when palpating a tender area.

Specific sites that should be palpated in the thoracic spine are discussed in other chapters of this text and will not be mentioned here. A few general guidelines are in order, however. First, knowledge regarding anatomy is the key to successful palpation. If you believe the old anatomy adage that structure subserves function, then a clear understanding of structure is necessary to both palpate it and recognize a dysfunctional state. Second, the palpation scheme used should be systematic in nature, so that all pertinent landmarks are examined. If the site of discomfort is immediately focused on, important related structures that may provide the key to the patient's problem may be overlooked. Third, examining the painful area last allows the clinician to examine the area with the patient relatively relaxed. If palpation of the involved area elicits pain and guarding, the majority of the examination will have been completed before this guarding. Finally, be sure to note related points such as effusion, edema, and tissue quality identified during the palpation.

Noteworthy Points Associated with Palpation

Muscle spasm is often annotated as a palpatory finding in response to pain and guarding. If spasm is conservatively defined as "a reversible state of sustained, involuntary contraction accompanied by muscle shortening and associated with electrical potential changes" [57], then the clinician needs to be aware that true spasm rarely occurs. In an elegant study in 1950 that involved both patients referred for spasm and subjects injected with a 6% hypertonic saline solution that caused hard, rounded lumps, electromyographic silence was demonstrated in the vast majority of cases [57]. This has been replicated more recently in 50 patients referred with "muscle spasm," with none of the patients demonstrating electromyographic evidence of muscular activity in the area of pain [58]. The exact mechanism associated with the change in tissue texture, for lack of a better term, has not been elucidated.

Laboratory Tests

Laboratory tests are part of the collaborative process of collecting information in an effort to ascertain the patient's problem. Rarely are they pathognomonic of a particular problem, indicating that they should be appropriately used to complement a thorough physical examination. Specific radiographic or laboratory tests are discussed elsewhere in this text and will not be covered here.

Assessment

The preceding examination should lead the clinician to a decision regarding a neuromusculoskeletal problem appropriate for physical or manual therapy treatment, or if the patient should be referred for medical treatment. As has been mentioned previously, the vast majority of patients with problems associated with the spine do not necessarily have a clear diagnosis, so it is not unusual to be working from a clinical hypothesis rather than a clear diagnosis [2]. This assessment should be based on the objective facts obtained during the evaluation, and it should be as precise as is reasonable. Having said that, the clinician is additionally obligated to determine if it is appropriate for him or her to handle the patient's dysfunction. Goodman and Snyder have indicated that "the hallmark of any health care professional is the ability to understand the limits of his or her professional knowledge" [59]. If the assessment is unclear or falls outside of a health care provider's scope of practice, then a medical referral is indicated. Additionally, at this point in the examination, potential red flags should be considered again.

Plans and Goals

While the typical SOAP note (subjective, objective, assessment, and plan) would suggest that the treatment plan should be developed before setting goals, this order should probably be reversed. If the clinician and patient together determine a set of mutually agreed upon goals, then this provides a map for the treatment plan. The goals should ideally be both short-term and long-term, and they should be measurable. Clearly stated goals will serve as the foundation for an optimal treatment plan.

Summary

The preceding material has presented the basics associated with a neuromusculoskeletal scan examination of the upper and lower quadrant. The scan examination's purpose is to be broad in scope and to clear adjacent areas of dysfunction or pathologic conditions, so that a focused regional examination may be undertaken without inadvertently overlooking the true cause of pain. Additionally, the scan examination provides a basis for a systematic, consistent assessment and serves to consider potentially serious pathologic entities. Whereas this chapter has focused on the scan examination and other chapters in this book deal with elements of the focused regional examination, recognize that they are typically seamless and are performed together as part of the total "patient examination."

References

1. Bourdillon JF, Day EA, Bookhout MR. Examination, General Considerations. In JF Bourdillon, EA Day, MR Bookhout (eds), Spinal Manipulation (5th ed). Boston: Butterworth-Heinemann, 1992;47–80.
2. Spratt KF, Lehmann TR, Weinstein JN et al. A new approach to the low-back physical examination. Spine 1990;15:96–102.
3. Boissonnault WG. Screening for Medical Disease. In WG Boissonnault (ed), Examination in Physical Therapy Practice. New York: Churchill Livingstone, 1991;17.
4. Saunders DH, Saunders R. Evaluation of the Spine. In DH Saunders (ed), Evaluation, Treatment and Prevention of Musculoskeletal Disorders (3rd ed). Bloomington, MN: Educational Opportunities, 1993;33–97.
5. Magee DJ. Principles and Concepts. In DJ Magee (ed), Orthopedic Physical Assessment (2nd ed). Philadelphia: Saunders, 1992;1–33.
6. Goodman CC, Snyder TK. Systemic Origins of Musculoskeletal Pain: Associated Signs and Symptoms. In CC Goodman, TK Synder (eds), Differential Diagnosis in Physical Therapy. Philadelphia: Saunders, 1990;327–345.
7. Goodman CC, Snyder TK. Introduction to the Interviewing Process. In CC Goodman, TK Snyder (eds), Differential Diagnosis in Physical Therapy. Philadelphia: Saunders, 1990;7–42.
8. Walton L. The Symptoms and Signs of Disease in the Nervous System. In L Walton (ed), Essentials of Neurology. New York: Churchill Livingstone, 1989;1–24.
9. Goodman CC. Red flags: recognizing signs and symptoms. Physical Therapy Magazine 1993;(September):55–62.

10. Mooney V, Cairnes D, Robertson J. A system for evaluation and treatment of chronic back disability. West J Med 1976;124:370–376.

11. Melzack R. The McGill pain questionnaire: major properties and scoring. Pain 1975;1:277–299.

12. Lawlis GF, Cuencas R, Selby D et al. The development of the Dallas pain questionnaire: an assessment of impact of spinal pain and behavior. Spine 1989;14:507–516.

13. Huskisson EC. Measurement of pain. Lancet 1974;2:1127–1131.

14. Jessell TM, Kelly DD. Pain and Analgesia. In ER Kandel, JH Schwartz, TM Jessell (eds), Principles of Neural Science (3rd ed). New York: Elsevier, 1991;385–399.

15. Barr ML, Kiernan JA. Visceral Innervation. In ML Barr, JA Kiernan (eds), The Human Nervous System—An Anatomical Viewpoint (6th ed). Philadelphia: Lippincott, 1993;364–376.

16. Fields HL. Pain from Deep Tissues and Referred Pain. In HL Fields (ed), Pain: Mechanisms and Management. New York: McGraw-Hill, 1987;79–98.

17. Tortora GJ. Sensory Structures. In GJ Tortora (ed), Principles of Human Anatomy (4th ed). New York: Harper & Row, 1986;487–526.

18. Mills KR, Newham DF, Edwards RHT. Muscle Pain. In PD Wall, R Melzack (eds), Textbook of Pain. New York: Churchill Livingstone, 1984;319–330.

19. Cyriax J. Referred Pain. In J Cyriax (ed), Textbook of Orthopaedic Medicine (7th ed). London: Baillière Tindall, 1978;30–54.

20. Stedman's Medical Dictionary (23rd ed). Baltimore: Williams & Wilkins, 1976.

21. Roberts WJ, Kramis RC. Sympathetic Nervous System Influence on Acute and Chronic Pain. In HL Fields (ed), Pain Syndromes in Neurology. Boston: Butterworth-Heinemann, 1990;85–106.

22. Payne R. Neuropathic pain syndromes, with special reference to causalgia and reflex sympathetic dystrophy. Clin J Pain 1986;2:59–73.

23. Raja SN, Meyer RA, Campbell JN. Hyperalgesia and Sensitization of Primary Afferent Fibers. In HL Fields (ed), Pain Syndromes in Neurology. Boston: Butterworth-Heinemann, 1990;19–41.

24. Lonstein JE. Natural history and school screening for scoliosis. Orthop Clin North Am 1982;19:227–237.

25. Keim HA. Scoliosis. Clin Symp 1972;24:1–30.

26. Medical Research Council of the United Kingdom. Aids to Examination of the Peripheral Nervous System. Memorandum No. 45. Palo Alto, CA: Pedragon House, 1978.

27. Florence JM, Pandya S, King WM et al. Intrarater reliability of manual muscle test (Medical Research Council Scale) grades in Duchenne's muscular dystrophy. Phys Ther 1992;72:115–126.

28. Goldberg S. The Four-Minute Neurologic Exam (3rd ed). Miami: MedMaster, 1992.

29. Cyriax J. The Diagnosis of Soft Tissue Lesions. In J Cyriax (ed), Textbook of Orthopaedic Medicine (7th ed). London: Baillière Tindall, 1980;64–103.

30. Magee DJ. Cervical Spine. In DJ Magee (ed), Orthopedic Physical Assessment (2nd ed). Philadelphia: Saunders, 1992;34–70.

31. Martin JH, Jessell TM. Anatomy of the Somatic Sensory System. In ER Kandel, JH Schwartz, TM Jessell (eds), Principles of Neural Science (3rd ed). New York: Elsevier, 1991;353–366.

32. Neurology Staff B. Basic Topics in Clinical Neurology. San Antonio, TX: U.S. Government Printing Office, 1990.

33. Hoppenfeld S, Hutton R. Evaluation of Nerve Root Lesions Involving the Upper Extremity. In S Hoppenfeld, R Hutton (eds), Orthopaedic Neurology. Philadelphia: Lippincott, 1977;7–44.

34. Hoppenfeld S, Hutton R. Evaluation of Nerve Root Lesions Involving the Trunk and Lower Extremity. In S Hoppenfeld, R Hutton (eds), Orthopaedic Neurology. Philadelphia: Lippincott, 1977;45–74.

35. Rothwell JC. Functional Consequences of Activity in Spinal Reflex Pathways. In JC Rothwell (ed), Control of Human Voluntary Movement. Rockville, MD: Aspen, 1987;126–157.

36. Mooney V, Robertson J. The facet syndrome. Clin Orthop 1976;115:149–156.

37. DeAndrade JR, Grant C, Dixon ASJ. Joint distension and reflex muscle inhibition in the knee. J Bone Joint Surg [Am] 1965;47:313–322.

38. Fahrer H, Rentsch HU, Gerber NJ. Knee effusion and reflex inhibition of the quadriceps. J Bone Joint Surg [Br] 1988;70:635–638.

39. Chusid JG. Reflexes. In JG Chusid (ed), Correlative Neuroanatomy and Functional Neurology (16th ed). Los Altos, CA: Lange, 1976;206–210.

40. Gilman S, Newman SW. Lesions of the Peripheral Nerves, Spinal Roots, and Spinal Cord. In S Gilman, SW Newman (eds), Clinical Neuroanatomy and Neurophysiology (8th ed). Philadelphia: FA Davis, 1992;84–95.

41. Greenman DE. Principles of High-Velocity, Low-Amplitude Thrust Technique. In DE Greenman (ed), Principles of Manual Medicine. Baltimore: Williams & Wilkins, 1989;94–100.

42. Cyriax J. Vertebral Manipulation. In PD Wall, R Melzack (eds), Textbook of Pain. New York: Churchill Livingstone, 1984;725–729.

43. Aspinall W. Clinical testing for the craniovertebral hypermobility syndrome. J Orthop Sports Phys Ther 1990;12:47–54.

44. Aspinall W. Clinical testing for cervical mechanical disorders which produce ischemic vertigo. J Orthop Sports Phys Ther 1989;11:176–182.

45. Kenneally M, Rubenach H, Elvey R. The Upper Limb Tension Test: The SLR Test of the Arm. In R Grant (ed), Physical Therapy of the Cervical and Thoracic Spine. New York: Churchill Livingstone, 1988;167–194.

46. Butler DS. Tension Testing—The Upper Limbs. In DS Butler (ed), Mobilisation of the Nervous System. New York: Churchill Livingstone, 1991;147–160.

47. Butler DS. Application, Analysis and Further Testing. In DS Butler (ed), Mobilisation of the Nervous System. New York: Churchill Livingstone, 1991;161–181.

48. Elvey RL. The Investigation of Arm Pain. In GP Grieve (ed), Modern Manual Therapy of the Vertebral Column. New York: Churchill Livingstone, 1986;530–535.

49. Goodman CC, Snyder TK. Overview of Cardiovascular Signs and Symptoms. In CC Goodman, TK Snyder (eds), Dif ferential Diagnosis in Physical Therapy. Philadelphia: Saunders, 1990;43–84.

50. Lord JW, Rosati LM. Thoracic outlet syndromes. Clin Symp 1971;23:1-32.

51. Phillips H, Grieve GP. The Thoracic Outlet Syndrome. In GP Grieve (ed), Modern Manual Therapy of the Vertebral Column. New York: Churchill Livingstone, 1986;359–369.

52. Toby BE, Koman LA. Thoracic Outlet Compression Syndrome. In RM Szabo (ed), Nerve Compression Syndromes: Diagnosis and Treatment. Thorofare, NJ: Slack, 1989;209–226.

53. Cloward RB. Cervical diskography—a contribution to the etiology and mechanism of neck, shoulder and arm pain. Ann Surg 1959;150:1052–1064.

54. Magee DJ. Lumbar Spine. In DJ Magee (ed), Orthopedic Physical Assessment (2nd ed). Philadelphia: Saunders, 1992;247–307.

55. Fahrni WH. Observations on straight-leg raising with special reference to nerve root adhesions. Can J Surg 1966;9:44–48.

56. Magee DJ. Hip. In DJ Magee (ed), Orthopedic Physical Assessment (2nd ed). Philadelphia: Saunders, 1992; 333–371.

57. Harell A, Mead S, Mueller E. The problem of spasm in skeletal muscle. JAMA 1950;143:640–644.

58. Johnson EW. The myth of skeletal muscle spasm. Am J Phys Med Rehabil 1989;68:1.

59. Goodman CC, Snyder TK. Introduction to Differential Screening in Physical Therapy. In CC Goodman, TK Snyder (eds), Differential Diagnosis in Physical Therapy. Philadelphia: Saunders, 1990;16.

60. Kendall FP, McCreary EK, Provance PG. Upper Extremity and Shoulder Girdle Strength Tests. In FP Kendall, EK McCreary, PG Provance (eds), Muscles: Testing and Function (4th ed). Baltimore: Williams & Wilkins, 1993;235–298.

61. Kendall FP, McCreary EK, Provance PG. Lower Extremity Strength Tests. In FP Kendall, EK McCreary, PG Provance (eds), Muscles: Testing and Function (4th ed). Baltimore: Williams & Wilkins, 1993;177–234.

Chapter 8

Evaluation of the Thoracic Spine and Rib Cage

Mark R. Bookhout

Evaluation of the thoracic spine and rib cage requires an appreciation of the anatomy and biomechanics of this unique spinal region. The thoracic region of the spine differs from the cervical and lumbar regions in that its spinal mechanics are directly influenced by the attachment of the ribs and sternum. The motion available in a particular region of the thoracic spine is also influenced by the changing orientation of the facet planes, with a more coronal facet orientation in the upper thoracic spine allowing a greater range of axial rotation and a more sagittal facet orientation at the thoracolumbar junction limiting axial rotation while allowing for the greatest range of flexion and extension in the thoracic spine (see Table 1.2). Biomechanically the thoracic spinal segments display motion characteristics similar to those of the lumbar spine, with coupling of rotation and side-bending occurring to the same side or to the opposite side depending on whether neutral or non-neutral mechanics exist and depending on whether side-bending or rotation is introduced first [1].

Pain complaints in the thoracic area are most often caused by dysfunctional spinal or rib cage mechanics [2], although midscapular pain can be referred from the lower cervical spine [3]. The cause of chest wall pain in patients with negative cardiopulmonary findings can often be attributed to dysfunctional vertebral or rib mechanics; conversely, the examiner should be alerted to the possibility of organic pathologic conditions in patients with thoracic or rib cage pain when mechanical findings are minimal (see Chapter 6).

Different biomechanical approaches have been advocated for the evaluation of the thoracic spine and rib cage. Although this chapter attempts to integrate some of these different schools of thought, the primary focus is based on a biomechanical model developed largely by the osteopathic profession. Inherent in any biomechanical evaluation process is the ability to clinically detect (diagnose) areas of abnormal function (dysfunction). From the osteopathic perspective, the art of structural diagnosis is to define the presence of somatic dysfunction (facilitated segment) and determine its significance, if any, to the patient's complaint or disease process at the time. The diagnostic findings that confirm the presence of somatic dysfunction include (1) asymmetry of position, (2) abnormalities in range of motion (usually hypomobility), and (3) tissue texture changes [1]. The provocation of pain is de-emphasized, because pain often arises from tissues and joints that are under compensatory strain secondary to neighboring hypomobility. However, pain provocation with active or passive mobility testing before and after treatment may be quite helpful in assessing the effectiveness of a given therapeutic intervention.

Barrier Concept

To detect the presence of somatic dysfunction, we must first understand normal range of motion. A normal joint has an available range of active movement limited by a physiologic barrier as tension de-

147

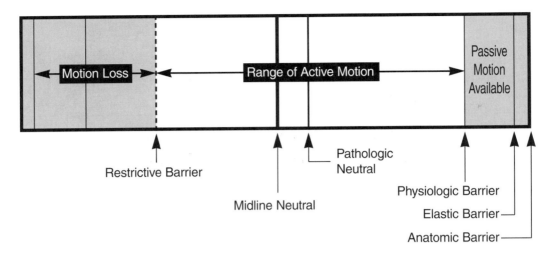

Figure 8.1. Illustration of active range of motion with a physiologic barrier and an anatomic barrier on the right and a restrictive barrier on the left.

velops within the joint capsule and supporting ligaments, surrounding musculature, and connective tissue structures. At the physiologic barrier there is an additional passive range of motion, known as accessory motion, available only when extraneously induced. Each joint has resistance at the end of its passive range of motion that is characteristic to that joint and the limiting tissue or tissues (end-feel). These normal end-feels have been described as muscular, soft-tissue approximation, ligamentous, cartilaginous, and capsular [4]. Beyond the available passive range of motion there exists an anatomic barrier that, if exceeded, disrupts the integrity of that joint. When a restrictive barrier exists, either the active range of motion is compromised from the expected normal or there is no passive range of motion available beyond the active range (Fig. 8.1). The nature of the resistance (end-feel) at the restrictive barrier again depends on the tissue at fault. Abnormal end-feels have been described as capsular, adhesions and scarring, bony block, bony grate, springy rebound, pannus, loose, empty, painful, and muscular [4]. The goal of treatment is to remove the restrictive barrier by selection of a treatment technique appropriate to that particular type of barrier. For example, muscle energy technique would be appropriate when hypertonic muscle is responsible for the limitation of motion, whereas a high-velocity thrust or joint mobilization technique might be indicated in the presence of a capsular restriction of motion.

Structural Diagnosis

Assessment for restrictive barriers to thoracic spinal motion can be made by a combination of any of the following tests: (1) active physiologic mobility tests in which the examiner either follows a pair of transverse processes as the patient actively flexes and extends through the thoracic spine or palpates the interspinous space for opening and closing as the patient moves through a flexion and extension arc, respectively; (2) positional testing with the operator assessing the transverse processes for asymmetry when the thoracic spine is in the hyperflexed, neutral, and hyperextended position; (3) passive physiologic mobility tests where the operator induces motion through the thoracic spine and assesses mobility with a palpating finger at the interspinous space; and (4) passive accessory mobility tests using unilateral posterior-to-anterior pressures applied to the transverse processes with the thoracic spine positioned in hyperflexion and hyperextension [5].

Active Physiologic Mobility Tests

An osteopathic approach to assessing the active range of motion of a thoracic spinal segment uses manual contacts, usually the thumbs, to palpate and follow a pair of transverse processes as they move during flexion and extension of the spine. Recall

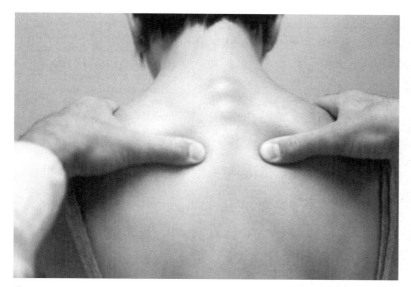

Figure 8.2. Active physiologic mobility testing for flexion. A. The examiner's thumbs are in contact with the transverse processes as the patient moves into flexion. B. Symmetric opening of facet joints during spinal flexion. The examiner's thumbs follow the transverse processes (T.P.) as flexion occurs.

A

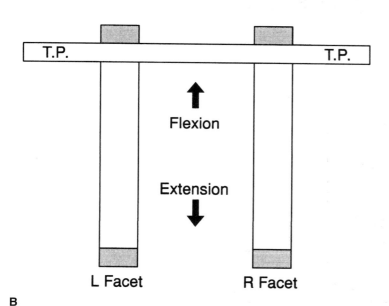

B

from Chapter 1 that the transverse processes are the longest at T1 and the shortest at T12, and the relationship between the location of the transverse processes relative to its spinous process is variable ("Rule of Three's"). Because of this relationship the examiner's palpating thumbs must be placed accordingly depending on the area of the thoracic spine being evaluated (see Table 1.1). On flexion of the spine the facet joints open bilaterally so that the examiner's thumbs, in contact with the transverse processes, should move an equal amount superiorly and anteriorly (Fig. 8.2). Conversely, with extension there is bilateral closing of the facet joints symmetrically so that the examiner's thumbs, in contact with the transverse processes, move an equal amount inferiorly and posteriorly (Fig. 8.3). This evaluation

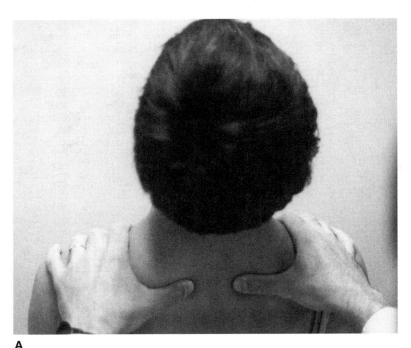

Figure 8.3. Active physiologic mobility testing for extension. A. The examiner's thumbs are in contact with the transverse processes as the patient actively extends through the upper thoracic spine. B. Symmetric closing of the facet joints during active spinal extension. The examiner's thumbs follow the transverse processes (T.P.) as extension occurs.

A

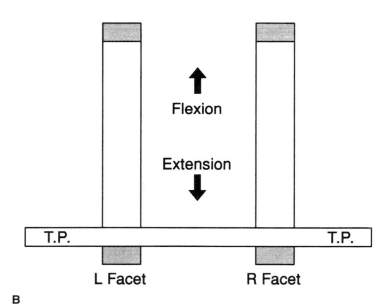

B

approach uses asymmetric movement of the transverse processes to detect motion restrictions within paired facet joints. The advantages of this approach are that only one plane of movement is introduced, the method does not put the segment through an articulatory procedure, and functional versus structural asymmetries are identified. For these reasons this evaluation approach is felt to be more consistent in

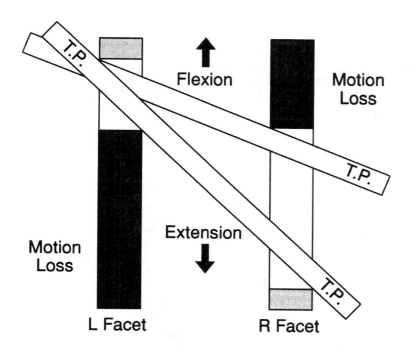

Figure 8.4. Behavior of the transverse processes with a bilateral restriction. There is a loss of facet opening on the right and facet closing on the left so that the transverse process remains rotated to the right throughout the range of flexion and extension.

terms of inter-rater reliability, although this remains to be proven. Structural asymmetries of the transverse processes can be ruled out by having the examiner follow what appears to be an asymmetric pair of transverse processes as the patient moves through a range of flexion and extension, noting whether the asymmetry of the transverse processes changes during the movement. If the transverse processes become symmetric either in flexion or extension, the asymmetry is functional in nature. However, if a transverse process is prominent because of asymmetric osseous development (structural) and the motion segment is normal, the transverse process will retain the same degree of prominence (asymmetry) throughout the full range of flexion and extension. The only exception occurs in the presence of a bilateral restriction when there is a loss of facet joint opening on one side and facet closing of the contralateral joint, so that asymmetry of the transverse processes is maintained throughout the range (Fig. 8.4). Intersegmental motion testing by palpation between spinous processes would confirm a loss of range of motion for both flexion and extension at that segmental level (Figs. 8.5 and 8.6).

Positional Tests

The patient is positioned in neutral, flexion, and extension while the examiner palpates for asymmetry between paired transverse processes to make a positional assessment (Fig. 8.7). Not only are paired transverse processes assessed for asymmetry but each spinal segment is evaluated relative to the segment below. This is performed with the patient in the sitting position for the upper thoracic spine. In the lower thoracic spine, flexion is assessed with the patient sitting, while neutral and extension are assessed in the prone lying and in the prone propped (sphinx) positions.

Passive Physiologic Mobility Tests

Assessment for restrictive barriers to motion at a given thoracic spinal segment can be made by passively flexing and extending the thoracic spine with the examiner palpating the interspinous spaces. Normally with flexion of the spine the examiner should feel a separation between the spinous processes, whereas with extension the spinous processes should

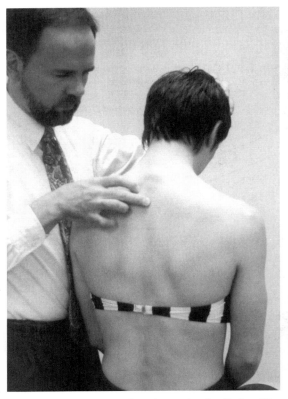

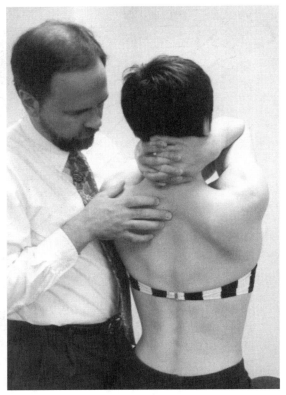

Figure 8.5. Intersegmental motion testing for flexion. The examiner's right middle finger is in the interspinous space palpating for opening as flexion is passively introduced through the head and neck into the upper thoracic spine.

Figure 8.6. Intersegmental motion testing for extension. The examiner's right middle finger palpates the interspinous space for closure as extension is passively introduced from the lower cervical spine into the upper thoracic spine.

approximate (see Figs. 8.5 and 8.6). Coupled motion of side-bending and rotation can also be assessed while the interspinous space is monitored. Three-dimensional assessment can be made by passively inducing side-bending and coupled rotation with the thoracic spine in a hyperflexed or hyperextended position, but this requires more technical skill by the examiner (Fig. 8.8). The problem with mobility tests is that each time motion is induced passively the joint is articulated, possibly changing the evaluative findings and adversely affecting interrater reliability [1].

Passive Accessory Mobility Tests

In addition to physiologic motion testing, passive accessory motions can be tested to complement and confirm the motion restrictions noted during the dynamic and static testing. The main accessory movements tested in the thoracic spine are posteroanterior (PA) central pressures, transverse vertebral pressures, and PA unilateral vertebral pressures [6]. Testing for accessory movements can be integrated with static positional testing by applying unilateral PA pressures on the transverse processes when the spine is hyperflexed or hyperextended to help confirm the positional diagnosis (Fig. 8.9). Posteroanterior central pressures performed with the patient prone assess translation at each thoracic spinal level. When applying a PA central pressure at T5, we assess the ability to bilaterally open the facet joints at T5–6 and also the ability to bilaterally close the paired facets at the level above—i.e., T4–5.

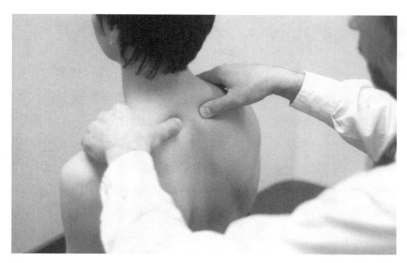

A

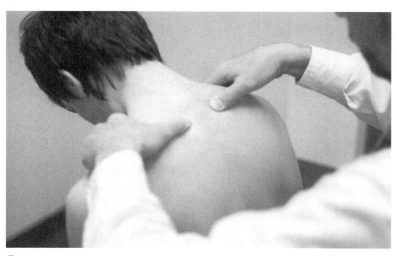

B

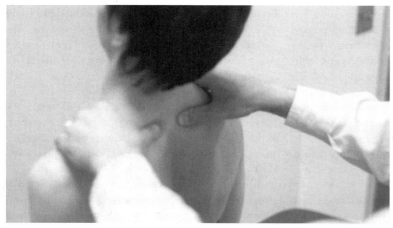

C

Figure 8.7. Positional testing. A. Neutral. B. Flexion. C. Extension.

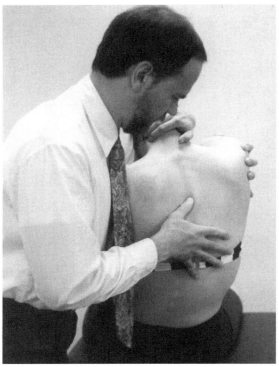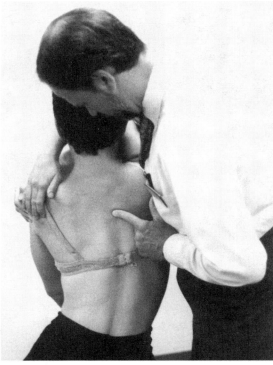

A   **B**

Figure 8.8. Passive physiologic mobility tests for combined movements. A. Flexion, left side-bending, and left rotation are passively introduced and an assessment of the available range of motion is made with the right thumb palpating at the interspinous space. B. Extension, left side-bending, and right rotation are introduced and mobility is assessed with palpation at the interspinous space.

Vertebral Structural Diagnosis

Single Segment Versus Multiple Segment Dysfunction

Vertebral dysfunctions in the thoracic spine can be either single segment dysfunctions or multiple (group) dysfunctions involving three or more vertebrae (Table 8.1). Single segment dysfunctions are traumatically induced, occur in flexion or extension, have coupling of side-bending and rotation to the same side, and need to be treated first. Because these dysfunctions occur in flexion or extension, they are referred to as non-neutral dysfunctions. The dysfunction is named by the position in which it is held. A segment that is held in a flexed, left-rotated, and left–side-bent position has a positional diagnosis of flexed, rotated, and side-bent left (FRS$_L$). The motion restriction for this dysfunctional segment is for extension, right rotation,

and right side-bending. The possibility exists for thoracic spinal segments to be positionally held in a flexed, rotated, and side-bent position (FRS) or an extended, rotated, and side-bent position (ERS), or to be bilaterally flexed or bilaterally extended (Table 8.2). When making a positional diagnosis, it is important to remember that the superior segment is always compared with the inferior segment in determining dysfunction—i.e., if T3 appears rotated to the right in flexion but T4 is also equally rotated to the right in flexion, then there is no difference between T3 and T4 and thus no dysfunction. However, if the T4 transverse processes were to appear symmetric in flexion, then T3 would be truly right rotated on T4 and dysfunctional—i.e., ERS right.

Multiple segment (group) dysfunctions involve three or more vertebral segments, are usually compensatory, have coupling of side-bending and rotation to the opposite side, and are treated last (see

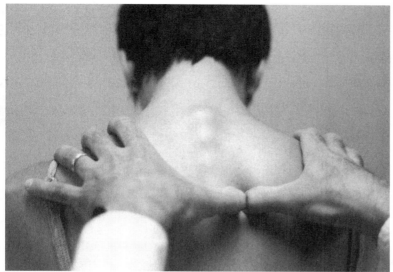

A

Figure 8.9. Passive accessory mobility tests. A. Unilateral posterior-to-anterior pressures on the right transverse process with the spine in flexion. B. Unilateral posterior-to-anterior pressures on the right transverse process with the spine in extension.

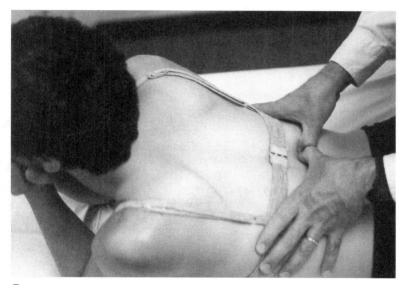

B

Table 8.1). Because these dysfunctions occur in neutral, they are referred to as neutral dysfunctions and are palpable in flexion, neutral, and extended positions of the spine with their primary restriction being side-bending and coupled rotation to the opposite side (Table 8.3).

C7 Through T4

In assessing the upper thoracic spine we have the opportunity to evaluate for restrictive barriers both statically (positional) and dynamically (active physiologic). Static positional findings are noted with the upper thoracic spine in neutral, hyperflexed, and hyperextended positions with the patient seated (see Fig. 8.7). The positional symmetry or asymmetry of the transverse processes at each successive level of the spine from C7 to T4 is recorded for each of the three positions. If no asymmetry is noted in a hyperflexed position from C7 to T4, the assumption is made that either no unilateral restrictive barrier to flexion or facet opening exists from C7–T1 to T4–5

Table 8.1. Types of Thoracic Spinal Dysfunction

Single Segment	Multiple Segment
Traumatic	Compensatory
Flexion or extension	Neutral
Side-bending and rotation coupled to the same side	Side-bending and rotation coupled to opposite side
Treat first	Treat last

or that a bilateral restriction for flexion may be present. When a bilateral restriction for flexion exists, a flat spot is noted at that dysfunctional segmental level of the thoracic spine during forward flexion. Passive intervertebral mobility testing during flexion confirms a failure to open at the interspinous space (see Fig. 8.5). Likewise, if extension of the upper thoracic spine shows no asymmetries of the transverse processes from C7 to T4, one can assume that there are no unilateral restrictive barriers to facet closure from C7–T1 to T4–5, or that a bilateral restriction for extension may exist. The examiner should suspect a bilateral restriction if there is a failure to reverse the thoracic kyphosis at a given segmental level during spinal extension. Confirmation of a bilateral restriction is made by performing passive intervertebral mobility testing into extension and noting a failure of the interspinous space to close (see Fig. 8.6).

In active physiologic mobility testing, the thumbs are placed on paired transverse processes and the patient is asked to move in sagittal-plane flexion and extension with the examiner's thumbs following the transverse processes. Normally the transverse processes should be felt to move in a symmetric manner superiorly and anteriorly with flexion of the spine and should move in a symmetric manner posteriorly and inferiorly on extension. When dysfunction exists, one transverse process will stop moving prematurely in the range, creating a rotational asymmetry. If, for example, there is a restrictive barrier for flexion or opening of the right facet joint between T3 and T4 and the examiner has his or her palpating thumbs on the transverse processes of T3, the right thumb will stop moving in comparison with the left during forward flexion, so that in a flexed position the T3 segmental level will appear to be right rotated in comparison with T4. On backward bending, since there is no restriction to facet closure in this example, the left thumb will travel posteriorly and inferiorly to become symmetric with the right thumb in full spinal extension (Fig. 8.10). The treatment approach would be directed at restoring facet opening on the right to regain flexion at the right facet of T3–4. Conversely, if there is a restriction to closure of the left facet joint, then the thumbs will appear to move in a symmetric manner superiorly and anteriorly during forward flexion, because there is no limitation to opening, but on backward bending or extension of the spine, the right transverse process will move posteriorly and inferiorly and the left transverse process will stop prematurely, resulting in a right-rotated T3 segment on T4 when the spine is in extension (Fig. 8.11). The restrictive barrier in this example is on the left side as the segment moves into extension and the treatment approach is directed at restoring facet closure on the left. Figure 8.12 represents the findings from a hypothetical patient and the thought process involved in determining which segments are dysfunctional.

Table 8.2. Single Segment Vertebral Dysfunction

Positional Dysfunction	Active and Passive Motion Restriction	Passive Accessory Restriction
FRS right	Extension, left rotation, left side-bending	Left facet will not close
ERS right	Flexion, left rotation, left side-bending	Right facet will not open
FRS left	Extension, right rotation, right side-bending	Right facet will not close
ERS left	Flexion, right rotation, right side-bending	Left facet will not open
Bilaterally flexed	Extension	Both facets will not close
Bilaterally extended	Flexion	Both facets will not open

Table 8.3. Multiple Segment Vertebral Dysfunction

Positional Dysfunction	Active and Passive Motion Restriction	Passive Accessory Restriction
Neutral, rotated right, side-bent left "convex right group"	Left rotation, right side-bending	Right facets will not close Left facets will not open
Neutral, rotated left, side-bent right "convex left group"	Right rotation, left side-bending	Left facets will not close Right facets will not open

T4 Through T12

In the lower thoracic spine we again use static positional testing with flexion assessed with the patient sitting, the neutral position assessed with the patient prone lying, and the extended position assessed with the patient prone lying propped on elbows (sphinx) (Fig. 8.13). Dynamic testing by monitoring the transverse processes through an active range of flexion and extension is not the preferred method of assessment, because it is more difficult in the lower thoracic spine as a result of the bulk of the spinal musculature. However, unique to evaluating the thoracic spine is the accessibility of the ribs for palpation both anteriorly and posteriorly. The ribs can be thought of as extensions of the transverse processes

and therefore reflect and enhance any vertebral dysfunction present, since rotational asymmetry becomes more discernible the further away one palpates from the axis of rotation. With the patient seated, the examiner palpates the rib angles, which are the most posterior and prominent bony landmarks of the ribs. The examiner's thumbs follow paired rib angles, noting any asymmetry, as the patient moves through a range of flexion and extension (Fig. 8.14). Palpation of the ribs anteriorly through a range of spinal flexion and extension can also be helpful in diagnosing non-neutral thoracic dysfunctions, particularly in the upper thoracic spine where posterior assessment may be difficult in the presence of increased tone of the midscapular musculature (Fig. 8.15). As with palpation of the transverse processes,

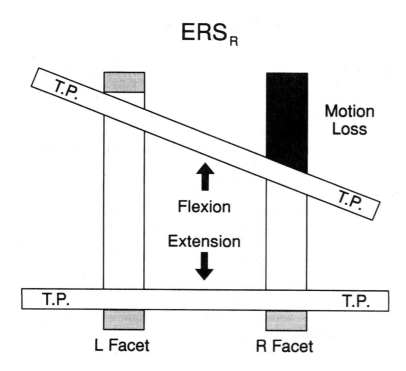

ERS$_R$

Motion Loss

Flexion

Extension

T.P.

T.P.

T.P.

L Facet

R Facet

Figure 8.10. Extended, rotated, and side-bent position (ERS), right. The response of the transverse processes (T.P.) when there is a loss of facet opening on the right. Note how the transverse processes appear symmetric in extension and asymmetric—i.e., rotated to the right—in flexion.

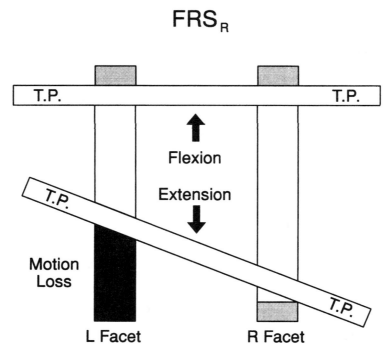

Figure 8.11. Flexed, rotated, and side-bent position (FRS), right. The response of the transverse processes (T.P.) when there is a loss of facet closure on the left. Note how the transverse processes appear symmetric in full flexion but become asymmetric—i.e., rotated to the right in extension.

one always compares any asymmetry of rib pairs to the rib pair below in order to determine dysfunction.

Passive physiologic mobility testing for flexion, extension, side-bending, and rotation and three-dimensional coupled motion of flexion or extension with side-bending/rotation can be introduced to confirm the findings noted during positional testing—i.e., with a positional diagnosis of an ERS_L at T9–10, one would expect to find a loss of passive coupled motion for flexion, right side-bending, and right rotation at T9–10 (Fig. 8.16A).

Treatment of the non-neutral dysfunctions—i.e., FRS or ERS—usually precedes evaluation of the rib cage. When using the ribs for mobility and positional testing for non-neutral vertebral dysfunction, the examiner should note that the asymmetric pair of ribs becomes symmetric in either flexion or extension depending on the type of nonneutral dysfunction—i.e., ERS or FRS. If the rib asymmetry does not change with flexion or extension of the trunk, then the rib itself may be dysfunctional and needs to be assessed and treated separately.

Rib Cage Structural Diagnosis

Structural diagnosis of the rib cage for somatic dysfunction also uses the diagnostic triad of asymmetry of position, alteration in range of motion, and tissue texture abnormalities. When the rib cage is evaluated and minimal restrictions are noted, particularly regarding excursion of the ribs during inhalation and exhalation, then the examiner may surmise that significant rib cage dysfunction probably does not exist. This approach can be a useful screening tool. Ribs 1–10 are initially evaluated while the patient is sitting; this avoids the influences that lying supine or prone would impose on the rib cage. The ribs are palpated anteriorly and posteriorly for contour, symmetry, and motion response to vertebral flexion and extension, and also are assessed for tissue texture changes and tenderness.

Posteriorly the key palpatory landmark for diagnosing rib dysfunction is the rib angle [1], which is the most posterior aspect of the rib and serves as the site of attachment for the iliocostalis thoracis muscu-

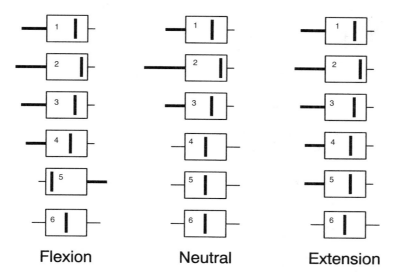

Figure 8.12. Positional findings from T1 through T6 in a hypothetical patient. In flexion, T6 is level, T5 is rotated right, T4 is rotated left, and T1, T2, and T3 represent a group curve rotated left and side-bent right. In neutral, T1, T2, and T3 appear even more rotated to the left and side-bent to the right with the apex of the curve at T2-3. T4, T5, T6 appear level. In extension T6 appears level, T5 appears rotated to the left relative to T6, T4 appears to be following T5 and is not dysfunctional, and T1, T2, and T3 represent a group dysfunction rotated to the left and side-bent to the right. Dysfunctions in this example include an ERS right at T5, an ERS left at T4, a FRS left at T5, and a neutral group left rotated, right side-bent from T1 through T3.

lature (see Fig. 1.11). Normally there is a posterior convexity to the rib angles, as well as a lateral flaring as one proceeds from cephalad to caudal. Identification of a rib angle that is out of the normal posterior convexity—e.g., it appears anterior or posterior—is a significant diagnostic finding of rib cage dysfunction. Associated with this change in the anterior/posterior displacement is the medial-to-lateral change in alignment of the rib angles from the expected normal. Also to be noted at the rib angle is the sharpness of the inferior border of the rib, which is usually more easily palpable than the superior border. A rib that appears to be flat with an inferior border that is difficult to palpate suggests that the rib is externally rotated about its long axis or "torsioned." This is another significant diagnostic finding for rib dysfunction. A change in the intercostal space between ribs such that the space below the rib is narrow and the space above the rib is wide indicates a change in the positional symmetry of the ribs and is associated with hypertonicity in the intercostal musculature either above or

below the rib. A change in tissue texture of the iliocostalis musculature as it attaches to the rib angle is highly suggestive of dysfunction of that rib.

The important findings in palpation posteriorly in diagnosing rib cage dysfunction are:

A. Position
   1. Assess the rib angle for the anterior/posterior relationship of each bilaterally paired set of ribs to the overall posterior convexity of the rib cage.
   2. Note the medial and lateral relationship of the rib angle, bearing in mind that the rib angles flare from medial to lateral as one proceeds from cephalad to caudal.
   3. Note the sharpness of the inferior versus superior border of the rib; normally the inferior border is more easily palpable.
   4. Note the intercostal space between the ribs—i.e., narrower intercostal space above a rib and wider space below.

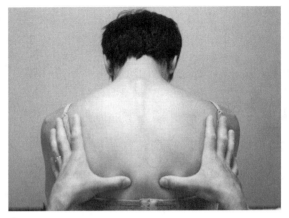

A

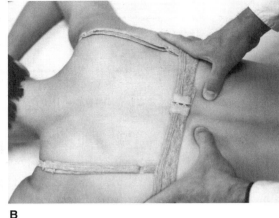

B

Figure 8.13. Positional testing of the lower thoracic spine. A. Flexion. B. Neutral. C. Extension (sphinx).

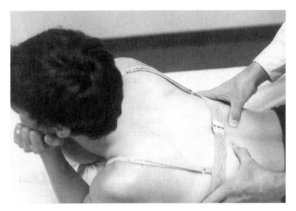

C

B. Mobility
1. With the thumbs on a pair of rib angles, assess the response of the ribs to flexion and extension of the thoracic spine, keeping in mind that the ribs serve as an extension of the transverse processes and can be helpful in diagnosing non-neutral vertebral dysfunctions as well as rib cage dysfunctions.
2. A situation in which asymmetric paired ribs never become symmetric throughout the range of spinal flexion or extension is indicative of structural rib dysfunction.
C. Tenderness
1. Palpate for tenderness and increased tone in the iliocostalis muscle; this tissue texture change is associated with somatic dysfunction of the rib.
2. Palpate for tenderness and tone in the intercostal muscles.

Anteriorly the thumbs are placed on paired ribs lateral to the costochondral junction and an assessment is made of the anterior convexity of the rib cage, noting positional asymmetries and the response of any asymmetry to thoracic spinal flexion and extension. Tissue texture abnormalities are detected by palpation of the intercostals and the costochondral junction for the presence of hypertonicity and tenderness.

The important findings in palpation anteriorly in diagnosing rib cage dysfunction are:

A. Position
1. With the thumbs placed lateral to the costochondral junction, an assessment is made relative to the anterior/posterior convexity of the chest wall (see Fig. 8.15A).
2. The sharpness of the superior versus inferior border of the rib is noted; normally the superior border is more easily palpated.

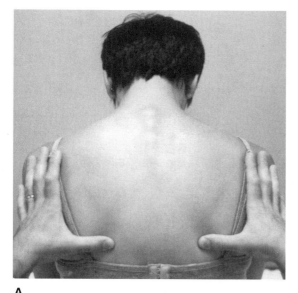

A

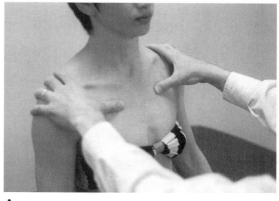

A

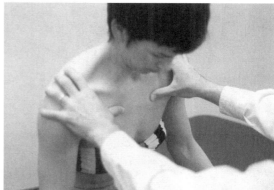

B

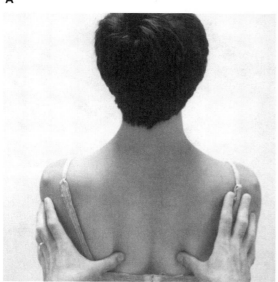

B

Figure 8.14. Active physiologic mobility testing using the ribs posteriorly. A. Flexion. B. Extension.

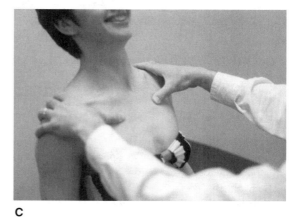

C

Figure 8.15. Active physiologic mobility testing utilizing the ribs anteriorly. A. Neutral. B. Flexion. C. Extension.

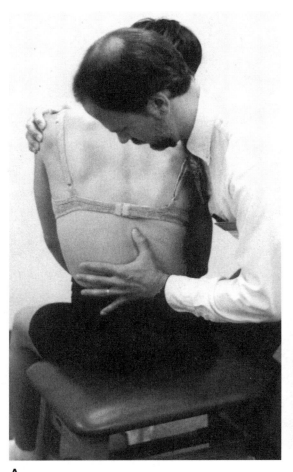

A

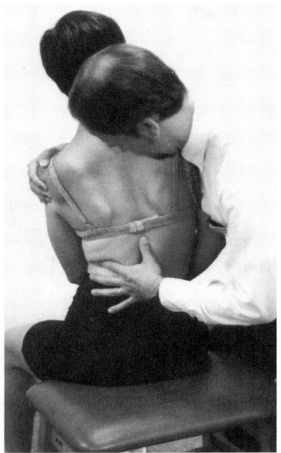

B

Figure 8.16. Passive physiologic mobility testing, lower thoracic spine. A. The examiner's left thumb palpates for motion at the interspinous space as the combined movements of flexion, right side-bending, and right rotation are intro-duced passively. B. The examiner's left thumb palpates the interspinous space as the combined movements of extension, left side-bending, and right rotation are introduced passively.

3. The intercostal space between the ribs is noted—i.e., narrower space above the rib and wider space below.

B. Mobility

1. With the thumbs placed on paired ribs anteriorly, note the response of each rib pair to thoracic spine flexion and extension. If any asymmetry exists during positional testing, does this asymmetry change during thoracic spinal movement? Note: Asymmetry of a pair of ribs may be a result of non-neutral vertebral dysfunctions, in which case the rib pair becomes symmetric when the non-neutral dysfunction becomes symmetric.

C. Tenderness

1. Palpation of the costochondral junction for tenderness confirms dysfunction, which is frequently misdiagnosed as costochondritis (Tietze's syndrome) [1, 7].

2. Palpation of the intercostals for tone and tenderness.

Rib Cage Dysfunction

Dysfunction of the ribs is classified as structural, torsional, or respiratory [1, 7]. Structural rib dysfunctions are true joint subluxations that are painful and result

Table 8.4. Structural Rib Dysfunctions

Dysfunction	Rib Angle	Midaxillary Line	Intercostal Space	Anterior Rib
Anterior subluxation	Less prominent	Symmetric	Tender, often with intercostal neuralgia	More prominent
Posterior subluxation	More prominent	Symmetric	Tender, often with intercostal neuralgia	Less prominent
Superior first rib subluxation	Superior aspect of first rib elevated (5 mm)	Hypertonicity of the scalene muscles on the same side	—	Marked tenderness of the superior aspect
Anterior-posterior rib compression	Less prominent	Prominent	Tender, often with intercostal neuralgia	Less prominent
Lateral compression	More prominent	Less prominent	Tender	More prominent
Laterally elevated	Tender	Prominent	Narrow above, wide below	Exquisitely tender at pectoral minor

in significant motion restrictions noted during both inspiratory and expiratory effort. Torsional ribs typically result from prolonged non-neutral thoracic dysfunction and, when they are not properly diagnosed and treated, are often the causative factor in recurrent thoracic spine dysfunction. Respiratory rib dysfunctions occur secondary to myofascial shortening of the intercostal musculature and other supporting muscles and are not the source of chest wall pain but are tender to palpation. Patients with chest wall pain or intercostal neuralgia without thoracic nonneutral dysfunction—i.e., ERS or FRS—or structural/torsional rib dysfunction are suspected of having a true organic pathologic condition—e.g., herpes zoster, cord tumors, or neoplastic disease, and should be appropriately referred for further workup (see Chapters 6 and 7).

Structural Ribs

As previously mentioned, structural rib dysfunctions are true joint subluxations that occur secondary to trauma and result in significant pain and motion restriction of the dysfunctional rib. Structural ribs are categorized as (1) anterior subluxation, (2) posterior subluxation, (3) superior first rib subluxation, (4) anterior posterior compression, (5) lateral compression, and (6) laterally elevated [1, 7] (Table 8.4).

Anterior Subluxation

The mechanism of injury in anterior subluxations is a blow to the back that shears the rib anteriorly at both the costotransverse and costovertebral articulations—e.g., a rear-end motor vehicle collision or a fall backwards landing over a railroad tie. Anterior subluxations are diagnosed by the following:

1. Less prominence of the rib angle posteriorly in the convexity of the chest wall and more prominence anteriorly. No change in the asymmetry of the rib anteriorly or posteriorly is noted with flexion or extension of the thoracic spine.
2. The rib angle appears to be medially displaced from its expected position in the normal contour of the rib cage.
3. Marked respiratory restriction of motion of both inhalation and exhalation.
4. Palpable tenderness and tension of the iliocostalis muscle.
5. Palpable tenderness at the costochondral junction anteriorly.

Posterior Subluxation

The mechanism of injury for posterior subluxations is a blow from the front that shears the rib posteriorly at both the costotransverse and costovertebral articulations—e.g., a motor vehicle collision in which the chest wall strikes the steering wheel. Posterior subluxations are diagnosed by the following:

1. More prominence of the rib angle posteriorly in the convexity of the chest wall and decreased prominence anteriorly. No change in the asymmetry of the rib anteriorly or posteriorly is noted

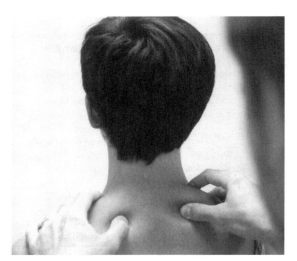

Figure 8.17. Palpation for a superior first rib. The examiner pulls the upper trapezius back and rests the tips of the index fingers on the superior surface of the first rib. The picture illustrates a superior first rib on the right.

with flexion or extension of the thoracic spine.
2. The rib angle appears to be laterally displaced from the expected position in the posterior convexity of the rib cage.
3. Marked respiratory restriction of motion of both inhalation and exhalation.
4. Palpable tenderness and tension of the iliocostalis muscle.
5. Palpable tenderness at the costochondral junction anteriorly.

Superior First Rib Subluxation

The mechanism of injury in superior first rib subluxation is repetitive overhead arm movements, sudden elevation of the shoulder girdle, or chronic tightness of the scalenes. It is diagnosed by the following:

1. Palpation of the superior aspect of the first rib just anterior to the trapezius muscle reveals the dysfunctional rib to be one finger width higher in relation to the contralateral side (Fig. 8.17).
2. Marked respiratory restrictions of motion for both inhalation and exhalation.
3. Hypertonicity of the scalene muscles on the dysfunctional side.
4. Marked tenderness of the superior aspect of the first rib.

Anteroposterior Compression

Th mechanism of injury in anteroposterior compression is a blow to the front of the chest with the back stabilized—e.g., a "sandwich" football tackle. Significant diagnostic findings are:

1. Flattening of the rib anteriorly and posteriorly.
2. Prominence of the rib shaft in the midaxillary line.
3. Marked respiratory restrictions for both inhalation and exhalation.
4. Associated with complaint of intercostal neuralgia [1].

Lateral Compression

The mechanism of injury in lateral compression is a blow laterally—e.g., in a broadside motor vehicle collision with the ribs striking the console or arm rest. Significant diagnostic findings are:

1. Prominence of the rib anteriorly and posteriorly.
2. Flattening of the rib shaft in the midaxillary line.
3. Significant restriction of motion for inhalation and exhalation at that rib.

Laterally Elevated

The mechanism of injury in a rib laterally elevated is similar to that of a superior subluxed first rib. Significant diagnostic findings are:

1. Frequently seen in ribs 2–4.
2. Ipsilateral shoulder is frequently held elevated with shoulder complaints and numbness and tingling reported in the upper extremity.
3. Very tender ipsilateral pectoralis minor.
4. Marked respiratory restrictions of that rib, particularly for exhalation.
5. Narrowing of the interspace above and a widening of the interspace below the dysfunctional rib in the midaxillary line.
6. Prominence of the rib shaft in the midaxillary line.

Torsional Ribs

Torsional rib dysfunctions occur as a sequelae to non-neutral thoracic vertebral dysfunction. During

Table 8.5. Torsional Rib Dysfunctions

Dysfunction	Rib Angle	Midaxillary Line	Intercostal Space	Thoracic Findings
External rib torsion	Superior border prominent and tender	Symmetric	Wide above, narrow below	ERS ipsilateral, level above
Internal rib torsion	Inferior border prominent and tender	Symmetric	Narrow above, wide below	FRS contralateral, level above

sagittal plane spinal flexion, the ribs bilaterally internally rotate, or torsion, and with extension the ribs bilaterally externally rotate, or torsion. With left rotation of the thoracic spine the ribs on the right side of the spine will internally rotate about their axes, and the ribs on the left side of the spine will externally rotate normally. In the presence of prolonged non-neutral thoracic vertebral dysfunctions—i.e., FRS or ERS—a rib may become torsioned and remain dysfunctional despite correction of the non-neutral vertebral dysfunction and may contribute to the recurrence of thoracic vertebral dysfunction. Rib torsions are classified as one of two types: external rib torsion or internal rib torsion, with the external rib torsion far more commonly seen and associated with an ERS dysfunction to the ipsilateral side at the level above. The internal rib torsion is less commonly seen and associated with FRS dysfunction to the contralateral side at the level above. Both types of torsioned ribs will result in respiratory restrictions for both inhalation and exhalation and will be the key rib of a respiratory group dysfunction (Table 8.5).

External Rib Torsion

External rib torsion is diagnosed by the following:

1. The rib appearing to be flat with the inferior border difficult to palpate and the superior border more prominent.
2. Significant tenderness and tension of the iliocostalis musculature at the attachment to the rib angle.
3. Increase in the intercostal space above and narrowing of the intercostal space below the dysfunctional rib.
4. Significant restriction of respiratory motion for both inhalation and exhalation.

5. Commonly associated with an ERS dysfunction to the ipsilateral side at the level above—e.g., external torsion of the sixth rib on the right associated with an ERS right at T5–6.

Internal Rib Torsion

Internal rib torsion is diagnosed by the following:

1. The rib appearing to be sharper at the inferior border than normal with an inability to palpate the superior border.
2. Significant tenderness and tension of the iliocostalis musculature at the attachment to the rib angle.
3. A decrease in the intercostal space above and an increase in the intercostal space below the dysfunctional rib.
4. Significant restriction of respiratory motion for both inhalation and exhalation.
5. Far less common than the external rib torsion, but seen with prolonged FRS dysfunction to the contralateral side at the level above—e.g., internal torsion of the sixth rib on the right associated with an FRS left at T5–6.

Respiratory Ribs

Respiratory rib dysfunctions occur in response to myofascial shortening of the intercostal muscles and are frequently related to poor postural habits. Respiratory rib dysfunctions occur singly or in groups and demonstrate restriction of either inhalation or exhalation movement (Table 8.6) [1]. There will often be a key rib that is responsible for a group of ribs not being able to move through their full range of motion during inhalation or exhalation. The key rib for an inhalation restriction is the top rib of the

Table 8.6. Respiratory Rib Dysfunction

Dysfunction	Restriction	Key Rib
Inhalation restriction	During inspiration the rib or group of ribs that cease rising	Top or superior rib
Exhalation restriction	During exhalation the rib or group of ribs that stop falling	Bottom or inferior rib

group, with intercostal muscle tightness and tenderness to palpation noted below the key rib. The key rib in exhalation restrictions is the bottom rib of the group, with increase in tone and tenderness to palpation noted in the intercostals above this dysfunctional rib. A structural or torsional rib dysfunction may be the key rib for both inhalation and exhalation group restrictions. Once the structural or torsional rib is successfully treated, the respiratory component can then be addressed if needed at a subsequent session. Since the key rib is restricting the ribs above or below it from moving through their normal excursion during inhalation or exhalation, the key rib needs to be identified for treatment purposes. Once the key rib is identified, a further determination is made whether the motion loss is greater in the sagittal plane, restricting pump handle motion, or whether the motion loss is greater in the frontal plane, limiting bucket handle motion. This is an important consideration that needs to be made before treatment is rendered.

Rib Cage Respiratory Diagnosis, Ribs 1–10

With the patient positioned supine, the examiner palpates between the intercostal spaces or directly over the ribs anteriorly and asks the patient to make a full inspiratory and expiratory effort (Fig. 8.18). The rib cage is divided into thirds, and an assessment is made of the respiratory excursion for the upper ribs, the middle ribs, and then the lower rib cage. With the dominant eye focused on the midline, the examiner identifies which group of ribs stops moving first during either inhalation or exhalation. Whichever group of ribs stops moving first is dysfunctional. Once this general screening has been done and an overall assessment of respiratory motion has been made, specific key ribs of dysfunction can be identified. As previously mentioned, the key rib for an inhalation restriction is the top rib of the group and the key rib for an exhalation restriction is the bottom rib of the group.

Therefore, for a group restriction of inhalation the examiner should start at the top of the group dysfunction and for an exhalation restriction the examiner should start at the bottom. Once the key rib has been identified, further determination is made whether more pump handle (anterior/posterior) versus bucket handle (lateral) movement is restricted for that key rib by palpating anteriorly and then laterally on the key rib to determine a greater restriction for pump handle versus bucket handle motion, respectively.

Rib Cage Respiratory Diagnosis, Ribs 11 and 12

To assess the eleventh and twelfth ribs, the patient is positioned prone with the examiner's hands lying over the eleventh and twelfth ribs posteriorly (Fig. 8.19). The patient once again makes a respiratory effort for both inhalation and exhalation and the examiner's hands, which are symmetrically placed over the ribs, palpate the movement, noting which group of ribs stops moving first, either during inhalation or exhalation. Remember, movement of the eleventh and twelfth ribs differs mechanically from the typical ribs with the motion defined as a caliper-type motion. For this reason bucket handle and pump handle motion restrictions do not occur.

Summary

Pain in the thoracic spine and rib cage is most often associated with somatic dysfunction (facilitated segment) involving the vertebral segment, the ribs, or both. This chapter provides an overview of the evaluation of this unique spinal region using an osteopathic biomechanical model complemented with mobility testing. Patients with vertebral or rib cage dysfunction as presented in this chapter respond well to manual therapy techniques that address the dysfunctions noted (see Chapters 9 and 10). Failure to

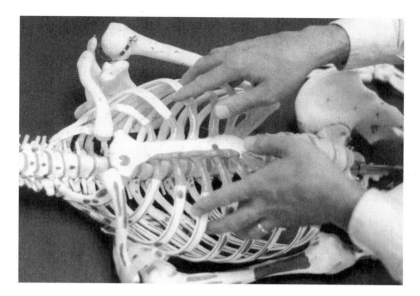

Figure 8.18. Palpation for respiratory rib diagnosis, patient supine. The fingers are placed between the ribs and the patient is asked to make a full inspiratory and expiratory effort. This is repeated for the upper ribs, middle ribs, and lower ribs.

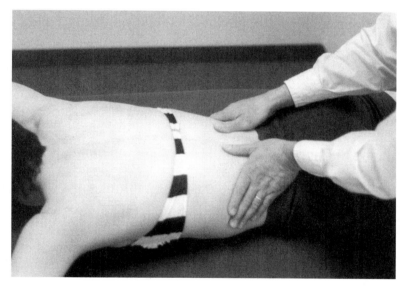

Figure 8.19. Respiratory rib diagnosis, ribs 11 and 12, patient prone. The hands are placed over the eleventh and twelfth ribs and the patient is asked to make an inspiratory and expiratory effort.

find significant mechanical dysfunction of either a rib or thoracic vertebral segment in a patient with thoracic pain raises concern of more serious organic pathologic conditions (see Chapter 6).

References

1. Greenman PE. Principles of Manual Medicine. Baltimore: Williams & Wilkins, 1989.
2. Stoddard A. Manual of Osteopathic Practice. London: Hutchinson, 1969.
3. Dwyer A, Aprill C, Bogduk N. Cervical zygapophyseal joint pain patterns 1: A study in normal volunteers. Spine 1990;15:453–457.
4. Paris SV, Patla C. E1 Course Notes. Extremity Dysfunction and Manipulation. St. Augustine: Patris, 1988.
5. Lee DG, Walsh MC. A Workbook of Manual Therapy Techniques for the Vertebral Column and Pelvic Girdle. Delta B.C.: Nascent, 1985.
6. Maitland GD. Vertebral Manipulation (5th ed). Londc Butterworth, 1986.
7. Bourdillon JF, Day EA, Bookhout MR. Spinal M' lation (5th ed). Oxford, England: Butterworth mann, 1992.

PART III

Treatment

Chapter 9

Direct Treatment Techniques for the Thoracic Spine and Rib Cage: Muscle Energy, Mobilization, High-Velocity Thrust, and Combined Techniques

Timothy W. Flynn

This chapter discusses "direct" approaches in the treatment of thoracic spine and rib cage dysfunction. "Direct" implies that the practitioner restores a loss of segmental movement by taking the dysfunctional or facilitated movement segment into its restricted range. For instance, consider a patient whose thoracic spine movement is restricted in extension, right side-bending, and right rotation. In this example, either the patient (muscle energy technique) or the practitioner (graded mobilization and high-velocity thrust [HVT] technique) will provide a force that will take the dysfunctional or facilitated movement segment "directly" into the barrier of extension, right side-bending, and right rotation.

Muscle Energy Technique

Origins

The muscle energy technique (MET) is a treatment modality in which the practitioner takes a dysfunctional or motion-restricted muscle-joint complex to its restrictive barrier and then requires the patient to perform an isometric action of either the agonist or an-

tagonist muscle followed by a complete relaxation. During this relaxation phase the practitioner moves the muscle-joint complex into the new restrictive barrier. The MET system developed in the 1940s and 1950s primarily from the work of Fred L. Mitchell, Sr. and was later documented by Mitchell, Moran, and Pruzzo [1]. An osteopathic physician, Mitchell used his detailed anatomic background in developing a patient-oriented system of introducing motion into a restricted joint segment without the use of a physician-introduced manipulative force. About a decade later in the physical therapy community the work of Kabot [2], Knott et al. [3, 4], and Voss et al. [5, 6] detailed a system of proprioceptive neuromuscular facilitation (PNF). The PNF system, which was more generalized in its implementation, incorporated a "hold-relax" isometric technique that is very similar to MET. Both systems relied on particular neurophysiologic principles. Foremost is the concept of reciprocal inhibition [7]. A restriction in segmental joint mobility can occur when there is an imbalance in the firing patterns of the deep segmental muscles. Reduction in the gamma efferent output to the facilitated antagonist muscle can be viewed in two simplistic ways (see Chapter 2 for a detailed neurophysiological discussion):

1. Controlled contraction of the agonist. This results in reflexive inhibition of the facilitated antagonist. Care must be taken to avoid too forceful of a contraction, which would result in a synergistic activity of the agonist and antagonist in an attempt to provide stabilization to the segment.
2. Controlled contraction of the antagonist. This is performed from an antagonist-lengthened position. This is followed by antagonist muscle lengthening during the postisometric relaxation phase. The majority of the METs in this chapter will use the second method, in which the restricted segment is taken to its barrier and the facilitated antagonist is fired and then repositioned into a further lengthened position.

Indications and Contraindications of the Muscle Energy Technique

The MET has many clinical uses, including lengthening a shortened or contracted muscle, strengthening a weakened muscle, reducing localized edema, mobilizing a restricted joint, and providing normal motor input into a weak or dysynchronous firing segment [8]. In the treatment of segmental spinal dysfunction, MET is generally the modality of first choice. There are several advantages in using MET:

- The patient is actively involved in the treatment.
- Performed correctly, the techniques are very safe.
- The patient is less likely to experience post-treatment symptom exacerbations.

The MET is most successful in acute and subacute conditions before prolonged joint changes have occurred. A MET is generally performed before a practitioner-introduced force. The rationale for this is that if the soft-tissue components of the muscle-joint complex are treated initially they are more likely to accept the introduction of a HVT technique and subsequently to maintain the correction once it is achieved.

The contraindications for using MET are:

- Articular instability at the level of treatment.

- Metastatic bone disease at the level of treatment.
- Long track cord signs.

Principles of the Muscle Energy Technique

The following are the general guidelines for MET that will be used consistently throughout this chapter:

1. The three-dimensional or tri-planar (i.e., flexion, rotation, side-bending) barrier will be precisely localized and engaged.
2. The practitioner maintains the three-dimensional barrier position and then has the patient gently fire the facilitated antagonist segment (occasionally the agonist segment is fired) in an isometric fashion. The direction of the contraction can be purely planar (i.e., right side-bending) or a diagonal pattern incorporating the three-directional antagonist components (i.e., flexion, right side-bending, and right rotation). The patient muscle effort should be minimal and no movement should take place.
3. After 3–5 seconds the patient is told to relax. The practitioner must wait for a complete relaxation of the patient. During the postisometric relaxation phase, the restricted muscle-joint complex is repositioned to the new barrier.
4. The technique is repeated three to five times and then the practitioner re-examines the motion of the segment.

Typical practitioner errors when using MET are (1) poor localization; (2) too much patient force; (3) allowing movement to occur instead of an isometric action; and (4) not allowing complete patient relaxation before repositioning the motion segment.

Translation for Localization

A very effective way of promoting localization to a restricted segment is by the use of translation. Translation is essentially moving a selected segment in any plane to produce localization at that level. It is possible to introduce right side-bending in the midthoracic spine by right side-bending the head and trunk down to the selected segment and right side-bending the lumbar and lower thoracic region up to the selected segment. A more effective way is

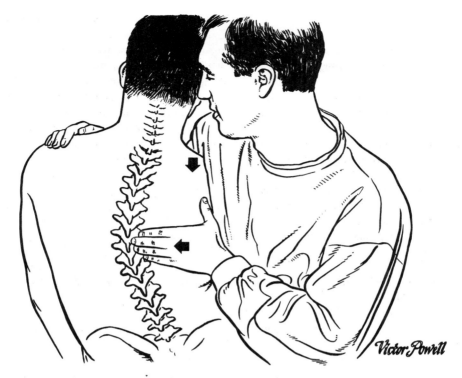

Figure 9.1. The use of translation to localize a convexity to a selected segment (example: Left translation introducing right side-bending).

by gently gliding or translating the selected segment from right to left while dropping the patient's right shoulder toward the right buttock, which results in a relative right side-bending of the selected segment (Fig. 9.1). This can be performed in all three planes of movement and is an effective method to localize when performing both MET and HVT procedures.

Mobilization

Origins

Mobilization is a treatment modality in which the practitioner introduces passive rhythmic oscillations within the segmental range of motion or at the restrictive barrier. Although this system has probably been used in various forms since ancient times, the refinement of this system was primarily from the work of Maitland [9] and Kaltenborn [10]. This system emphasizes passive accessory mobility testing and treatment as a method of restoring pain-free segmental spinal motion.

Indications and Contraindications of Mobilization

The clinical uses of mobilization include restoring passive accessory motion, reducing pain, and increasing segmental and total spinal range of motion. Depending on the grade of mobilization used, it can be effective in acute, subacute, and chronic conditions.

There are certain contraindications to mobilization that result from the fact that the practitioner is introducing an external force into the patient's musculoskeletal system. These include:

- Articular instability in the direction of mobilization.
- Segmental hypermobility at the level of treatment.
- Inflammatory joint disease at the level of treatment.
- Metastatic bone disease at the level of treatment.
- Long track cord signs.

Principles

Mobilization and articulation procedures are generally graded in the following manner:

Grade 1. A small-amplitude movement or oscillation at or near the starting position of the range of motion.
Grade 2. A large-amplitude movement or oscillation that is into the restricted range of motion but does not engage the barrier.
Grade 3. A large-amplitude movement or oscillation that is into the restricted range of motion and engages the barrier.
Grade 4. A small-amplitude movement or oscillation at the restrictive barrier.

The grades 1 and 2 mobilizations are most effective in the treatment of acute conditions. The grades 3 and 4 mobilizations are most effective in the treatment of subacute and chronic conditions. In the thoracic spine region, the classic mobilization system of Maitland generally applies oscillations in the prone position. In this chapter the principles of graded mobilizations will be used, but they will be performed from the same position as the HVT procedures. This has several advantages: It allows the practitioner to improve his or her skills in HVT through graded mobilization; it minimizes patient position changes during treatment; and it allows the practitioner to progress from a graded mobilization to an HVT easily during treatment.

High-Velocity Thrust Technique

Origins

The HVT is a treatment modality in which the practitioner moves the motion-restricted muscle-joint segment into the early point of the restrictive barrier followed by the practitioner introducing a very specifically directed force of high velocity and low amplitude (range of motion) that guides the segment through the restrictive barrier. The HVT has been termed the most useful and the most abused weapon in the manipulative arsenal [11]. The appropriate and selective use of HVT can, however, greatly improve treatment outcomes in patients with thoracic spine and rib cage dysfunction.

In various forms, HVT has been used in medicine since ancient times. However, techniques often were forceful and nonspecific in their direction and localization. In the last half of this century many individuals have contributed to refining the appropriateness and specificity of the HVT technique [8–10, 12, 13]. Notably, it was Mennell [14, 15] who introduced the concept of joint play and the importance of these small involuntary movements in the normal pain-free movement of joints and the importance of loss of these movements in the etiology of joint and muscle pain. Furthermore, Mennell elaborated on the importance of therapeutic joint manipulation (HVT) in restoring loss of segmental joint play.

Indications and Contraindications to the High-Velocity Thrust Technique

The HVT technique is most appropriate when treating subacute and chronic segmental dysfunction of the thoracic spine and rib cage. Its clinical uses include lengthening a shortened muscle, reducing localized edema, mobilizing a restricted joint (restoring normal joint play), and normalizing the motor input to a dyssynchronous firing segment.

There are certain contraindications to HVT that result from the fact that the practitioner is introducing a force into the patient's musculoskeletal system. These include:

- Articular instability at the level of treatment
- Segmental hypermobility at the level of treatment
- Inflammatory joint disease at the level of treatment
- Metastatic bone disease at the level of treatment
- Long track cord signs

Certain conditions, such as osteoporosis and degenerative joint disease, are relative contraindications to HVT [8, 12]. The use of HVT in these instances depends on the practitioner's ability to introduce a very precise and low-force thrust. The practitioner should also be cautioned that HVT potentially increases the sympathetic outflow and can result in visceral symptoms such as gastrointestinal discomfort.

Principles of the High-Velocity Thrust Technique

The following are the general guidelines that will be used consistently throughout this chapter for the HVT techniques described:

1. The three-dimensional barrier will be precisely localized at the point of minimal resistance or the initial barrier point. In other words, the restricted segment is not locked; it must be free to move.
2. The segments above and below the restricted segment must be locked. The locking is accomplished via a ligamentous lock (when flexion is used), a facet lock (when extension is used), or a combination of a ligamentous and a facet lock (rotation with contralateral side-bending). For example, if the practitioner is performing a HVT to increase flexion at T4, the localization of flexion would come from above downward to T4 and from below upward to T5; this allows the T4–5 segment freedom to move.
3. The velocity of the HVT must be high. It is essential that the practitioner apply a quick thrust rather than a slow push.
4. The amplitude or magnitude of the thrusting force is minimal. If the barrier is well localized, minimal force is required to achieve a therapeutic result. The HVT is not a forceful technique; rather, it is a quick, low-force technique applied in a precise direction.

Patient Activation

Several of the HVT techniques in this chapter will use patient activation. Patient activation is an adjunct used to assist the practitioner in freeing the restrictive barrier and to assist in patient relaxation. When patient activation is used, the patient is told to fire the muscles that would move the segment into the barrier. This results in a reflex inhibition of the antagonist restrictors. For example, if the practitioner is trying to move the T4 segment to the left, the patient will be told to look left just before the HVT is introduced; the moment the practitioner senses movement at the T4 segment, the HVT is performed. The use of patient activation is extremely helpful in overcoming patient guarding and allowing a painless HVT procedure.

Combined Technique

In several instances in this chapter the practitioner will use both MET and mobilization or HVT within one technique. This is termed a *combined technique.*

Sequencing

The order in which areas of dysfunctional regions are addressed can influence the patient's response to treatment and the incidence of recurrence of symptoms. In the management of thoracic spine and rib cage dysfunction the following sequencing guidelines can improve the treatment success rate: (1) A nonneutral (type 2) mechanical dysfunction is treated before a neutral (type 1) dysfunction. (2) Thoracic spine dysfunction is treated before the rib cage is treated. The exception is torsional rib dysfunction, which is treated concurrently with the thoracic spine. (3) In the rib cage, structural and torsional ribs are treated before respiratory rib restrictions are addressed.

Chapter Format

The remainder of this chapter will demonstrate techniques used in the treatment of mechanical dysfunction of the thoracic spine and rib cage. The techniques presented should be modified in a way that conforms to individual body size and flexibility. The practitioner should always feel balanced and firmly in control of the patient's segments during treatment. Restriction in movement of the spine should be viewed in the same manner as any other joint in the body. For example, when the knee joint has a 10-degree limit or block from terminal extension, it has an extension restriction. It could also be said that the knee joint position is flexed. The spinal segments are no different. For example, if T4 is limited in full backward bending, it has an extension restriction. It could also be said that T4 is positioned flexed. In this chapter the motion restriction will be presented, followed by the type of treatment technique demonstrated, and the level of the example. Finally, the positional diagnosis in the three cardinal planes will be stated. Generally, the MET will be demonstrated followed by the mobilization and HVT technique together. Table 9.1 provides the practitioner with general guidelines for determining

Table 9.1. General Indications for Treatment Selection Based on Onset Time of Symptoms

	Acute	Subacute	Chronic
Muscle energy	Strongly indicated	Strongly indicated	Use to prepare tissue for high-velocity thrust and prevent recurrence of dysfunction
Mobilization	Grade 1—small-amplitude movements in early range Grade 2—large rhythmic movements stopping prior to end-range	Grade 2—large rhythmic movements stopping prior to end-range Grade 3—large rhythmic movements into end-range	Grade 3—large rhythmic movements into end-range Grade 4—small-amplitude movement at end-range
High-velocity thrust	Rarely indicated	Moderate to strong indication if muscle energy technique not effective	Strong indication if muscle energy technique not effective

treatment technique selection based on the length of time from symptom onset or injury.

Flexion Restriction (Extended, Rotated, Side-Bent [ERS] Dysfunctions)

A flexion restriction or ERS dysfunction is a non-neutral mechanical dysfunction. It is more commonly seen in the T3–T5 region as well as in the lower thoracic spine but can occur at any level. The T3–T5 segments are frequently problematic in women, whose bra straps can cause a fulcrum between the shoulder straps and back strap resulting in an extension moment occurring above the back strap. This tends to cause the T4 and T5 segments to be maintained in a prolonged extended position that eventually limits flexion motion of these segments. During the palpatory examination these areas are flattened. Restrictions are noted in flexion and can be bilaterally restricted at the same segment.

Flexion Restriction of T1–T4 (Example: MET-Sitting, T3 ERS Right)

Position

The patient is seated with the practitioner standing behind. The practitioner's left hand guides and supports the patient's head, while the practitioner's right

hand monitors motion at the T3-4 and T4-5 interspinous spaces and for muscle contraction at the T3-4 intertransverse space (Fig. 9.2).

Engaging the Barrier

The practitioner slightly rotates the patient's head to the left and tells the patient to slump into the fingers of the practitioner's left hand. Left side-bending is introduced by translating the patient to the right.

Treatment

The patient is told to gently look backward over the right shoulder. After 3–5 seconds the patient is told to relax, and a translatory motion to increase flexion, left side-bending, and left rotation is introduced at the T3-4 segment. This is repeated three to five times followed by the practitioner re-examining the motion segment.

Flexion Restriction of T1–T4 (Example: HVT-Sitting, T2 ERS Left "Opening the Left Facet")

Position

The patient is seated with the practitioner standing behind. The practitioner's left forearm supports and protects the patient's head (Fig. 9.3). The practitioner's right thumb contacts the spinous process of T2.

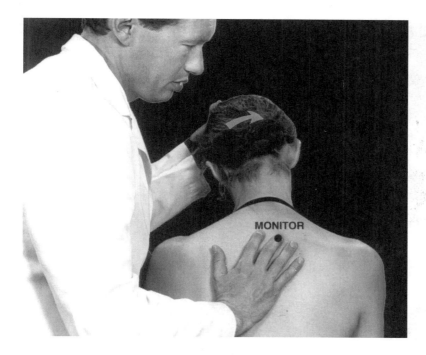

Figure 9.2. A sitting muscle energy technique for a T3 segment that is restricted in flexion, left rotation, and left side-bending (ERS right T3). The practitioner monitors muscle contraction at the right T3-4 intertransverse space.

Localization to the Barrier

The patient is told to slump into the practitioner's left hand, which produces flexion to the barrier. A combination of right rotation and right side-bending to the restricted barrier is achieved by a diagonal translatory movement.

Mobilization or Thrust

The patient is told to gently tilt the left ear toward the left shoulder to ensure localization. This is followed by a complete relaxation. At complete relaxation, the practitioner introduces graded mobilizations or an HVT with the right arm through the right thumb in a right-to-left translatory direction (Fig. 9.4). The motion segment is re-examined.

Flexion Restriction of T4–T12 (Example: MET-Sitting, T10 ERS Left)

Position

The patient is seated with the practitioner's right arm cradling the patient's shoulders. The practitioner's

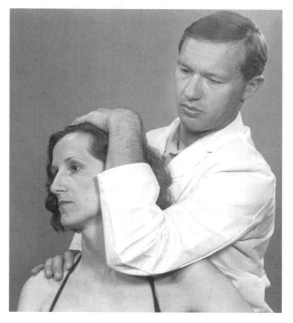

Figure 9.3. The practitioner using the forearm to support and protect the patient's cervical spine. This allows the practitioner to introduce motion from above down to the involved segment.

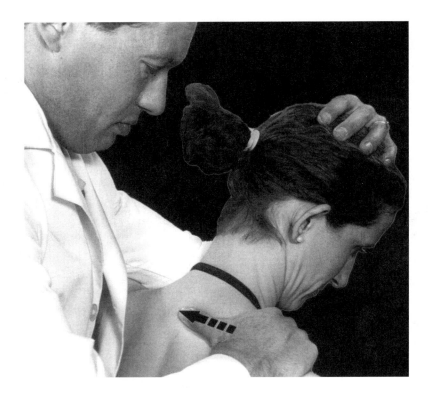

Figure 9.4. A sitting high-velocity thrust technique for a T2 segment that is restricted in flexion, right rotation, and right side-bending (ERS left T2). The aim of treatment is an opening of the left T2-3 facet and stretching of the periarticular structures on the left side.

chest wall guides the patient's trunk. The practitioner's left hand monitors the T10 motion segment and the T10-11 intertransverse space for muscle contraction.

Engaging the Barrier

The practitioner tells the patient to slump into the practitioner's hand to introduce the flexion barrier. The practitioner drops the right shoulder to introduce side-bending down to the segment followed by slight right rotation of the trunk.

Treatment

The patient is told to gently lift the right shoulder and drop the left shoulder against the practitioner's unyielding resistance, which isometrically fires the left side-benders (Fig. 9.5). After 3–5 seconds the patient is told to relax, and a translatory motion to increase flexion, left side-bending, and left rotation is introduced at the T10-11 segment. This is repeated three to five times followed by the practitioner re-examining the motion segment.

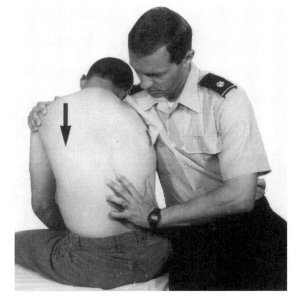

Figure 9.5. A sitting muscle energy technique for a T10 segment that is restricted in flexion, right rotation, and right side-bending (ERS left T10). The practitioner monitors muscle contraction at the left T10-11 intertransverse space.

Supine High-Velocity Thrust Techniques

In the supine HVT techniques demonstrated throughout the remainder of this chapter, several variations of both the patient's and the practitioner's arm and hand positions will be used. When treating the T4–T10 segments, the crossed arm technique is preferred where the patient's arm opposite the practitioner is placed on top and the patient's arm nearest the practitioner is placed underneath (Fig. 9.6). When treating the lower segments (T10–T12), the patient clasps both hands behind the base of the neck (Fig. 9.7). The practitioner's hand placement requires stabilization of the bottom vertebral segment via the transverse process (Fig. 9.8). For instance, treatment of a T4 FRS would require the practitioner to stabilize the T5 segment and move the T4 segment on it. There is a wide variety of hand placements for contacting the inferior vertebral segment, including an open hand, a fisted hand, or, as demonstrated in Fig. 9.9, where the thenar eminence is contacting one transverse process and the practitioner's flexed second digit is on the transverse process on the contralateral side. To protect the practitioner's interphalangeal joints, a piece of rubber tubing or a rolled-up towel can be placed inside the flexed second digit.

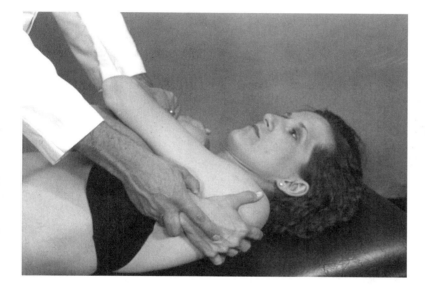

Figure 9.6. The patient's arm position for a supine high-velocity thrust technique. The patient's arm that is farthest away from the practitioner is placed on top.

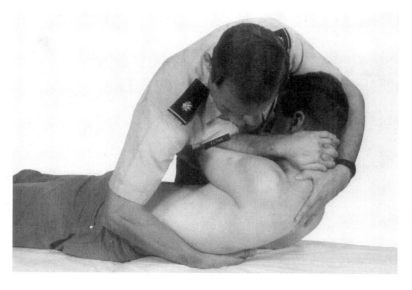

Figure 9.7. The patient's arm position for supine high-velocity thrust techniques in the lower thoracic region. The patient's hands are interlaced on the neck, not on the head.

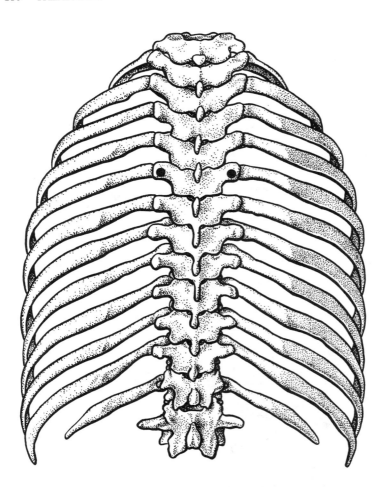

Figure 9.8. Points of contact for stabilization of a vertebral segment in a supine high-velocity thrust technique.

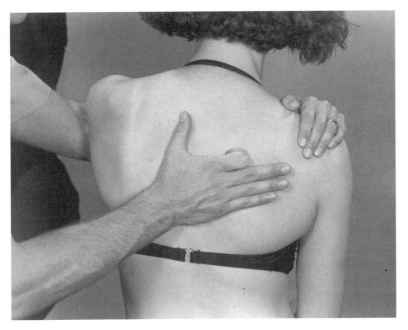

Figure 9.9. Contacting paired transverse processes with the practitioner's thenar eminence and a flexed second digit.

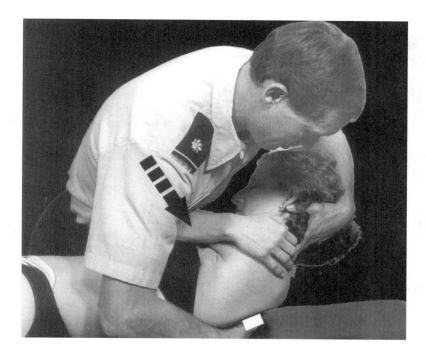

Figure 9.10. A supine high-velocity thrust technique for a T4 segment that is restricted in flexion, right rotation, and right side-bending (ERS left T4). The aim of the technique is an opening of the left T4-5 facet and a stretching of the periarticular structures on the left side. The vector of force should be directed at T5.

Flexion Restriction of T4–T12 (Example: HVT-Supine, T4 ERS Left "Opening the Left Facet")

Position

The patient is supine with arms crossed and the practitioner stands on the patient's right side. The practitioner rolls the patient toward him or her and contacts the T5 vertebral segment.

Localization to the Barrier

The practitioner's left arm cradles the patient's head and upper back. The practitioner flexes the patient's head and shoulders down to the T4–5 segment followed by a slight right side-bending and a right rotation to the three-dimensional barrier.

Mobilization or Thrust

The patient is told to take a deep breath in and let it all out. As the patient nears the end of the exhalation phase, the patient is asked to look over the right shoulder. As the practitioner senses the movement nearing the practitioner's right hand, an HVT is provided with the chest wall through the patient's elbows in a vector toward T5 (Fig. 9.10). This will

introduce a flexion moment at the T4-5 segment. Graded mobilizations can also be performed from this position. The motion segment is re-examined.

Extension Restrictions (Flexed, Rotated, Side-Bent [FRS] Dysfunctions)

An extension restriction or FRS dysfunction is a non-neutral mechanical dysfunction. It is frequently encountered in the T1–T2 and the T11–T12 regions but can occur at any level. When palpating the thoracic spine, look for regions where bumps occur. Segments that are bilaterally restricted can be treated on one side, then the other.

Extension Restriction of T1–T3 (Example: MET-Sitting, T3 FRS Left)

Position

The patient is seated with the practitioner standing behind. The practitioner's left arm supports the patient's head, while the right hand monitors for interspinous motion and for muscle contraction in the left intertransverse space of T3-4.

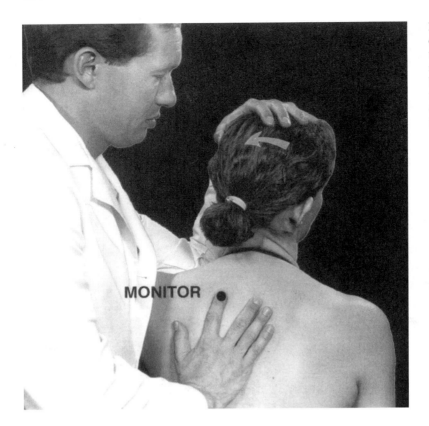

Figure 9.11. A sitting muscle energy technique for a T3 segment that is restricted in extension, right rotation, and right side-bending (FRS left T3). The practitioner monitors muscle contraction at the left T3-4 inter-transverse space.

Engaging the Barrier

The practitioner slightly rotates the patient's head to the right and then translates the trunk forward by gently pushing forward with the right hand while asking the patient to sit up straight to concurrently introduce extension from above and below.

The side-bending component is taken up by the practitioner's translating the patient to the right side-bending barrier. Finally, a small amount of right rotation engages the right rotation barrier.

Treatment

The patient is told to gently look to the left, gently push the left ear to the left, or to gently look to the floor (Fig. 9.11). After 3–5 seconds the patient is told to relax and a translatory motion to increase extension, right rotation, and right side-bending is introduced to the T3 segment. This is repeated three to five times, and the motion segment is re-examined.

Extension Restriction of T1–T4 (Example: HVT-Sitting, T3 FRS Left "Closing the Right Facet")

Position

The patient is seated. The practitioner stands behind with the left foot on the table and the patient's left arm draped over the practitioner's left thigh. The practitioner's left arm supports and protects the patient's head and neck, while the practitioner's right thumb contacts the spinous process of T3.

Localization to the Barrier

The practitioner slightly rotates the patient's head to the right and then translates the trunk forward by gently pushing forward with the right hand to introduce extension from above and below.

The side-bending component is taken up by the practitioner translating the patient into the right side-bending barrier. Finally, the right rotation barrier is engaged with slight head rotation.

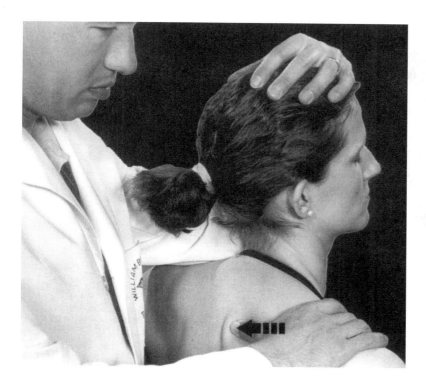

Figure 9.12. A sitting high-velocity thrust technique for a T3 segment that is restricted in extension, right rotation, and right side-bending (FRS left T3). The aim of the technique is a closing of the right T3-4 facet.

Mobilization or Thrust

The patient is told to gently look left, while the practitioner monitors to ensure localization to the barrier. After relaxation, the patient is told to take a deep breath in and let it all out. At the end of exhalation an HVT is introduced through the practitioner's right hand and thumb in a right-to-left and slightly ventral direction. Graded mobilizations can be performed from this same position by oscillation of the practitioner's right hand (Fig. 9.12). The motion segment is re-examined.

Extension Restriction of T1–T4 (Example: HVT-Prone, T2 FRS Left "Closing the Right Facet")

During this technique the practitioner will contact the inferior segment of the dysfunctional motion segment. The technique requires moving the inferior segment under the superior segment (i.e., move T3 to affect the dysfunctional T2 segment).

Position

The patient is prone with the chin resting on the table and the practitioner standing at the head of the table. The practitioner lifts the patient's head and moves it into a right–side-bent and right-rotated position down to T2 (Fig. 9.13).

Localization to the Barrier

The practitioner stabilizes the patient's head with the right hand and contacts the right transverse process of T3 with his or her left pisiform.

Mobilization or Thrust

While maintaining the patient's head position, the practitioner's left pisiform applies a graded mobilization or HVT in a downward and slightly caudal direction on the T3 right transverse process (Fig. 9.14). This moves the T3 segment into left rotation resulting in a relative extension and right rotation of T2. The practitioner should never thrust through the

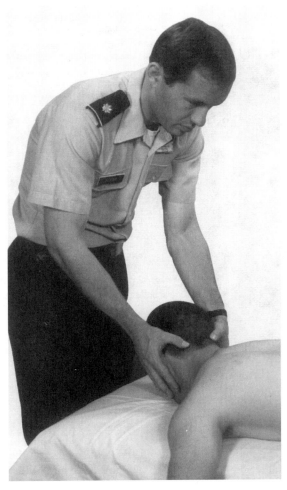

Figure 9.13. Positioning the patient's head for a prone high-velocity thrust technique of a T2 segment restricted in extension, right rotation, and right side-bending (FRS left T2). The practitioner introduces right side-bending and right rotation down to the T2-3 segment.

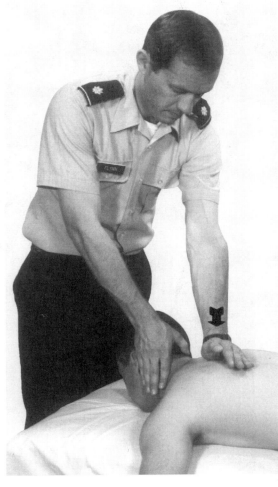

Figure 9.14. A prone high-velocity thrust technique for a T2 segment restricted in extension, right rotation, and right side-bending (FRS left T2). The mobilization or high-velocity thrust is on the right transverse process of T3.

head and neck. This area is stabilized only. The motion segment is re-examined.

Extension Restriction of T7–T12 (Example: MET-Sitting, T10 FRS Right)

Position

The patient is seated with the practitioner sitting on the table and the practitioner's left arm over the pa-

tient's left shoulder. The practitioner's right hand monitors the motion segment.

Localization to the Barrier

The patient is told to slowly stick out the stomach, which introduces extension to the barrier. Side-bending is introduced by lowering the patient's left shoulder toward the left buttock. This is followed by a slight left rotation of the trunk to the barrier.

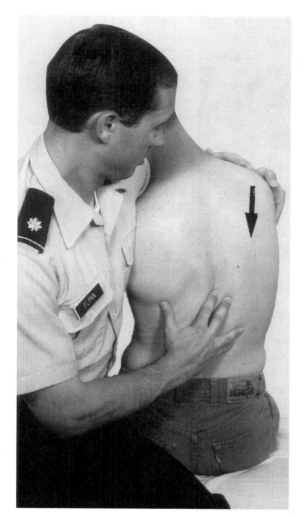

Figure 9.15. A sitting muscle energy technique for a T10 segment that is restricted in extension, left rotation, and left side-bending (FRS right T10). The practitioner monitors muscle contraction at the right T10–11 intertransverse space.

Treatment

The patient is told to gently drop the right shoulder and lift the left, while the practitioner resists this motion (Fig. 9.15). After 3–5 seconds the patient is told to relax, and a translatory motion to increase extension, left rotation, and left side-bending is introduced to the T10 segment. This is repeated three to five times, and then the practitioner re-examines the motion segment.

Extension Restrictions of T4–T12 (Example: HVT-Prone, T6 FRS Right "Closing the Left T6-7 Facet")

Position

The patient is prone with the head turned toward the left and the practitioner standing on the patient's left side.

Localization to the Barrier

The practitioner's right hypothenar eminence contacts the right T6 transverse process and loads it ventrally, thus introducing left rotation of T6. The practitioner's left hypothenar eminence contacts the left T6 transverse process and exerts a caudal pressure.

Mobilization or Thrust

The patient is told to take a deep breath in and let it all out. The practitioner follows the expiration and applies either graded mobilizations or a HVT directly toward the table (Fig. 9.16). The motion segment is re-examined.

Extension Restrictions of T4–T12 (Example: HVT-Supine, T4 FRS Right "Closing the Left T4-5 Facet")

Position

The patient is supine with the arms crossed and the practitioner standing on the patient's right side. The practitioner rolls the patient to the right and contacts the transverse processes of T5 with his or her right hand.

Localization to the Barrier

The practitioner's left arm cradles the patient's head and upper back. The practitioner flexes the patient up and slightly past the T4 segment, followed by a

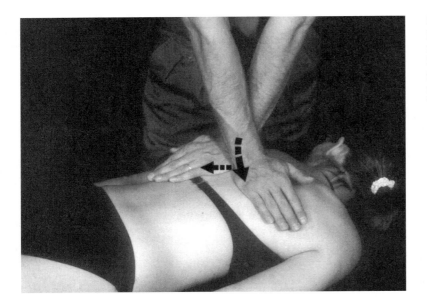

Figure 9.16. A prone high-velocity thrust for a T6 segment that is restricted in extension, left rotation, and left side-bending (FRS right T6). The aim of the technique is closing the left T6-7 facet.

slight left side-bending of the patient's upper back down to the T4 segment.

Mobilization or Thrust

The patient is told to take a deep breath in and let it all out. Near the end of exhalation, the practitioner tells the patient to look left. As the practitioner feels movement nearing his or her right hand, he or she drops the patient back into extension and with the chest wall performs a gentle HVT through the patient's elbows in a vector toward the left T4-5 facet (Fig. 9.17). The motion segment is re-examined.

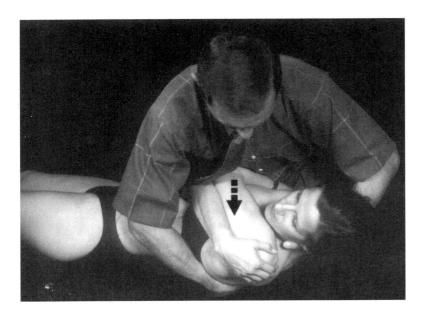

Figure 9.17. A supine high-velocity thrust for a T4 segment that is restricted in extension, left rotation, and left side-bending (FRS right T4). The aim of treatment is a closing of the left T4-5 facet. The vector of force is directed at T4.

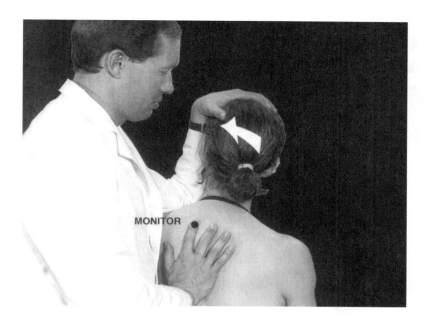

Figure 9.18. A sitting muscle energy technique for the T2–T4 segments, which are restricted in right side-bending and left rotation (convex right T2–T4). The practitioner monitors muscle contraction at the left T3-4 intertransverse space.

Neutral Group Restrictions (Convex Groups)

When three or more vertebral segments are involved in a motion restriction, a frontal plane asymmetry is present (i.e., a convex lateral curvature). A fullness along several transverse processes will be noticeable. This is a type 1 neutral mechanical dysfunction. Therefore, rotation and side-bending are coupled to opposite sides. The convex side is always the side toward which the vertebrae are rotated. In neutral or convex group restrictions typically the greatest restriction is in the side-bending and rotational components with minimal flexion or extension components.

Rotation and Side-Bending Restriction of T1–T4 (Example: MET-Sitting, T2–T4 Convex Right)

Position

The patient is seated with the practitioner standing behind. The practitioner's left forearm guides and supports the patient's head and the practitioner's right hand monitors for muscle contraction.

Engaging the Barrier

The practitioner introduces right side-bending followed by left rotation of the patient's head to the T3-4 segment barrier while maintaining a neutral (neither flexed nor extended) posture.

Treatment

The patient is told to gently tilt the left ear toward his or her left shoulder (Fig. 9.18). After 3–5 seconds the patient is told to relax and a translatory motion to increase right side-bending followed by left rotation to the new T3 barrier is introduced. This is repeated three to five times and then the segment is re-examined.

Rotation and Side-Bending Restriction of T1–T4 (Example: HVT-Sitting, T2–T4 Convex Right)

Position

The practitioner sits behind the patient with the left leg on the table underneath the patient's left armpit. The practitioner supports and guides the

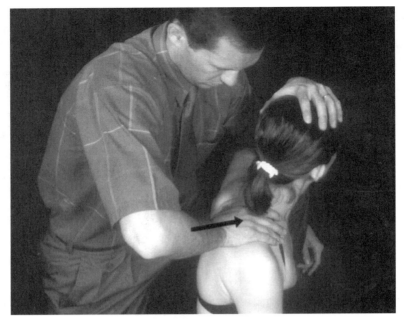

Figure 9.19. A sitting high-velocity thrust for the T2–T4 segments, which are restricted in right side-bending and left rotation (convex right T2–T4).

patient's head using the left forearm and contacts the right *intertransverse space* of the T3–4 segment with the right thumb while allowing the web space of the right hand to drape over the patient's shoulder.

Localization to the Barrier

While maintaining the patient in a neutral (neither flexed nor extended) position the practitioner translates the patient into right side-bending via the practitioner's right hand followed by left rotation to the barrier. The patient is told to gently drop the left ear to the left to ensure localization to the segment and then relax.

Mobilization or Thrust

The patient is told to breathe in and exhale completely. At the point of maximum relaxation, an HVT is introduced through the practitioner's right hand in a right-to-left and anterior direction, which

will cause a right side-bending and left rotation force to the segment (Fig. 9.19). Graded mobilizations can be performed from the same position. The motion segment is re-examined.

Rotation and Side-Bending Restriction of T1–T4 (Example: HVT-Prone T2–T4 Convex Right)

Position

The patient is prone with the practitioner standing at the head of the table.

Localization to the Barrier

The patient's head is lifted into right side-bending down to the T3–4 segment, and then the practitioner's right hand rotates the patient's head to the left. The practitioner's left hand contacts the right *intertransverse* space of the T3–4 segment and exerts a downward and medial pressure to the barrier.

Mobilization or Thrust

The patient is told to inhale and exhale completely and an HVT is given through the practitioner's left hand while the right hand stabilizes the head (Fig. 9.20). The practitioner should never thrust through the head and neck; this area is stabilized only. The motion segment is re-examined.

Side-Bending and Rotation Restrictions of T6–T12 (Example: MET-Sitting, T6-T8 Convex Left Group)

Position

The patient is seated with the practitioner's left arm over the patient's left shoulder and grasping the right shoulder. The practitioner's chest wall guides the trunk, while the right hand monitors the T7–8 motion segment for movement and muscle contraction.

Engaging the Barrier

While maintaining a neutral (neither flexed nor extended) position, the practitioner introduces left side-bending by dropping his or her left shoulder and translating to the barrier. The patient's trunk is then slightly right rotated to the barrier.

Treatment

The patient is told to gently lift the left shoulder and drop the right (Fig. 9.21). After 3–5 seconds the patient is told to relax, and a translatory motion to increase right rotation and left side-bending is introduced to the T6–T8 segments. This is repeated three to five times and then the practitioner re-examines the motion segment.

Side-Bending and Rotation Restriction of T4–T12 (Example: HVT-Supine, T4–T6 Convex Left)

Position

The patient is supine with the arms crossed and the practitioner standing on the patient's right side.

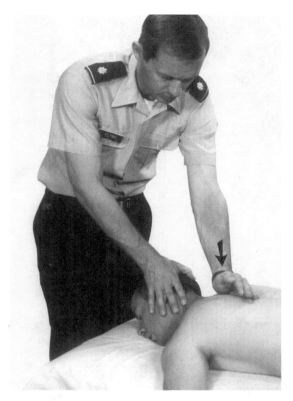

Figure 9.20. A prone high-velocity thrust for the T2–T4 segments, which are restricted in right side-bending and left rotation (convex right T2–T4). The mobilization or high-velocity thrust is on the right intertransverse space of T3-4.

The practitioner rolls the patient to the right and contacts the transverse processes of T6 with the right hand.

Localization to the Barrier

The patient is rolled back firmly onto the practitioner's right hand followed by the practitioner exerting a downward pressure toward the stabilizing right hand.

Mobilization or Thrust

The patient is told to take a deep breath and let it all out (Fig. 9.22). As full exhalation nears, the patient is asked to look right and, as the practitioner feels movement nearing the right hand, he or she applies an HVT with the chest wall in a vector toward the T6 segment. The motion segment is re-examined.

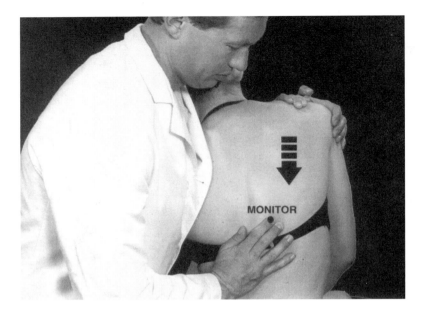

Figure 9.21. A sitting muscle energy technique for the T6–T8 segments, which are restricted in left side-bending and right rotation (convex left T6–T8). The practitioner monitors muscle contraction at the right T7-8 intertransverse space.

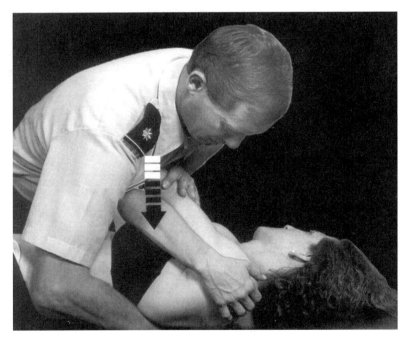

Figure 9.22. A supine high-velocity thrust for the T4–T6 segments, which are restricted in left side-bending and right rotation (convex left T4–T6). The vector of force is directed at T6.

Rib Cage (Costovertebral) Technique

The remainder of this chapter is directed at the treatment of costal vertebral or rib cage dysfunction. The rib cage dysfunctions will be divided into three categories: structural dysfunction, torsional dysfunction, and respiratory restrictions.

Structural Rib Dysfunction

Structural rib dysfunctions include anterior subluxed rib, posterior subluxed rib, superiorly subluxed first rib, anterior-posterior rib compression, lateral rib compression, and a laterally elevated rib. Structural ribs are trauma induced and are hyper-

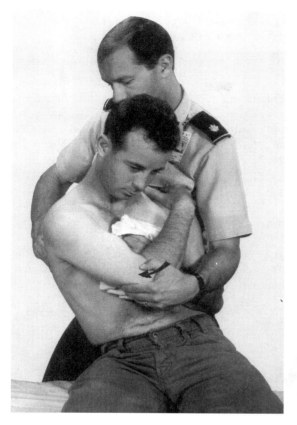

Figure 9.23. Treatment position for a right anteriorly sub-luxed sixth rib viewed from the front. A rolled up towel and the patient's left fisted hand are placed over the anterior aspect of the sixth rib.

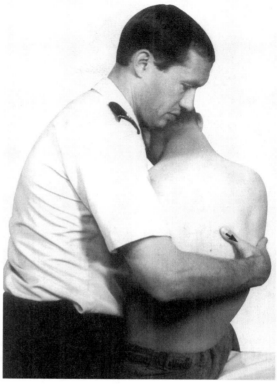

Figure 9.24. A sitting muscle energy technique for a right anteriorly subluxed sixth rib viewed from the back. The practitioner attempts to glide the sixth rib in a posterolateral direction.

mobile by nature. Mobilization and HVT techniques should not be used in the treatment of these conditions. The preferred treatment approach is with MET.

Anterior Subluxed Rib (Example: MET-Sitting, Right Sixth Rib)

Position

The patient is sitting with the right arm across the chest. A rolled up towel and the patient's left fist are placed firmly over the costochondral junction of the right sixth rib (Fig. 9.23). The practitioner stands behind the patient, right thumb medial to the angle of the sixth rib and left hand reaching over the patient and grasping the patient's right elbow.

Engaging the Barrier

The patient is told to slump into the practitioner's right hand, which facilitates the right sixth rib into a posterior glide movement (Fig. 9.24). A slight lateral and posterior pull is introduced through the practitioner's right thumb.

Treatment

The patient is told to gently lift the right elbow up and out. This facilitates the right serratus anterior. With the arm fixed, the right serratus anterior will produce a posterior translatory motion on the right sixth rib. After 3–5 seconds the patient is told to relax, and the practitioner engages the new barrier by (1) increasing the slump of the patient, (2) applying a lateral pull on the rib angle, and (3) compress-

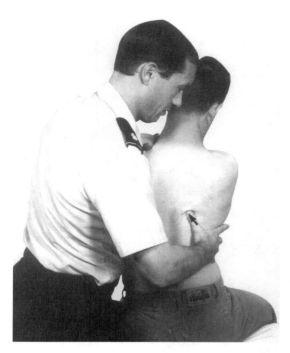

Figure 9.25. A sitting muscle energy technique for a right posteriorly subluxed sixth rib viewed form the back. The practitioner attempts to glide the sixth rib in an anteromedial direction.

ing the patient's right elbow into the patient's chest wall. The procedure is repeated three to five times followed by re-examination of the segment.

Posterior Subluxed Rib (Example: MET-Sitting, Right Sixth Rib)

Position

The patient is seated with the right arm across the chest. The practitioner stands behind the patient, right thumb lateral to the angle of the sixth rib and left hand reaching over and grasping the patient's right elbow.

Engaging the Barrier

The patient is told to stick out the stomach and drop the right shoulder. This facilitates an anterior glide of the right sixth rib (Fig. 9.25). A slight anterome-

dial push is introduced with the practitioner's right thumb on the sixth rib angle.

Treatment

The patient is told to gently pull his or her right elbow down and to the left. This facilitates the right pectoralis major muscle, which will promote an anterior translatory movement of the ribs. If the dysfunctional rib is lower (ribs 7–10), the command is to flex the trunk in order to facilitate the abdominals.

After 3–5 seconds the patient is told to relax, and the practitioner engages the new barrier by (1) increasing the patient's thoracic extension and right side-bending; and (2) applying a medial push on the rib angle. This is repeated three to five times followed by re-examination of the segment.

Superior Subluxed First Rib (Example: MET-Sitting, Right First Rib)

Position

The patient is seated with the left arm draped over the practitioner's left leg. The practitioner stands behind the patient with the left leg on the table and the left forearm supporting the patient's head.

Engaging the Barrier

The practitioner's right second and third fingers contact the superior aspect of the right first rib anterior to the trapezius. The practitioner's right thumb contacts the posterior aspect of the first rib (Fig. 9.26). The practitioner right side-bends the patient's trunk and neck to release tension off the right first rib.

Treatment

The patient is told to gently tilt the left ear to the left. This facilitates the left scalenes to contract with a reflex inhibition of the right scalenes. After 3–5 seconds the patient is told to relax, and the practitioner pushes slightly anterior with the right thumb and applies a caudal traction force through the right second and third fingers to release the first rib. The segment is re-examined.

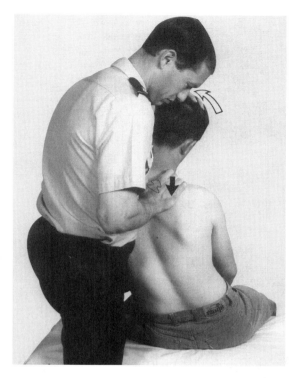

Figure 9.26. A sitting muscle energy technique for a right superior subluxed first rib. The practitioner disengages the rib by an anterior directed force through the thumb and then glides the rib inferiorly.

Anterior-Posterior Rib Compression (Example: MET-Sitting, Right Seventh Rib)

Position

The patient is seated with the right hand resting on the left shoulder. The practitioner stands on the patient's left side and reaches around to interlace his or her fingers and contact the prominent right seventh rib in the midaxillary line.

Engaging the Barrier

The practitioner translates the patient into right side-bending while applying a compressive force on the lateral aspect of the rib.

Treatment

The patient is told to gently drop the left shoulder. This facilitates left trunk side-bending (Fig. 9.27).

After 3–5 seconds the patient is told to relax, and the practitioner increases the compression on the seventh rib and increases the patient's right side-bending. This is repeated three to five times and the segment is re-examined.

Lateral Rib Compression (Example: Right Fourth Rib)

Position

The patient is seated on the edge of the treatment table with the right arm draped over the practitioner's left shoulder. The practitioner stands on the patient's right side and contacts the patient's right fourth rib anteriorly at the costochondral junction with the right hand and posteriorly contacts the angle of the right fourth rib with the left hand.

Engaging the Barrier

The practitioner compresses the right fourth rib anteriorly and posteriorly in an attempt to flare the rib in the midaxillary line. The practitioner then left side-bends the patient's trunk with the apex at the fourth rib.

Treatment

The patient is told to take a deep breath in and drop the right shoulder. This facilitates right trunk side-bending (Fig. 9.28). After 3–5 seconds the patient is told to relax, and the practitioner increases the anterior-posterior compression and the left trunk side-bending. This is repeated three to five times and the segment is re-examined.

Laterally Elevated Rib (Example: Combination MET and Myofascial Mobilization, Left Second Rib)

Position

The patient is supine on the treatment table with the practitioner standing on the patient's right side. The practitioner places the palm of the right hand along the patient's left midaxillary line and slowly works the finger pads up the axilla to the patient's second rib.

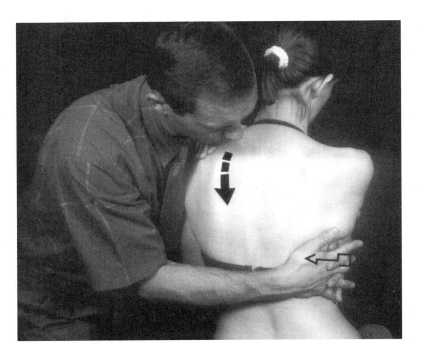

Figure 9.27. A sitting muscle energy technique for a anteroposterior compression of a right seventh rib.

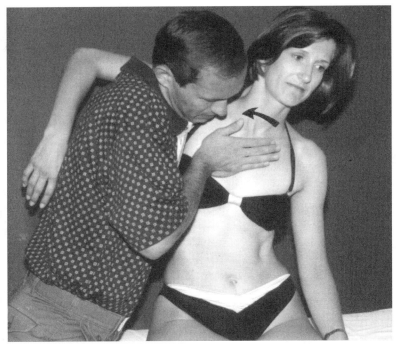

Figure 9.28. A sitting muscle energy technique for a lateral compression of the right fourth rib.

Engaging the Barrier

To assist the practitioner in grasping the patient's left second rib, the practitioner left side-bends the patient's head and upper trunk (Fig. 9.29).

Treatment

The patient is told to exhale and reach the left hand toward the left knee. This increases the left side-bending and should be repeated five times. After

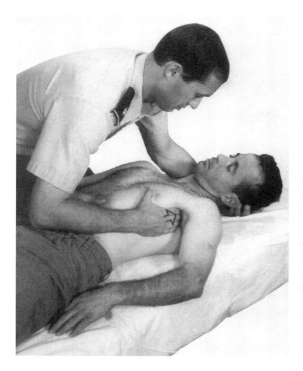

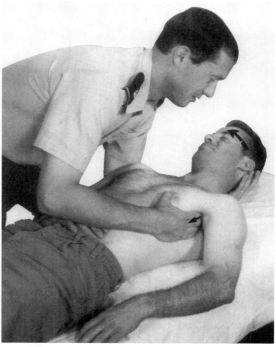

Figure 9.29. Treatment starting position to facilitate grasping a left laterally elevated second rib.

Figure 9.30. A combination technique for treatment of a left laterally elevated second rib (end position).

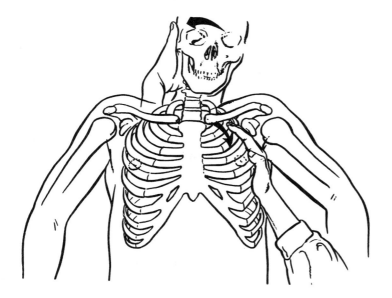

Figure 9.31. Diagrammatic representation of the treatment of a left laterally elevated second rib.

the fifth exhalation phase, the practitioner firmly grasps the superior aspect of the left second rib with the right finger pads and slowly straightens the patient's head and neck into right side-bending (Figs. 9.30 and 9.31). This will restore the superior subluxed rib to a neutral position and stretch the adaptively shortened tissue on the superior aspect of the second rib.

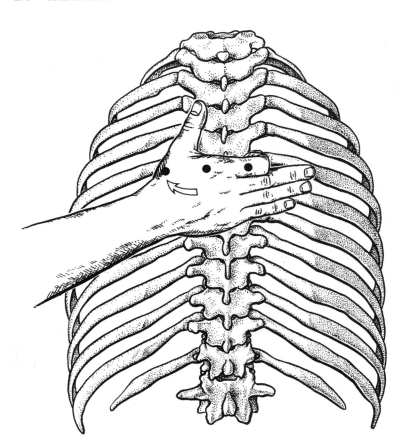

Figure 9.32. Hand contact for the supine high-velocity thrust technique used in the treatment of an externally torsioned fifth rib with T4 ERS left. The thenar eminence contacts the inferior border of the fifth rib at the rib angle and lifts the rib angle superiorly; the remainder of the first and second digits stabilize T5.

Torsional Rib Dysfunction

Torsional ribs generally occur in response to a chronic nonneutral (FRS and ERS) thoracic dysfunction. As noted in Chapter 1, during flexion of the thoracic spine the coupled rib segment rotates internally, and during extension of the thoracic spine the rib segment rotates externally. In this chapter the torsional ribs will not be treated as separate entities; rather the ribs will be treated in combination with the frequently seen concurrent thoracic spine nonneutral dysfunction.

Externally Torsioned Rib with Thoracic Flexion Restriction (Example: HVT-Supine, Left Fifth Rib Externally Torsioned with T4, ERS Left)

The most common rib torsional dysfunction is the external rib torsion coupled with an extended vertebral segment one level above (i.e., T4 ERS left with an externally torsioned fifth rib). This is a common

cause of recurrent thoracic spinal pain and dysfunction. If the practitioner only addresses the thoracic ERS component, the externally torsioned rib will tend to drive the thoracic spine back into an extended position. Therefore, the practitioner should treat both the thoracic and the rib components when this entity is noted on physical examination. The aim of this technique is to open the left T4-5 facet and open and internally rotate the left fifth rib at the costotransverse joint.

Position

The patient is supine with the arms crossed and the practitioner standing on the patient's right side. The practitioner rolls the patient to the right and contacts the T4 segment and the left fifth rib as noted in Fig. 9.32. The practitioner's right hand rotates as noted in Fig. 9.33. This drives the rib into an internal torsional movement. The patient is rolled firmly back onto the practitioner's right hand and pressure is given by the practitioner through the patient's arms.

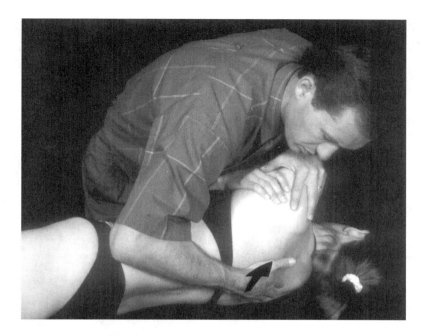

Figure 9.33. Hand contact emphasizing a rotation of the practitioner's right hand. Used in the treatment of an externally torsioned left fifth rib with a concurrent T4 ERS left.

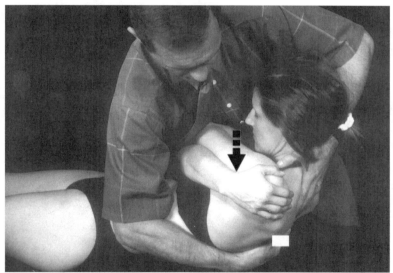

Figure 9.34. A supine high-velocity thrust used in the treatment of an externally torsioned left fifth rib with a concurrent T4 ERS left. The vector of force is directed to the left T5 transverse process.

Localization to the Barrier

The practitioner's left arm cradles the patient's head and upper back. The practitioner flexes the patient's head and shoulders down to the T4-5 segment, followed by slight right side-bending and right rotation to the three-dimensional barrier. The practitioner applies additional pressure through the chest wall to ensure the segment is loaded.

Mobilization or Thrust

The patient is told to take a deep breath and let it all out. As the patient nears the end of the exhalation phase, the patient is asked to look over the right shoulder. As the practitioner senses the movement nearing the right hand, he or she provides a HVT with the chest wall through the patient's elbows in a vector toward the costotransverse joint of the fifth rib (Fig. 9.34). This will introduce a flexion movement at the T4-5 segment and an internal torsional movement of the fifth rib. The segment is re-examined.

Exercise

Because of the recurrent nature of this dysfunction, the patient is typically instructed to perform the following barrel hug exercise. Have the patient reach around a large Swiss ball (Fig. 9.35) or have the patient imagine that a 55-gallon drum is on his or her lap and that he or she should attempt to get the arms all the way around it (Fig. 9.36). For this example, the patient should be in flexion, right side-bending, and right rotation. The apex should be at the left T4-5 segment. Have the patient reach until a firm stretch is felt at the appropriate level and then hold that position for 30–90 seconds. This should be repeated three times for three to five sets per day.

Internally Torsioned Rib with Thoracic Extension Restriction (Example: HVT-Supine, Left Fifth Rib Internally Torsioned with T4, FRS Right)

A less frequently encountered torsional dysfunction is the internally torsioned rib with concurrent FRS thoracic dysfunction. If the practitioner only addresses the thoracic FRS component, the internally torsioned rib will tend to drive the thoracic spine forward into a flexed position. Therefore, the practitioner should treat both the thoracic and the rib components when this entity is noted on physical examination. The aim of this technique is to close the left T4-5 facet and open and externally rotate the left fifth rib at the costotransverse joint.

Position

The patient is supine with the arms crossed and the practitioner standing on the patient's right side. The practitioner rolls the patient toward the right and contacts the T5 vertebral segment and the superior border of the angle of the left fifth rib as shown in Fig. 9.37. The practitioner rotates his or her right hand to initiate an external torsional movement of the fifth rib (Fig. 9.38).

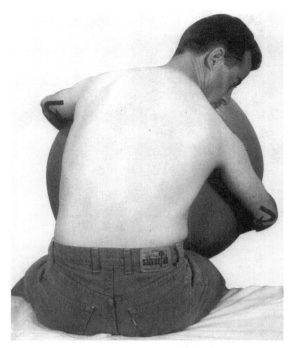

Figure 9.35. The barrel hug stretch with a Swiss ball used to facilitate flexion, right rotation, and right side-bending in the midthoracic spine.

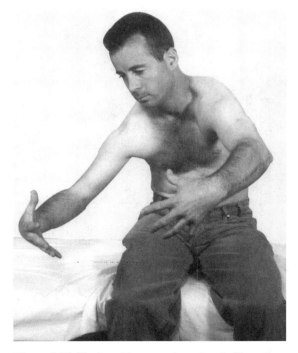

Figure 9.36. The barrel hug stretch used to facilitate flexion, right rotation, and right side-bending in the midthoracic spine.

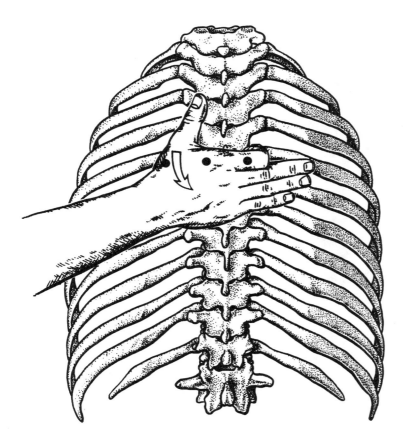

Figure 9.37. Hand contact used in the treatment of an internally torsioned left fifth rib with a concurrent T4 FRS right. The thenar eminence contacts the superior border of the fifth rib at the rib angle and guides the rib angle inferiorly. The remainder of the first and second digit stabilize T5.

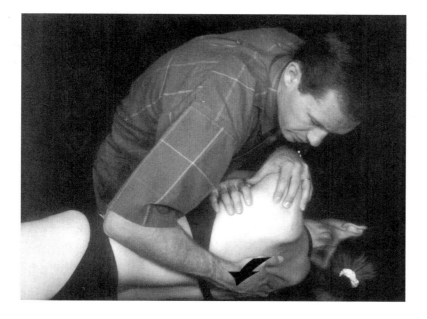

Figure 9.38. Hand contact emphasizing a rotation of the practitioner's right hand. Used in the treatment of an internally torsioned left fifth rib with a concurrent T4 FRS right.

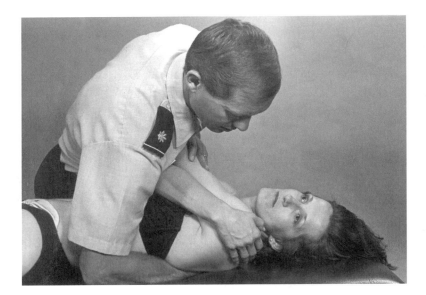

Figure 9.39. A supine high-velocity thrust for an internally torsioned left fifth rib with a concurrent T4 FRS right. The vector of force is directed to the left T4 transverse process.

Localization to the Barrier

The practitioner's left arm cradles the patient's head and upper back. The practitioner flexes the patient up and slightly past the T4 segment followed by a slight left side-bending of the patient's upper back down to the T4 segment.

Mobilization or Thrust

The patient is told to take a deep breath in and let it all out. Near the end of exhalation the practitioner tells the patient to look left. As the practitioner feels movement nearing his or her right hand, the patient is dropped back into extension over the right-hand fulcrum, and, with the chest wall, the practitioner performs a gentle HVT through the patient's elbows in a vector toward the costotransverse joint of the left fifth rib (Fig. 9.39). This will introduce an extension movement at the T4-5 segment and an external torsional movement of the fifth rib. The segment is re-examined.

Respiratory Rib Restrictions

Restrictions in respiratory motion of the rib cage can be noted in both inhalation and exhalation. Respiratory rib restrictions present as a group of ribs with limited respiratory excursion. The key rib is the rib that is at the top of the group in an inhalation re-striction and at the bottom of the group in an exhalation restriction. The key rib may be a structural or torsional rib dysfunction, in which case it would need to be appropriately treated before the respiratory component is addressed. Treating a structural or torsional key rib often will restore any respiratory restrictions; however, if the structural or torsional rib has been present for some time (more than 4–6 weeks), adaptive changes have most likely occurred in the myofascial components of the adjacent ribs and may manifest as respiratory rib restrictions.

Inhalation Restrictions

The key rib will be the top rib in the group and the following techniques are directed at the key rib segment.

Inhalation Restriction of the First Rib (Example: MET-Supine, Left First Rib)

Position

The patient is supine with the practitioner on the patient's left side. The practitioner's right arm slides under the patient and with the finger pads of two to four digits contacts the posterior-superior aspect of the patient's left first rib. The practitioner's left hand is placed on the left side of the patient's forehead.

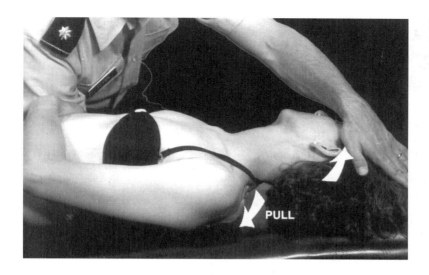

Figure 9.40. A supine muscle energy technique used in the treatment of a left first rib inhalation restriction.

Engaging the Barrier

The practitioner pulls his or her right arm in a diagonal to promote a left side-bending apex at the C7–T1 segment. The practitioner rolls the second to fourth fingers on the right back, which encourages an elevation of the right anterior aspect of the left first rib.

Treatment

The patient is told to take a deep breath in and hold it. At maximum inhalation, the patient is asked to gently lift the head off the table, promoting a left scalene contraction that will increase the inspiratory motion of the left first rib (Fig. 9.40). After 3–5 seconds the patient is told to relax and the practitioner takes up the slack by a combination of rolling the fingers back and pulling his or her right arm diagonally. The procedure is repeated three to five times and the segment re-examined.

Inhalation Restriction of the First Rib (Example: HVT-Supine, Left First Rib)

Position

The patient is supine with the practitioner on the patient's right side. The hand placement is very similar to that for the first rib MET just described, where the practitioner's right hand contacts the left first rib. How-

ever, in the HVT technique the practitioner's left hand cradles the patient's head underneath the occiput.

Localization to the Barrier

The practitioner's right arm pulls in a diagonal to promote left side-bending at the C7-T1 segment and rolls the right second to fourth fingers backward.* The practitioner right rotates the patient's head and neck until movement is felt by the practitioner's right hand.

Thrust

At the point of maximum patient relaxation, the practitioner maintains the right rotation and introduces an HVT by an exaggeration of the left side-bending (Fig. 9.41). The segment is re-examined.

Inhalation Restriction of the Second Rib (Example: MET-Supine, Left Second Rib)

The technique for inhalation restriction of the second rib is the same as that described for a first rib inhalation restriction (see Fig. 9.40). However, the practitioner contacts the patient's left second rib posteriorly; all other components of the technique are the same.

---

*This technique can also be modified for a first rib exhalation restriction. The only change is that the practitioner rolls the fingers forward to promote exhalation.

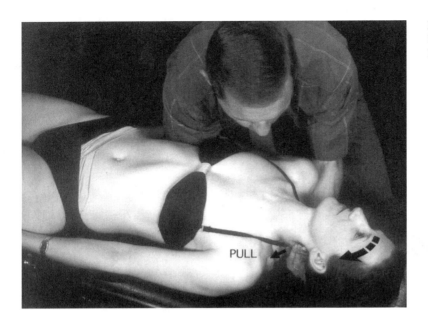

Figure 9.41. A supine high-velocity thrust for treatment of a left first rib inhalation restriction.

Inhalation Restriction of the Second Rib (Example: HVT-Sitting, Right Second Rib)

Position

The patient is seated with the practitioner standing behind. The patient's left arm is draped over the practitioner's left leg, while the practitioner's left arm protects the patient's head and neck. The practitioner's right thumb contacts the shaft of the second rib just lateral to the T2 transverse process.

Localization to the Barrier

The patient is translated to the barrier using neutral vertebral mechanics by introducing right side-bending and left rotation at the T2 segment.

Mobilization or Thrust

When all the slack is taken out, an anterior and caudal thrust is applied through the shaft of the second rib, which will promote a cephalic rise of the anterior portion of the rib, thereby increasing the inhalation (Fig. 9.42)*. The motion segment is re-examined.

---

*This technique can be modified for a second rib exhalation restriction. The only modification is that the thrust is in an anterior and cranial direction, which will promote a caudal drop of the anterior portion of the second rib, thus increasing exhalation.

Inhalation Restriction of the Third to Tenth Ribs (Example: MET-Supine, Right Ribs 3–10)

Position

The patient is supine with the practitioner standing on the patient's right side. The practitioner's left arm reaches over the patient and, with the finger pads of the second to fourth digits, contacts the posterior-superior aspect of the key rib. The practitioner's right hand placement depends on the chosen level of treatment (Figs. 9.43 and 9.44).

Engaging the Barrier

The practitioner's left arm pulls in a lateral and caudal direction to disengage the costovertebral segment and encourage an elevation of the anterior aspect of the key rib.

Treatment

The patient is told to take a deep breath and hold it. At maximum inspiration the patient is asked to either lift the elbow off the table (see Fig. 9.43), promoting a right pectoral contraction if ribs 3–5 are being treated, or to pull the elbow to the side (see Fig. 9.44), for a latissimus dorsi contraction if treating ribs 6–10. After 3–5 seconds the patient is told to relax, and the practitioner takes up the slack by

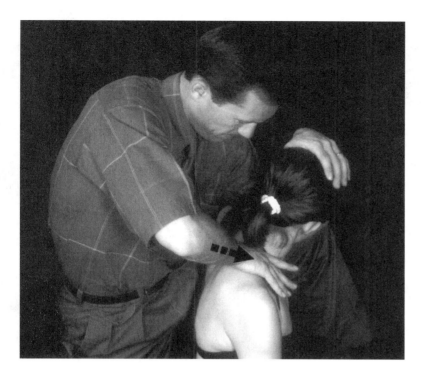

Figure 9.42. A sitting high-velocity thrust for use in the treatment of a right second rib inhalation restriction. The practitioner's right thumb is on the shaft of the second rib.

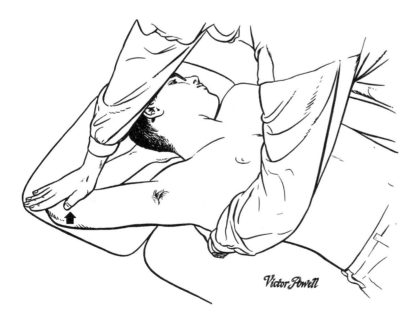

Figure 9.43. A supine muscle energy technique for treatment of inspiratory restriction of ribs 3–5 on the right.

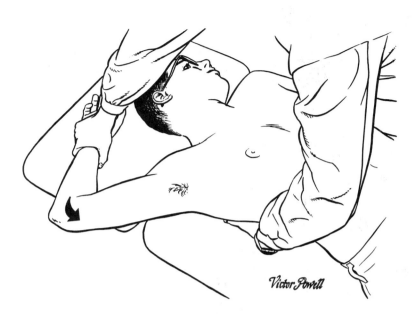

Figure 9.44. A supine muscle energy technique for treatment of inspiratory restriction of ribs 6–10 on the right.

Victor Powell

pulling his or her left arm in a lateral and caudal direction. The procedure is repeated three to five times and the segment re-examined.

Inhalation Restriction of the Third to Tenth Ribs (Example: HVT-Supine, Left Ribs 5–7)

Position

The patient is supine with arms crossed and the practitioner standing on the patient's right side. The practitioner reaches over the patient and contacts the angles of left ribs 5–7 with the palm and rotates the hand down and medially (Fig. 9.45). This encourages a cranial rise of the anterior aspect of the rib.

Localization to the Barrier

The patient is rolled completely over onto the practitioner's right hand.

Thrust

At the point of maximum patient relaxation, an HVT is introduced through the practitioner's chest wall in a vector toward the angles of left ribs 5–7 (Fig. 9.46). The motion segment is re-examined.

Inhalation Restriction of Ribs 11–12 (Example: MET and HVT-Prone, Left Eleventh and Twelfth Ribs)

The motion of the eleventh and twelfth ribs is described as a caliper motion and requires a treatment approach modified from that for the typical ribs. The MET and HVT are similar and will be described together. The positioning will be the same for each technique. The difference will be the introduction of a HVT at the completion of the MET.

Position

The patient is prone with the trunk side-bent to the right and the practitioner standing on the patient's right side. The practitioner's left hand grasps the patient's anterior-superior iliac spine, and the hypothenar eminence of the practitioner's right hand contacts the eleventh and twelfth ribs just lateral to the transverse processes.

Engaging the Barrier

The practitioner's right hand applies a lateral and slightly cranial force. The practitioner lifts the patient's pelvis off the table to engage the barrier.

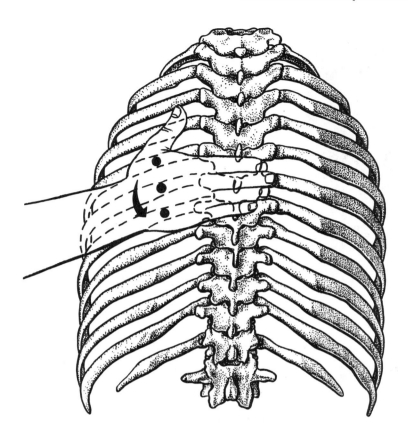

Figure 9.45. Hand contact showing a rotation of the practitioner's right hand. Used in the treatment of an inhalation restriction of ribs 5–7 on the left.

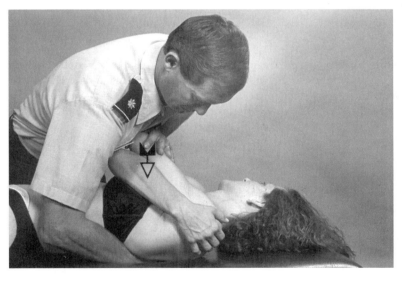

Figure 9.46. A supine high-velocity thrust used in the treatment of an inhalation restriction of ribs 5–7 on the left. The vector of force is directed at the rib angles 5–7.

Treatment/Thrust

The patient is told to take a deep breath in and hold it followed by the command to pull the left hip toward the table. The practitioner holds this position

for 3–5 seconds, then allows full exhalation while maintaining the previously gained inspiratory motion (Fig. 9.47). This is repeated three to five times and the motion segment is re-examined. An HVT can be introduced through the practitioner's right

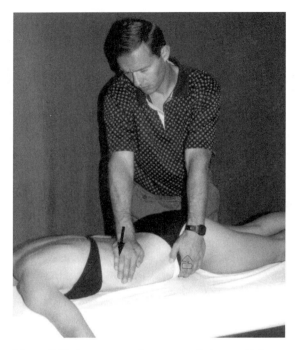

Figure 9.47. A prone muscle energy technique or high-velocity thrust technique for the treatment of an inhalation restriction of the left eleventh and twelfth ribs.

hand just before full patient inhalation. The motion segment is re-examined.

Rib Cage Exhalation Restrictions

Exhalation Restriction of the First Rib (Example: MET-Supine, Left First Rib)

Position

The patient is supine with the practitioner sitting at the head of the table. The practitioner's left thumb is placed on the superior border of the left first rib either just anterior to the trapezius for a bucket-handle restriction or just posterior to the clavicle for a pump-handle restriction. The practitioner's right hand supports the patient's head.

Engaging the Barrier

The practitioner flexes and left side-bends the patient's head to promote a downward movement of the left first rib.

Treatment

The patient is told to take a small breath in and exhale completely. During the exhalation phase, the practitioner's left thumb guides the first rib in a caudal direction while flexion and side-bending of the patient's head are increased. This is repeated three times while the gained expiration range of motion of the rib is maintained (Fig. 9.48). After the third complete exhalation effort, the practitioner holds the left first rib down and returns the patient's head to a neutral position. The motion segment is re-examined.

Exhalation Restriction of the First Rib (Example: HVT-Sitting, Left First Rib)

Position

The patient is seated with the practitioner standing behind with his or her right foot on the table. The patient drapes the right axilla over the practitioner's right leg. The practitioner's right arm protects the patient's head and neck while the web space of the practitioner's left hand contacts the superior aspect of the left first rib.

Engaging the Barrier

The practitioner's left hand rolls to contact the rib slightly anterior to promote exhalation.* The practitioner introduces a left side-bending motion to the C7-T1 segment via translation of the practitioner's hands to the barrier.

Mobilization or Thrust

An HVT of the practitioner's left hand in a caudal and medial direction is performed at the point of maximal patient relaxation (Fig. 9.49). The motion segment is re-examined.

---

*This technique can also be modified for use in a first rib inhalation restriction. The only difference is that the practitioner rolls the thrusting hand posteriorly, which will promote inhalation of the first rib (Fig. 9.49).

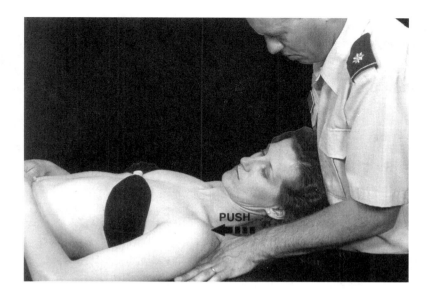

Figure 9.48. A supine muscle energy technique for the treatment of an exhalation restriction of the left first rib.

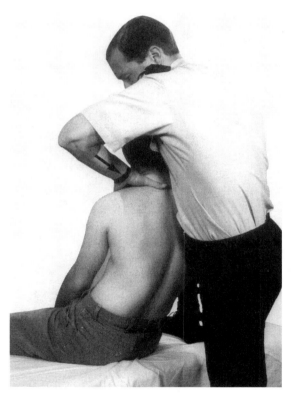

Figure 9.49. A sitting high-velocity thrust for the treatment of an exhalation restriction of the left first rib.

Exhalation Restriction of the Second to Eighth Ribs (Example: MET-Supine, Left Third Rib)

The technique is similar to that described for the first rib supine MET except the contact of the practitioner's hand is on the anterior-superior aspect of the dysfunctional left third rib (Fig. 9.50).

Exhalation Restriction of the Eighth to Tenth Ribs (Example: MET-Supine, Left Ninth Rib)

Position

The patient is supine with the practitioner standing at the head of the table. The practitioner's left hand contacts the superior border of the left ninth rib in the midaxillary line and the right hand is placed under the patient's neck and upper back.

Engaging the Barrier

The practitioner left side-bends the patient's trunk down to the ninth rib.

Treatment

The patient is told to take a small breath in, exhale completely, and reach with the left hand toward the left knee. The practitioner follows the rib into exha-

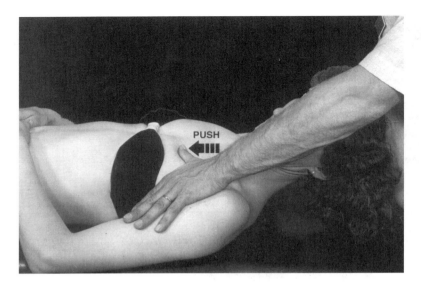

Figure 9.50. A supine muscle energy technique for the treatment of an exhalation restriction of the left third rib.

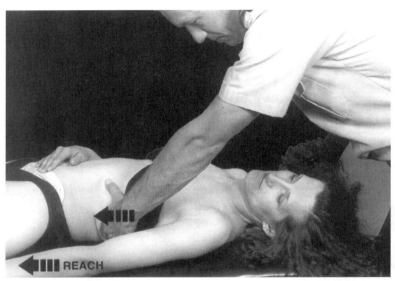

Figure 9.51. A supine muscle energy technique for the treatment of an exhalation restriction of the left ninth rib.

lation and holds the exhalation position (Fig. 9.51). This is repeated three times. After the third repetition, the practitioner holds the rib down while returning the patient's head and trunk to a neutral position. The motion segment is re-examined.

Exhalation Restriction of Ribs 3–10 (Example: HVT-Supine, Left Ribs 5–7)

This technique is similar to the technique described for the inhalation HVT except that the practitioner rotates the stabilizing hand superiorly and medially

(Fig. 9.52). This encourages a caudal drop of the anterior aspect of the rib. The HVT is directed at the angles of left ribs 5–7 as noted in Fig. 9.46.

Exhalation Restriction of the Eleventh and Twelfth Ribs (Example: MET and HVT, Left Eleventh and Twelfth Ribs)

The motion of the eleventh and twelfth ribs is described as a caliper motion and requires a treatment approach modified from that for the typical ribs. The MET and HVT are similar and will be described to-

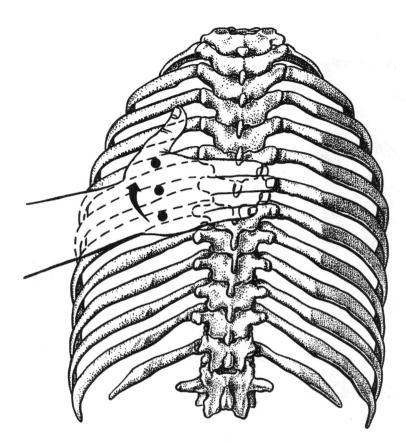

Figure 9.52. Hand contact showing a rotation of the practitioner's right hand. Used in the treatment of an exhalation restriction of ribs 5–7 on the left.

gether. The positioning will be the same for each technique. The difference will be the introduction of a HVT at the completion of the MET.

Position

The patient is prone with the trunk side-bent to the left and the practitioner standing on the patient's right side. The practitioner's left hand grasps the patient's anterior-superior iliac spine, and the hypothenar eminence of the practitioner's right hand contacts the eleventh and twelfth ribs just lateral to the transverse processes.

Engaging the Barrier

The practitioner's right hand applies a lateral and slightly caudal force. The practitioner lifts the patient's pelvis off the table to engage the barrier.

Treatment/Thrust

The patient is told to take a breath in and blow it out, followed by the command to pull the left hip toward the table. The practitioner holds this position for 3–5 seconds and allows full exhalation while following the rib into exhalation (Fig. 9.53). This is repeated three to five times and the motion segment is re-examined. An HVT can be introduced through the practitioner's right hand just before full patient exhalation. The motion segment is re-examined.

Summary

This chapter provides the principles of several direct methods for restoring normal pain-free mobility of the thoracic spine and rib cage. The examples and figures are provided to allow visualization of the po-

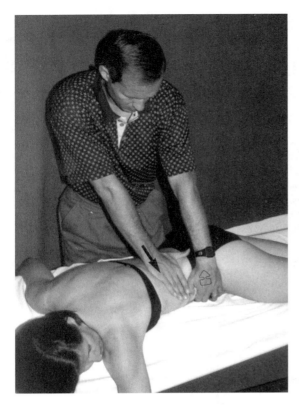

Figure 9.53. A prone muscle energy technique or high-velocity thrust for the treatment of an exhalation restriction of the left eleventh and twelfth ribs.

sition and direction of the techniques. As long as the practitioner adheres to the principles of the techniques, modifications can be made that best suit the individual practitioner.

References

1. Mitchell FL, Moran PS, Pruzzo NA. An Evaluation and Treatment Manual of Osteopathic Muscle Energy Procedures. Valley Park: Mitchell, Moran, and Pruzzo, 1979.
2. Kabot H. Proprioceptive Facilitation in Therapeutic Exercise. In S Licht (ed), Therapeutic Exercise (2nd ed). New Haven: Elizabeth Licht, 1961.
3. Knott M, Barufaldi D. Treatment of whiplash injuries. Phys Ther Rev 1961;41:753–577.
4. Knott M, Voss DE. Proprioceptive Neuromuscular Facilitation Patterns and Techniques. New York: Harper & Row; 1968.
5. Voss DE, Knott M. The application of neuromuscular facilitation in the treatment of shoulder disabilities. Phys Ther Rev 1953;33:536–541.
6. Voss DE. Proprioceptive Neuromuscular Facilitation: The PNF Method. In HE Bouman (ed), An Exploratory and Analytical Survey of Therapeutic Exercise. Baltimore: Williams & Wilkins, 1966;839–898.
7. Sherrington C. The Integrative Action of the Nervous System. New Haven: Yale University Press, 1961.
8. Greenman PE. Principles of Manual Medicine. Baltimore: Williams & Wilkins, 1989;88–100, 150–203.
9. Maitland GD. Vertebral Manipulation (4th ed). London: Butterworth, 1977;82–167.
10. Kaltenborn EM. Mobilization of the spinal column. Wellington, NZ: New Zealand Press, 1970.
11. Blackman J. Manipulation: A Personal View. In GP Grieve (ed), Modern Manual Therapy of the Vertebral Column. New York: Churchill Livingstone, 1986;656–660.
12. Bourdillon JF. Spinal Manipulation. London: Butterworth, 1970.
13. Cyriax J. Textbook of Orthopaedic Medicine (6th ed). Vol. 1. London: Baillière Tindall, 1975.
14. Mennell JM. Back Pain. Boston: Little, Brown, 1960.
15. Mennell JM. Joint Pain. Boston: Little, Brown, 1964.

Chapter 10

Myofascial Considerations in Somatic Dysfunction of the Thorax

Jeffrey J. Ellis and Gregory S. Johnson

Somatic dysfunction is defined as impaired or altered function of related components of the somatic (body framework) system; that is, the skeletal, arthrodial, and myofascial structures and related vascular, lymphatic, and neural elements [1]. The specific identification and timely amelioration of this dysfunction has been the challenge and goal of manual medicine since its inception.

Somatic dysfunction of the thoracic spine and rib cage is ubiquitous in nature with respect to patients complaining of spinal pain and produces a myriad of subjective and objective findings that challenge the clinician to arrive at a concise and accurate diagnosis. In fact, the thoracic vertebral column has been termed "one of the elusive frontiers in spine research" [2]. Recognition of the neuromusculoskeletal and biomechanical attributes and potentials of this region is very helpful in formulating appropriate treatment protocols as well as prognoses. As concepts of vertebral and rib cage motion, both normal and abnormal, are challenged, and even redefined by some [2, 3], increasing attention is being paid to the "driving force" behind this movement—the myofascial system and its potential role in creating and perpetuating somatic dysfunction [4–9].

Long recognized as a potential source of pain in biomechanical somatic dysfunction of the vertebral column [9–15], numerous terms and classifications have been proposed as designates for primary myofascial dysfunction (MFD), including muscular rheumatism [16–18], myalgia [19–21], interstitial myofibrositis [22], myofascial pain syndrome [23], myofaciitis [24–27], and fibrositis [28]. More recently, the myofascial system has received attention because of its causative or primary role in creating biomechanical sources of somatic dysfunction as opposed to its being intrinsically the direct source of pain [5, 6, 29–31].

Myofascial structures are those tissues that are either musculoskeletal (in this case) or connective in makeup and origin. The interrelationship between these tissues and the mechanical dysfunction that can be directly linked to their aberrant function demands the closest attention.

In the thoracic spine and rib cage, structural lesions can be defined through biomechanical nomenclature and include non-neutral type II, FRS (flexed, rotated, and side-bent) or ERS (extended, rotated, and side-bent) dysfunctions of a single vertebral segment; type I, neutral vertebral dysfunctions; and structural, torsional, and respiratory rib cage lesions. The myofascial system frequently provides insight into the identification and causation of underlying somatic dysfunction and presenting symptomatology. Myofascial structures may be observed from four specific perspectives with respect to thoracic spine and rib cage somatic dysfunction (Table 10.1).

First, their diagnostic value should be considered. In the presence of aberrant positional and motion dysfunction of the vertebral column or rib cage, adjacent myofascial structures will often have tissue texture abnormalities. These findings have been de-

Table 10.1. The Role of Myofascial Tissue in the Evaluation, Pathogenesis, and Treatment of Structural Somatic Dysfunction of the Thorax

---

Diagnostic role
    Facilitated segment
    Tissue texture abnormality
Primary motion restrictor
    Cause of structural dysfunction
Use in MET/PNF
    Primary activation force
Source of entrapment/tunnel syndrome
    Myofascial/fiber-osseous tunnels

---

scribed in the osteopathic literature as being consistent with the presence of a "facilitated segment" [1, 32–37]. Korr [34], Mitchell et al. [35], Greenman [1], and others have described the myofascial changes that represent a facilitated segment, including hypertonicity, increased temperature, hyperesthesia, and concomitant fascial dysfunction of the immediate surrounding tissues. These changes are commonly present in the muscles of a single segment of the vertebral column (including the transversospinalis groups located in the anatomic groove between the transverse and spinous process) and of the rib cage (including the levator costae and intercostal muscles). These changes may, however, be analogous to an "idiot light" on a car (e.g., the oil gauge), which when lit, although meriting attention, belies a problem elsewhere. Tissue texture abnormalities in these regions often reflect underlying biomechanical dysfunction and should warrant further investigation. Undue preoccupation with these "lights" and the correlative subjective complaints that accompany biomechanical dysfunction elsewhere, frequently misguide and detract the clinician from formulating an appropriate diagnosis and implementing proper treatment. However, in the presence of a chronic facilitated segment, compensatory myofascial dysfunction may develop, become symptomatic, and warrant treatment in combination with the primary source of dysfunction.

Second, myofascial structures should be recognized for their potential role as primary motion restrictors in somatic dysfunction [7, 38–40]. In the presence of aberrant myokinematics of the thorax with respect to increased muscle tone, deficient muscle play/accessory mobility, changes in strength or neuromuscular responsiveness, and subsequent alteration in functional excursion/length, motion dysfunction of the related articular structures may result. This diminished functional capacity of the correlative articular structures (thoracic vertebral and rib segments) provides the environment for aberrant arthrokinematics, precipitating the occurrence of a cascade of possible chronic, degenerative changes [41].

In addition, because of the initial myofascial dysfunction, the neuromuscular system commonly functions inefficiently and is unable to provide the proper motor control and intrinsic stabilization necessary to protect and produce efficient function at these related segments [42]. This furthers the degenerative cascade through the repeated trauma of inefficient and improper movement patterns, both segmentally (arthrokinematically) and as an entire kinetic chain (osteokinematically).

Third, myofascial tissues are the operational focus during corrective treatment procedures such as muscle energy technique (MET) and proprioceptive neuromuscular facilitation (PNF) techniques. Lever principles (short and long) are used during METs to localize and normalize articular structures. These techniques, however, require tremendous specificity and rely on the presence of normal kinematics of related myofascial tissues for appropriate localization and to be efficacious. Normalization of MFD of these tissues may be required before their utilization in MET.

Finally, consideration must be given to the role myofascial tissues play in entrapment or tunnel syndromes of the neurovascular structures that pass through or reside in the thorax [13, 43, 44]. As they emerge from their origin in the spinal cord and until they reach their effector organs, nerves must pass through bony, fibrous, osteofibrous, and fibromuscular tunnels, where they risk potential compression, damage, and impairment of their end function [45]. Careful assessment of related myofascial tissues in combination with specifically selected neural tension tests [43, 44] will allow specific identification and isolation of causative myofascial dysfunction.

The purpose of this chapter is to recognize the varied influence and diagnostic information the myofascial tissues of the thorax can provide in managing somatic dysfunction of this region. In particular, the reader will be exposed to:

1. The relevant anatomic and biomechanical attributes of the myofascial structures of the thoracic spine and rib cage.

2. An enumeration and correlation of the specific myofascial structures that characterize nonresponsiveness to treatment, or recurrence in thoracic spine and rib cage articular (position/motion) dysfunctions.
3. An algorithmic methodology for evaluating and enumerating specific myofascial structural dysfunction.
4. An organized framework, methodology, and principles for treating myofascial dysfunction.
5. Relevant case studies that demonstrate the effectiveness of addressing myofascial dysfunction in the presence of movement dysfunction of the thoracic spine and rib cage.

Myofascial Tissue

The body is composed of four primary soft tissues: epithelial, muscle, nerve, and connective [46–48]. The interrelationship of muscle and connective tissue (i.e., myofascial tissue) provides for both normal biomechanics, which support static and dynamic activities (9), and pathomechanics in the dysfunctional state.

Connective tissue chiefly comprises ligaments and tendons (regular or dense) as well as aponeuroses, fascia, synovial membranes, joint capsules, and intrinsic elements of muscle (dense and loose irregular) [47, 48]. Continuous throughout the entire body, the fascial system interconnects with tendons, aponeuroses, ligaments, capsules, peripheral nerves, and intrinsic elements of muscle [49].

Connective Tissue: Fibrous Component

Connective tissue may be organized into two distinct components: fibrous and nonfibrous. The fibrous components consist primarily of collagen and elastin fibers. Irregular and regular connective tissues are distinguished by the periodicity and direction of fibers within each. Irregular connective tissue is recognized by its multidirectional fiber orientation, which provides the necessary strength, in all directions, required for structures such as capsules, aponeuroses, synovial membranes, and fascia. Regular connective tissue is distinguished by a uniplanar or linear fiber orientation, which provides the tensile strength required by ligaments and tendons [46–48, 50].

Connective Tissue: Nonfibrous Component

The nonfibrous portion of connective tissue consists primarily of amorphous ground substance, which is a viscous gel composed of long chains of carbohydrate molecules called mucopolysaccharides, known as glycosaminoglycan (GAG), bound to a protein and water (60–70% of net content). Collectively termed proteoglycan aggregate [48, 51], the nonfibrous portion of connective tissue plays a key role in providing a lubricous state in which collagen and elastin fibers can coexist and thrive. In addition, the proteoglycan aggregate provides appropriate spacing, described as critical fiber distance (CFD), between the fibrous elements and is necessary for normal mobility.

Viscoelastic Properties of Connective Tissue

Collagen fibers are relatively inextensible; however, they have the biomechanical attribute of being able to withstand high tensile forces [47, 48]. Fascia is composed of wavy, multidirectional, multiplanar collagen fibers and elastin fibers and is therefore highly extensible as well as strong. Force, or the load applied to the tissue, is defined as *stress*, whereas the tissue deformation realized is termed *strain* [48, 52]. This stress/strain relationship (Fig. 10.1) depicts the viscoelastic response connective tissue undergoes when force is applied and includes the initial toe region elastic, plastic, and, finally, failure ranges. This collagenous elongation or deformation is known as *creep* and occurs through the process of hysteresis (Fig. 10.2) [52–54].

It is through these physiologic and biomechanical properties that soft-tissue mobilization techniques are purported to demonstrate their efficacy. Collagen has in fact been found to realign, strengthen, and orient its fibroblasts and the resulting newly synthesized fibers in response to the type, amount, duration, and frequency of the stress applied [55–57]. In short, newly deposited collagen fibers become oriented in the direction of stress [58–61]. This process of remodeling in accordance with stresses imposed is known as Wolf's Law of C.T. [55–58] and will be a prime consideration in our attempts to influence the connective tissue system with myofascial mobilization technique.

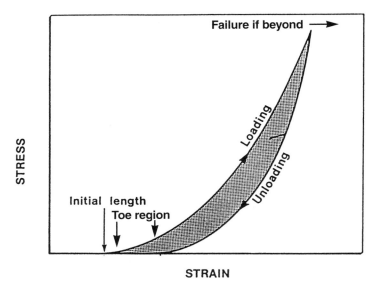

Figure 10.1. Stress/strain curve. This curve demonstrates the viscoelastic behavior and resulting deformation of connective tissue to externally applied stress. (Reprinted with permission from N Bogduk N, LT Twomey. Clinical Anatomy of the Lumbar Spine. New York: Churchill Livingstone, 1987.)

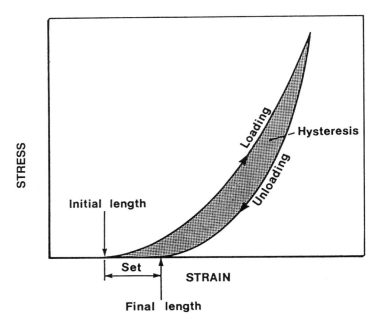

Figure 10.2. Hysteresis. This curve demonstrates tissue deformation with loading and the permanent length changes realized after stress is removed "set." (Reprinted with permission from N Bogduk, LT Twomey. Clinical Anatomy of the Lumbar Spine. New York: Churchill Livingstone, 1987.)

Effects of Immobilization

The effects of immobilization of articular capsules have been well documented [48, 50, 62–64], and the information provided may be extrapolated for use in observing what occurs to other connective tissues including fascia. The chief effects of immobilization are summarized in Table 10.2.

These changes equate to stiffer, harder tissues, a reduction in muscle play and functional elongation, and an overall diminution in fascial mobility secondary to biomechanical aberrancies. Myofascial mobilization efforts are directed at normalizing these aberrancies while keeping in mind the histologic and biochemical reasons for this presentation.

Table 10.2. Effects of Immobilization on Connective Tissue

Reduction in glycosaminoglycan (especially hyaluronic acid, which maintains a high affinity for H_2O
Subsequent reduction in H_2O
Thixotropic state according to dehydration
Increased tissue rigidity and stiffness
Production of abnormal cross-link formation
Decreased and altered spacing between collagen fibers (decreased critical fiber resistance)
Diminished fiber glide
Fatty infiltrate within spaces, which potentially matures to become scar tissue
Random orientation and deposition of newly synthesized collagen fibers

Muscle

Three types of muscles are found in the human body: cardiac muscle; smooth (nonstriated or involuntary) muscle, which lines the hollow internal organs; and skeletal (striated or voluntary) muscle, which attaches to the skeleton via tendons, causes movement to occur and accounts for 40–45% of total body weight [52].

Performing both static and dynamic activities, skeletal muscle, which will be our focus, consists of two basic components: muscle fibers (the contractile component), and connective tissue (the noncontractile component) [52]. The fiber, the structural unit of skeletal muscle, is virtually sheathed in connective tissue, first as a single fiber covered with loose endomysium, then as various sized bundles or fascicles covered with dense perimysium, and finally as muscle bellies covered with epimysium [47].

An intimate relationship exists between the contractile and noncontractile elements of skeletal muscle. The contractile portion provides force production, relaxation, and extensibility, whereas the noncontractile portions provide for space, the lubrication of the contractile elements, and the elasticity required by muscle for appropriate broadening, lengthening, and muscle play.

Numerous authors have written about the histologic and biomechanical effects of trauma and immobilization in the form of microscopic and macroscopic changes to the myofascial unit [63, 65–67]. These dysfunctions include alteration of tone (secondary to impaired peripheral and central innervation); hypertonicity with localized trigger points (contraction) [14]; diminution of motor recruitment and control [39, 41, 68]; a decrease in functional excursion/muscle length secondary to sarcomere loss [62, 66, 67, 69, 70]; diminished accessory motion of connective tissue elements (contracture); and decreased muscle play. It is these microscopic and macroscopic changes that combine to create abnormal tension vectors and levers that alter the normal homeostatic balance that exists in the biokinetic chain.

Myofascial Dysfunction: Contracture/Contraction/Cohesion-Congestion (Fluidochemical)

In the consideration of motion dysfunction of the thoracic spine and rib cage, as well as the entire vertebral column, careful attention must be placed on defining the causative or contributory barriers to normal movement. Three theoretical models for the manifestation of MFD are contracture, contraction, and cohesion-congestion. Elements of each of these categories are presented in Table 10.3.

Table 10.3. Theoretical Models for the Manifestation of Myofascial Dysfunction

Contracture	Contraction	Cohesion-Congestion
Inert/noncontractile	Muscle contraction	Fluidochemical
Capsular/fascial fibrotic	Muscle holding	Edematous/dehydrated
Abrupt/firm end-feel	Hypertonicity/spasm	Boggy/stiff/reactive
Chronic	Acute/distress	Acute/chronic

Contracture

Contracture describes those myofascial structures (particularly connective tissues) that have undergone some degree of fibrotic alteration that makes their end-feel stiffer, harder, and less resilient or elastic, with associated shortening [5, 14, 58]. This may be secondary to various and numerous biomechanical and biochemical causes but yields as its end result specific characteristics including microscopic cross-linking of collagen fibers with diminution of fiber glide; alterations in tissue creep capacities [71]; alterations in tissue layer mobility, resulting in adhesion to underlying myofascial or osseous structures [29]; a change in mobility of intramuscular septum; and posttraumatic scarring. This definition of contracture should be distinguished from other works that classify "contracture" as the sustained intrinsic activation of the contractile mechanism of muscle fibers [72].

Contraction

The classification *contraction* may be used synonymously with spasm and is defined as increased tension with or without shortening of a muscle caused by involuntary motor nerve activity that cannot be stopped by voluntary relaxation [73]. This hypertonicity is usually associated with an increased level of tissue reactivity to palpation and often correlates with articular dysfunction at the same level. The tissue end-feel encountered is described as reactive, firm, painful, and frequently accompanied by increased tissue temperature. In addition, there may be localized signs of inflammation including swelling or edema.

Cohesion-Congestion

Webster's New Collegiate Dictionary [74] defines cohesion as "the act or process of sticking together tightly" and congestion as "to bring together, to concentrate in a small or narrow space." "This category includes macro- and microcirculatory changes affecting fluidochemical transport and exchange (such as altered chemical exchange on a cellular level, impaired lymphatic flow, vascular stasis or ischemia, etc.), and considers various chemical substances which may influence myofascial tissue such as metabolites, electrolytes, hormones, neurotransmit-

ters, neurogenic and nonneurogenic pain mediators, etc." [71]. This category includes those fluidochemical changes related to a diminution in tissue hydration that may go on to provide the foundation for biomechanical dysfunction as a sequela to ground substance dehydration and resulting changes within the fibrous and nonfibrous elements of connective tissue. It also, however, encompasses those situations in which there is an overabundance of tissue hydration with resulting biomechanical alteration.

Myofascial Anatomy of the Thorax

The myofascial tissues of the thorax, although multipurpose, maintain the distinction of providing one overriding function—respiration (Table 10.4). Together, the various tissues of the thoracic wall constitute a strong yet delicately regulated pump or bellows, providing the rigidity capable of resisting surrounding pressure, the mobility that allows active expansion and aspiration of air, and a resilience that imparts properties of elastic recoil [46]. In addition, these muscles act in an orchestrated fashion with the back musculature of the thoracolumbar and cervicothoracic regions to initiate and control functional movements of the thoracic spine and rib cage.

Understanding the anatomic topography and myokinematics of all of these muscles allows their normal and dysfunctional states to be more easily identified and managed. In addition, the pathomechanics of this region secondary to aberrant muscle function may be more commonly attributed to specific dysfunctional myofascial tissues as their anatomic presentation is understood. These muscles are listed topographically and in accordance with their function in Tables 10.4 through 10.10 (for further details, see Chapter 1).

Table 10.4. Muscles of the Thorax

Diaphragm
Intercostales externi
Intercostales interni
Intracostales
Triangularis sterni
Levatores costarum

Source: Adapted from H Gray. Anatomy, Descriptive and Surgical. Philadelphia: Running Press, 1974.

Table 10.5. Topographical/Layer Orientation of the Back Muscles of the Cervical, Thoracic, and Lumbar Spine

First Layer	Second Layer	Third Layer	Fourth Layer	Fifth Layer

Trapezius
Latissimus dorsi
	Levator anguli
	  scapulae
	Rhomboideus minor
	Rhomboideus major
		Serratus posticus
		  superior
		Serratus posticus
		  inferior
		Splenius capitis
		Splenius colli
			Sacral and lumbar
			  regions:
			    Erector spinae
			Dorsal region:
			  Ilio-costalis
			  Musculus accessorius
			    ad iliocostalem
			  Longissimus dorsi
			  Spinalis dorsi
			Cervical region:
			  Cervicalis ascendens
			  Transversalis cervicis
			  Trachelo-mastoid
			  Complexus
			  Biventer cervicis
			  Spinalis colli
				Semispinalis dorsi
				Semispinalis colli
				Multifidus spinae
				Rotatores spinae
				Supraspinales
				Interspinales
				Extensor coccygis
				Intertransversales
				Rectus capitis posticus
				  major
				Rectus capitis posticus
				  minor
				Obliquus capitis inferior
				Obliquus capitis superior

Source: Adapted from H Gray. Anatomy, Descriptive and Surgical. Philadelphia: Running Press, 1974.

The musculature of the back (cervicothoracic, thoracolumbar) must receive equal consideration because it exerts a significant influence on the overall static and dynamic posturing of the thoracic spine and rib cage. Although the postvertebral muscles show little if any rhythmic activity in quiet respiration, their chief function is primarily postural, maintaining erect posture against gravity. Dysfunction of these tissues (i.e., increased muscle tone, decreased play, alteration in strength or neuromuscular responsiveness, or changes in functional excursion) may produce significant postural changes and resultant dysfunction of the rib cage [75]. These muscles may be identified topographically from a larger perspective (see Table 10.5).

Muscles of respiration may also play a key role in the structural, torsional, or respiratory rib dysfunctions (see Chapter 8). These muscles have been categorized as primary and accessory muscles of inspiration and primary and accessory muscles of expiration (see Tables 10.6, 10.7) [11, 76].

Finally, the muscles of the abdomen must be considered because they exert influence on and support for the thoracolumbar region and the rib cage. These muscles are topographically divided into superficial and deep groups (see Table 10.8).

Although not discussed in this text, additional consideration should also be given to the muscles of the

Table 10.6. Muscles of Inspiration

Primary
  Diaphragm
  Levator costarum
  External intercostals
  Internal intercostals (anterior)
Accessory
  Scaleni
  Sternocleidomastoid
  Trapezius
  Serratus anterior and posterior superior
  Pectoralis major and minor
  Latissimus dorsi
  Thoracic spine extensors
  Subclavius

Source: Adapted from HO Kendall, FP Kendall, DA Boynton. Posture and Pain. Huntington, NY: Robert E. Krieger, 1977.

upper extremities, particularly the rotator cuff musculature, because dysfunction of the upper extremity can directly affect the scapula and clavicle and indirectly the rib cage and thoracic spine. Each muscle group of the thorax, back, abdomen, and upper extremity and their related fascial attachments should be considered in somatic dysfunction of this region.

Table 10.7. Muscles of Expiration

Primary
    Abdominal muscles
    Internal oblique, external oblique, rectus abdominis
    Transversus abdominis
    Internal intercostals, posterior
    Transversus thoracis
Accessory
    Latissimus dorsi
    Serratus posterior inferior
    Quadratus lumborum
    Iliocostalis lumborum

Source: Adapted from HO Kendall, FP Kendall, DA Boynton. Posture and Pain. Huntington, NY: Robert E. Krieger, 1977.

Table 10.8. Abdominal Muscles

Superficial
    Obliquus externus
    Obliquus internus
    Transversus abdominis
    Rectus abdominis
Deep
    Psoas major
    Psoas minor
    Iliacus
    Quadratus lumborum

Source: Adapted from H Gray. Anatomy, Descriptive and Surgical. Philadelphia: Running Press, 1974.

Pathomechanics and Sequelae of Myofascial Dysfunction

Kinetic Chain Principles

A kinetic chain is a series of interconnecting segments that affects the position, movement, potential for movement and shock absorption, and attenuation of forces that are transmitted through those segments. Intimately linked and supportive of the skeletal structures, the myofascial tissues play a key role in the way this chain functions.

Myofascial Joints "Above and Below"

The axiom that thorough assessment of an individual articulation demands examination of the immediate articulations above and below the dysfunctional articulation [63] is equally germane to the soft-tissue system. Through a series of direct and indirect attachments or junctions, all myofascial tissues maintain an interrelationship that allows biomechanical influence on one another. Dysfunction in one myofascial structure may have a profound effect on the functional ability of a distant, but related, second myofascial structure.

Gratz's Functional Joint

Gratz defined the space that exists within and between these junctions as well as all structures of the human body as "functional joints" [77]. He went on to define a functional joint as "a space built for motion." From a functional and biomechanical basis, the mobility provided by the presence of this "space" [77] has been designated "muscle play" [29]. This concept will be critical in understanding the subtle yet profound impact that loss of accessory motion within the myofascial structures can have on the entire kinetic chain. The aberrance, or loss of normal "functional joint mobility" as defined by Gratz, should prompt one to consider the mechanical interface that exists between virtually all structures in the body. From a microscopic, cellular perspective to a macroscopic observation of structures such as muscle bellies, fascial sheaths, and underlying bony structures, the available spacing and mechanical interface relationship that exists must be considered, especially when attempting to restore normal mobility to the kinetic chain.

Myofascial Dysfunction in Primary and Compensatory Vertebral and Rib Dysfunction

Of primary importance in determining and sequencing treatment is whether presenting myofascial dysfunction represents the primary cause of a movement dysfunction or is a component of compensatory dysfunction. Primary sources of movement dysfunctions of the vertebral column, classified as type II non-neutral FRS or ERS dysfunctions (see Chapter 8), and of the rib cage, classified as structural, torsional, or respiratory, represent the causative agents of both aberrant position and motion of the involved motion segment. In the vertebral column, unisegmental muscles have been implicated as the possible source of

Table 10.9. Proposed Myofascial Sources of Thoracic Spine and Rib Cage Motion Dysfunction

Myofascial Structure	Potential Structural Dysfunction
Anterior scalenes	Superior subluxation of the first rib segment
	Exhalation restriction
Medial scalenes	Superior subluxation of the first rib segment
	Exhalation restriction
Posterior scalenes	Superior subluxation of the second rib
	Exhalation restriction
Pectoralis minor	Exhalation restriction
	External torsion
Transversospinalis muscles	Type II FRS/ERS dysfunction
Respiratory diaphragm	Inhalation restriction
Quadratus lumborum	Inhalation restriction
	12th rib structural dysfuntion
Serratus posterior superior	Internal torsion ribs 2–4
Serratus posterior inferior	External torsion ribs 9–12
Latissimus dorsi	Exhalation restriction more frequent than inhalation restriction
	Lateral bucket-bail
Serratus anterior	Upper fibers: Inhalation restriction
	Lower fibers: Exhalation restriction, lateral bucket-bail
Internal intercostals (anterior)	Exhalation restriction
External intercostals	Exhalation restriction
Abdominals	Inhalation restriction
Iliocostalis lumborum	External torsion

myofascial dysfunction in primary movement dysfunction. These include the transversospinalis, multifidus, and rotatores muscles [1, 3, 7, 36, 78]. In the rib cage, the anterior and medial scalenes, the levatores costarum, the intercostals, the pectoralis minor, the serratus posterior superior and inferior, the serratus anterior, and the latissimus dorsi muscle groups are common sources of primary movement dysfunction. Specifically, these muscles may contribute to primary vertebral or rib dysfunction by compensatorily shortening (secondary to increased tone-contraction or connective tissue shortening contracture), thereby producing a significant impact on the possibility of structural correction through MET or mobilization efforts alone. Table 10.9 provides a list of muscles and their possible myokinematic influence on thoracic spine and rib cage dysfunction. It must be remembered, however, that the respective tone and length of a muscle do not constitute the only considerations for possible dysfunction; the entire surrounding fascial structures must be considered as well.

In response to type II non-neutral vertebral dysfunction of the thoracic spine and structural rib cage dysfunction, compensatory responses of the vertebral column, described as type I neutral dysfunctions, are expected (see Chapter 8). Spanning three or more vertebral levels with osteokinematic sidebending to one side and concurrent rotation to the opposite side, myofascial dysfunction with adaptive shortening often occurs concomitantly. This is particularly true in cases of chronicity (Fig. 10.3).

These myofascial adaptations frequently include aberrant muscle play and functional excursion/length on the concave side of the type I curve and alteration of neuromuscular responsiveness/strength on the convex side. These compensatory changes typically include multisegmental muscles such as the iliocostalis and longissimus groups. Changes in muscle length, tone, play, or accessory motion responsible for the causation or perpetuation of type I vertebral dysfunctions must be addressed because they often contribute to nonresponsive or recurrent lesions elsewhere in the kinetic chain.

Although type I dysfunction often correlates with concomitant myofascial dysfunction in this region, it may also be related to and demands differentiation from at least 13 other possible causes (see Table 10.10).

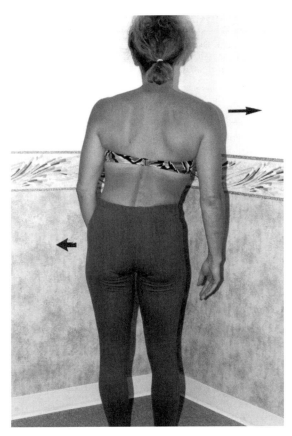

Figure 10.3. Type I neutral dysfunction of the thoracolumbar spine with thoracic sidebending to the left and concurrent rotation to the right.

Sequencing Treatment Strategies

Of paramount importance in determining treatment strategies are the identification and amelioration of myofascial sources of primary movement dysfunction. In the acute phase, these will typically be related to those sources of dysfunction classified as contraction, cohesion-congestion, or both (see Table 10.3) and will be most evident at or immediately adjacent to the dysfunctional vertebral or rib dysfunction. Correction of these dysfunctions should yield immediate changes in both position and motion characteristics of the involved motion segment. In addition, when these dysfunctions are present in the acute phase and are not associated with longstanding myofascial changes, compensatory myofascial dysfunctions (i.e., increased tone, muscle holding, superficial fascial dysfunction) will also normalize.

Equally important, however, is the identification of myofascial dysfunction associated with chronic, compensatory vertebral dysfunction (type I neutral dysfunction), which is often classified as "contracture" in nature (see Table 10.3). Because they are accompanied by adaptive myofascial changes, particularly alteration in muscle length/elongation and play/accessory mobility, failure to address these aberrancies may allow for poor correction of osteokinematic movement dysfunctions (i.e., type II non-neutral vertebral dysfunction or structural rib dysfunction). In addition, failure to normalize the myofascial structures associated with

Table 10.10. Thirteen Causes for the Presence of Type I, Neutral Dysfunction of the Vertebral Column, with Sidebending and Rotation Opposite

Type II nonneutral, vertebral dysfunction (FRS/ERS) below the type I dysfunction
Type II nonneutral, vertebral dysfunction (FRS/ERS) above the type I dysfunction
Subcranial dysfunction (particularly at the O/A articulation)
Rib cage dysfunction (structural or torsional)
MFD of the abdomen
Idiopathic scoliosis
Sacral base unleveling (sacroiliac joint dysfunction)
Innominate or iliosacral dysfunction
Structural leg length assymetries
Functional leg length assymetries (rearfoot pronation/supination deformities)
Adverse neural tension signs, upper extremity
Adverse neural tension signs, lower extremity
Visceral dysfunction

Source: JJ Ellis. LPI—Lumbo-Pelvic Integration, A Course Manual. Patchogue, NY: 1990.

compensatory vertebral dysfunction may provide the "environment" for primary movement dysfunctions to recur (i.e., recurrent tendencies).

Myofascial Assessment: CHARTS Methodology of Evaluation

Evaluation of somatic dysfunction of the thoracic spine and rib cage requires careful attention to detail. The use of an algorithmic approach will help the clinician avoid overlooking the smallest yet perhaps most significant of details. One such approach is the CHARTS methodology of evaluation [6] (Table 10.11). This system builds on the osteopathic evaluative acronym ART, which stands for *a*symmetry of bony landmarks, *r*ange of motion/mobility alteration, and *t*issue texture abnormalities [1, 36, 79]. In the CHARTS model, chief complaints, history (particularly recent biomechanical and systems review), and special tests (e.g., radiologic, blood analysis) are added for thoroughness and precision in arriving at a diagnosis. (See Chapters 3–7 for a thorough discussion of history and special tests.) In addition, tissue texture abnormalities, "T," have been embellished in keeping with this chapter's emphasis of the importance of this area.

Evaluation and General Screening Procedures

Evaluation of myofascial tissues, "T" within the CHARTS methodology, requires consideration of several specific characteristics. These elements are assessed through static, dynamic, and physiologic movement patterns using a layer approach, which assesses tissues from the most superficial to the deepest—i.e., those inserting into bony contours (Table 10.12).

Static Postural Assessment

Static evaluation takes place with the patient standing, seated, prone, supine, and on all fours (quadruped). The evaluative process begins at the moment of initial visual contact with the patient. A keen sense of observation as the patient walks to the evaluative suite and then throughout the static pos-

Table 10.11. CHARTS Methodology of Evaluation

C: Chief complaint
H: Histories
Family history
Social/recreational history
Past medical history
Pharmacologic history
Current history/presenting dysfunction
A: Asymmetries of bony landmarks
Orthostatic postural assessment
Specific spinal/costal/extremity landmarks
R: Range of motion/mobility testing
Osteokinematic spinal/costal/extremity ROM
Arthrokinematic spinal/costal/extremity ROM
Special mobility testing
T: Tissue texture/tension/tonal abnormalities
Skin/fascial layer assessment
Muscle play/accessory mobility
Bony contour assessment
Functional excursion/length
Neuromuscular control/functional strength
S: Special tests
Neurologic screen
Vertebrobasilar clearance testing
Ligamentous integrity testing
Gait assessment
Radiologic screen
Laboratory profiles
Functional capacity/work hardening screen

Source: JJ Ellis. LPI—Lumbo-Pelvic Integration, A Course Manual. Patchogue, NY: 1990.

tural screen will yield much information regarding static and dynamic postures, reactivity levels, muscle guarding/holding, gait deviations, tolerance to certain functional postures (e.g., sitting, standing), and perhaps appropriateness and psychological state. Ideally, the practitioner should provide an environment suitable for patient comfort and privacy, while allowing for unobstructed visual observation from a distance of 8–12 feet. Evaluation suites should be carpeted, adequately heated to allow disrobing, and have lighting arranged to avoid unnecessary shadowing or glare.

The static postural examination often yields valuable information regarding underlying osseous/articular structures as well as asymmetries and aberrancies within myofascial structures. This may directly correlate with altered motion and positional dysfunction within the thoracic vertebral column and

Table 10.12. Myofascial Assessment

A. General screening procedures
   1. Static postural assessment
     a. Skeletal observation
     b. Soft tissue observation
   2. Dynamic postural assessment
     a. Vertical compression testing (VCT)
   3. Physiologic movement patterns
     a. Thoracic movement patterns
     b. Upper extremity movements
     c. Respiratory movements
     d. Functional movement patterns (FMP)
B. Skin and superficial fascial assessment
   1. Palpation
   2. Soft-tissue contours
   3. Skin condition
   4. Skin mobility
   5. Scar tissue
   6. Superficial/deep fascia
C. Bony contours
   1. Thoracic spine
     a. Vertebral segments
   2. Rib cage
     a. Sternum
       i. Manubrium
       ii. Body
       iii. Xiphoid
     b. Clavicle
     c. Rib segments 1–12
   3. Scapula
D. Muscle assessment
   1. Muscle tone
   2. Muscle play/accessory
   3. Muscle length/functional
   4. Neuromuscular control

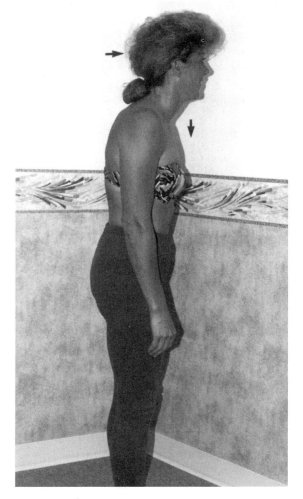

Figure 10.4. Forward head postural dysfunction with accompanying bilaterally protracted shoulders, depressed sternum, and thoracic kyphosis.

the rib cage. An example of this is a patient with forward head posture (FHP), bilaterally protracted shoulders with one greater than the other (the right shoulder in this example), a depressed sternum, and myofascial dysfunction of the pectoralis minor/major muscle complex (right greater than left) (Fig. 10.4).

This aberrant condition of the myofascial structures may be the primary cause of the resulting respiratory, exhalation dysfunction of the third, fourth, and fifth ribs on the right (see Chapter 8). In addition, asymmetric myofascial tightness may directly correlate with type I dysfunction in the thoracic spine.

Skeletal Observation

Beginning with posterior, anterior, and, finally, lateral views, static postural assessment should proceed in a caudal to cranial direction and include careful inspection of both skeletal and soft-tissue structures. Skeletal structures are evaluated with respect to symmetry from side to side and should include observation of aberrant position, spacing, size, and relative support. Anterior and posterior perspectives will provide information regarding skeletal and soft-tissue deviations of the cranioverterbral structures, rib cage, pelvis, and extremities in the coronal plane. Lateral shifts, type I dysfunctions, relative torsional and rotational patterns of the rib cage, pelvis and upper and lower extremities will be visualized in these postures. Lateral perspectives will yield information regarding sagittal deviations and include forward head posture (FHP), excessive cervicothoracic angulation ("dowager's deformity") or diminished, or absent cervical lordosis, sternal and sternomanubrial positions, shoulder posturing (protracted, retracted), rib cage resting position (exhalation, inhalation pattern), thoracolumbar and lumbopelvic angles, and genu recurvatum and/or flexion deformities.

The thoracic spine should have a smooth, uninterrupted curve reflecting a sagittal kyphosis with little or no coronal shift or lateral displacement. Sharp breaks or angulation in this contour often correlate with areas of focal hypermobility [80] and may present with increased muscle hypertonicity in the immediate surrounding tissues. In addition, these areas may reflect the presence of type II vertebral dysfunction or occur at transitional zones between two groups of type I vertebral dysfunction. Flattened areas within the thoracic sagittal kyphosis may relate to areas of hypomobility. Lateral deviations or alteration in the coronal plane may reflect the presence of type I multisegmental dysfunction.

In addition, inspection and side-to-side comparison of the individual relationships of rib segments (including spacing and superior, inferior, anterolateral and posterolateral contours), the scapula, and the clavicle should be considered. Asymmetric contours of the rib cage may yield valuable information regarding underlying somatic dysfunction (respiratory, torsional, or structural) in this region.

Soft-Tissues Observation

Soft tissues are also observed in the static postural screen from the posterior, anterior, and lateral perspectives. Beginning with a global view, the general patterns, types, and contours of soft tissues should be assessed. Initial impressions will often provide the direction of soft-tissue evaluation as central areas of dysfunction are discovered. Soft-tissue dysfunction of the thoracic spine and rib cage often has a proclivity for spiral and diagonal patterns, which course from a central, focal location of somatic dysfunction. These dysfunctions may zig-zag throughout the ki-

netic chain and provide a visual and palpatory link to primary sites of dysfunction. Observations should focus on several characteristics of the soft-tissue system including general contours, girth, muscle mass and development, symmetry from side to side, and three-dimensional relationships including depth, width, height, and length. Specifically, soft-tissue structures are evaluated for the presence of bands, restrictions, adhesions, and depressions within the superficial and deep fascial tissues. These characteristics may yield valuable information regarding underlying or adjacent osseous and articular somatic dysfunction as well as the functional characteristics and movement potential they possess. The presence of asymmetric contours or muscular development may provide valuable information regarding aberrant patterns of use, habitual postures, prior trauma, or improper training emphasis. Bands, contours, adhesions, and restrictions in the superficial tissues, often appearing as depressions or puckering of the dermis or epidermis, may direct attention to the possibility of aberrant superficial and deep fascial tissues, which often accompany or are responsible for underlying vertebral and rib cage dysfunction.

In addition, the examiner should look for and evaluate areas of focal neuromuscular activity or muscle holding because of their role as protective or pain avoidance mechanisms, or as part of aberrant postural or segmental mechanics. This is commonly seen in the scapulocostal region in the presence of forward head posture with abnormal muscle holding/neuromuscular activity of the levator scapulae muscle. In the chronic dysfunctional state, several aberrant static and dynamic dysfunctions may be seen in the sequelae that result from this abnormal muscle holding. These findings include cranial tilt to the ipsilateral side of increased muscle activity, elevated ipsilateral shoulder girdle, altered scapulocostal posturing with possible suprascapular and dorsal scapular nerve entrapment syndrome [43, 81], upper rib cage dysfunction, and upper thoracic spine dysfunction (Fig. 10.5).

Dynamic Postural Assessment

Vertical Compression Testing

Vertical compression testing (VCT) [29] is used to further assess the position, integrity, and force atten-

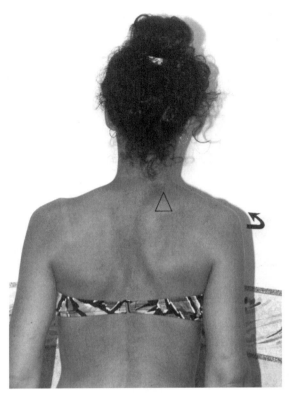

Figure 10.5. Myofascial dysfunction of the right levator scapulae muscle with increased muscle holding (contraction) secondary to postural dysfunction including forward head posture, protracted shoulders, cranial side tilting, and depressed sternum.

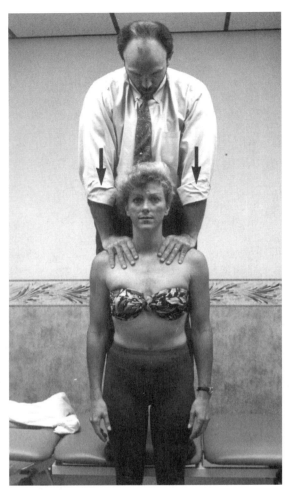

Figure 10.6. Vertical compression testing in the standing posture to assess postural dysfunction including the presence of type I and II vertebral dysfunctions.

uation characteristics of the vertebral column, pelvis, and lower extremities in various weight-bearing postures (i.e., standing and sitting). Aberrant positional dysfunction of the spine (i.e., type I and II) is both palpated and visually magnified through the vertical compression test. In addition, this testing procedure provides kinesthetic feedback to the patient regarding aberrant positional and motion dysfunction by emphasizing malalignment and then serving as positive feedback after correction and retesting. This often proves invaluable in enlisting the patient's support, understanding, and participation in a rehabilitation program.

The VCT is performed with the patient both standing and sitting and is accomplished by applying a gently increasing vertical compressive load through the shoulders and rib cage in a cranial-to-caudal direction (Figs. 10.6 and 10.7). This load may vary from ounces to several pounds as the clinician localizes to various levels of the vertebral column and lower extremity.

Vertical Compression Testing with Somatic Dysfunction

Observation of buckling, shearing, torsion, translation, or exaggeration of type I rotoscoliosis and increases in thoracolumbar kypholordosis should be noted (Fig. 10.8).

Sharp, acute apexes may indicate areas of focal hypermobility/instability and warrant further inves-

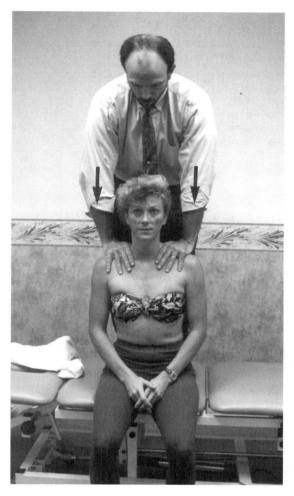

Figure 10.7. Vertical compression testing in the seated posture.

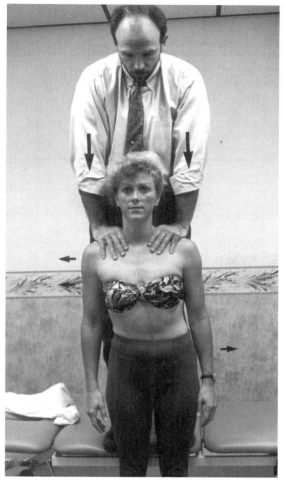

Figure 10.8. Vertical compression testing with shearing to the right secondary to the presence of a type I neutral dysfunction.

tigation (e.g., passive intevertebral motion testing [PIVMT], spring/translational testing and radiologic motion testing). These areas may also be related to type II non-neutral FRS/ERS vertebral dysfunctions and are frequently accompanied by tissue texture abnormalities (including increased muscle tone and decreased muscle play). Finally, these areas may occur at transitional zones in the vertebral column (i.e., cervicothoracic, thoracolumbar, and lumbosacral junctions) or at a rotoscoliotic curve. Left untreated, these areas may become sites of aberrant static and dynamic postural mechanics, resulting in neuromuscular imbalances with altered patterns of functional movement and, ultimately, focal areas of degenerative articular changes.

Although the emphasis of this diagnostic test is objective observation, the patient should also be encouraged to provide subjective feedback regarding symptoms during the procedure. Patients with a history of being "load sensitive" should be evaluated with caution, as this test may be provocational to them.

Physiologic Movement Testing

Dynamic postures used in assessing active range-of-motion (AROM)/combined movement testing include physiologic AROM of the thoracic spine in all planes (i.e., flexion, extension, side-bending, and rotation), AROM of the upper extremities, and respi-

Table 10.13. Observations During Active/Passive, Physiologic Motion Testing, and Functional Movement Patterns (FMP)

Excursion of movement
Quality of movement
Barriers to movement
Coordination of movement
Freedom of movement (both articular and soft tissue)
Substitutions to normal movement patterns
Subjective complaints before, during, and following

Table 10.14. Functional Movement Patterns (FMPs)

Pelvic clock
Unilateral hip rotation in various positions
Quadruped (arch/sag)
Unilateral lower extremity extension in prone
Lower trunk rotation in prone
Diagonal breathing
Sidelying arm circles

ratory patterns of breathing. Combined movement patterns are also performed and include lateral glide/translatory shear and quadrant patterns (i.e., combined flexion, side-bending, and concurrent rotation to the same side followed by extension, side-bending, and concurrent rotation to the same side). Assessment should include observation of both arthrokinematic and myokinematic function throughout each particular movement and should focus on several components (Table 10.13).

Functional movement patterns (FMPs) are defined as any functional motion that may be used to evaluate function, functional capacity, integration of movement segments, differentiation of individual segments, and sequencing of motion including both passive and active ranges of motion [4, 30]. In addition, motor recruitment and neuromuscular control can be assessed throughout the FMP. Aspects of these evaluative movements are derived from the proprioceptive neuromuscular facilitation (PNF) diagonal movement patterns [38, 82] and from the work of Feldenkrais and his Awareness Through Movement (ATM) lessons [83]. These patterns are applicable to both the spine and extremities and are listed in Table 10.14.

Once dysfunctions are identified, treatment is administered during the performance of a portion of or throughout the entire FMP. An example of an FMP, sidelying arm circle, is a pattern that is appropriate for both patients with a cervicothoracic upper quarter dysfunction, and patients with a lumbopelvic lower quarter dysfunction. This pattern is accomplished as follows:

With the patient in the sidelying position, the trunk is stabilized by the inferior hand holding the superior leg while movement occurs through the superior arm scribing the widest circle possible around the axis of the shoulder. In the efficient state, the hand maintains contact with the floor throughout the full arc of motion. This occurs through the orchestrated movement of the shoulder, shoulder girdle, rib cage, and thoracic and lumbar spine. In the presence of restrictions in any of the articulations or soft tissues of this region, hand contact to the floor will be altered, as will the synchronous motion throughout the arc. The practitioner should observe and palpate for specific motion and dysfunctional tissue barriers. Treatment is begun while the patient performs the FMP, moving in and out of the restricted range while soft-tissue mobilization is concurrently performed. During physiologic movement patterns (both passive and active), several variables, including response to treatment, should be observed while concurrently palpating the respective tissues for additional points of restriction and aberrant motion (Fig. 10.9).

Skin Assessment

Palpation

Whereas the observational evaluation is used to identify myofascial structures that may be dysfunctional and contributing to symptomatology, manual palpation is the primary modality used to assess the condition of the myofascial tissues. Developing and refining one's skill in palpation is paramount in both the successful evaluation and the treatment of somatic dysfunction. Specific distinctions of myofascial dysfunction are identified most commonly via digital compression, shear, and specifically appropriated tension on soft tissues. Firm yet gentle pressure should be directed with a specific tissue depth in mind and with a three-dimensional perspective.

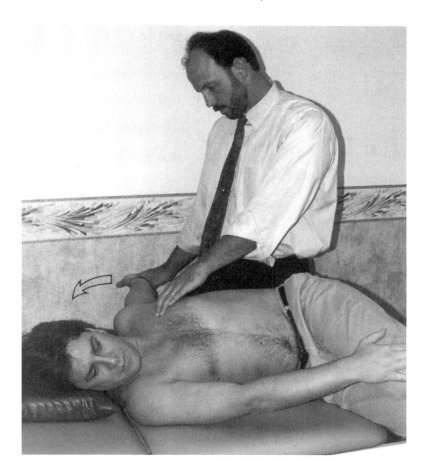

Figure 10.9. Functional movement pattern—arm circles. Performed in a right sidelying position with the inferior arm supporting the superior knee while the superior arm and shoulder are evaluated in a 360-degree circular motion. Myofascial structures are palpated during the entire pattern.

Subtle alterations in tone, excursion, end-feel, fibrous content, contours, reactivity, elasticity, recoil, and response to active contraction and passive lengthening should be assessed. Although emphasis should be placed on objective variables, the patient's subjective response to palpation may also provide insight into biomechanical dysfunction and the relative level of reactivity. Numerous contacts may be used during palpation and include the finger tips, finger pads, thumb, open palm, knuckles, heel of hand, elbow, and forearm. Specifically, the evaluation of myofascial somatic dysfunction of the thoracic spine and rib cage should include careful attention to the components listed in Table 10.15. These elements must be evaluated in both static and dynamic postures (including physiologic, combined movement, and functional movement patterns) and correlated with associated articular dysfunction.

Evaluation of the myofascial tissues should logically begin with the most superficial tissues and

Table 10.15. Elements of Emphasis During Myofascial Examination

Skin mobility
Superficial/deep fascia
Bony contours
Muscle play (accessory mobility)
Muscle tone (hypertonicity/trigger points)
Muscle length/functional excursion
Functional strength/neuromuscular responsiveness

progress inward toward deeper layers. The most superficial tissues include the outer epidermis of ectodermal origin and the deeper dermis of mesodermal origin [8]. The superficial epidermis, the dermis, and the superficial fascia are continuous with the deeper fascia and underlying structures via direct attachment to the basement membrane [47]. Arbitrary compartmentalization of the fascia has been pro-

Table 10.16. Fascial Layers

Dermis/epidermis
Superficial fascial layer
Potential space (between superficial and deep fascial layers)
Deep fascial layer
Subserrous fascia (over body cavities)

Source: Adapted from RF Becker. The Meaning of Fascia and Fascial Continuity. New York: Insight Publishing, 1975.

posed based on anatomic disposition and function [84] and is provided in Table 10.16. The recognition of these layers may assist the practitioner in appreciating the various and varying depths of restrictions during both the evaluation and treatment of MFD.

The skin and superficial tissues of the thorax are assessed with a combination of open palmar and digital contacts (Figs. 10.10 and 10.11) for:

1. Soft-tissue contours, symmetry, bulk, draping, and proportions.
2. Skin condition.
3. Skin mobility, excursion, and recoil.
4. Superficial and deep fascia.

5. Scar tissue mobility, extensibility, and adherence to underlying and surrounding structures.

Contact

Soft-Tissue Contours, Symmetry, Bulk, Draping, Proportions

Visual as well as palpatory evaluation of the myofascial structures will often yield vital information regarding the underlying bony or articular somatic dysfunction. Puckered or adherent myofascial contours commonly accompany muscle play deficiencies and tonal abnormalities. In addition, these may correlate with areas of diminished or altered function such as in the case of long-standing respiratory rib cage dysfunction. This is particularly true of the "key rib" (see Chapter 8). Changes in symmetry, bulk, and proportions frequently occur concurrently with tonal or strength deficiencies and may also reveal chronic, compensatory patterns of movement or function. Observation of how myofascial tissue drapes over its underlying osseous and articular structures may also yield information regarding its relative viability and movement potential in addition to the functional capacity of the immediate associated articular structures.

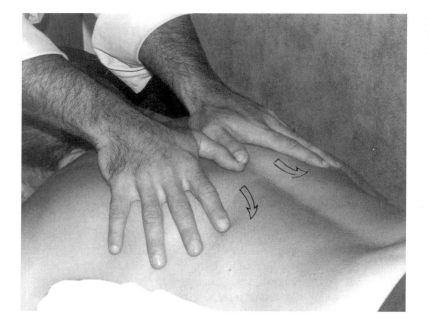

Figure 10.10. Open palmar contact for evaluation of superficial tissues.

Skin Condition

Light palpation of the skin and superficial fascia will reveal much regarding the health and vitality of the tissues being assessed. Tissues should be palpated for their relative dryness, moistness, warmth, coolness, or flaking. Textural abnormalities such as dry, shiny, smooth, or flaking skin will often accompany chronic conditions such as psoriasis, seborrhea, and scleroderma. Elevated skin temperatures with commensurate increases in skin moisture may indicate an active inflammatory process, whereas cool skin temperatures may accompany chronic tissue or articular dysfunction.

Skin blemishes, rashes, moles, and nodules should also be identified. Particular scrutiny should ensue if these alterations are of recent onset, are progressive in nature, or demonstrate adhesions to underlying structures. Subcutaneous nodules or fatty lipomas are common; however, they should be monitored for their role in creating aberrant myofascial kinematics.

Skin Mobility, Excursion, and Recoil

With the patient positioned in the prone and supine positions on an imaginary clock face (i.e., 12 o'clock cranially, 6 o'clock caudally), objective criteria for defining directions of fascial dysfunction are pro-vided. Beginning with a light, open palmar contact, with the hands placed on either side of the vertebral column, tissues are evaluated in a multidirectional fashion with side-to-side comparison. This process is continued in a cranial-to-caudal direction from the cervicothoracic junction to the thoracolumbar junction. Note that complete assessment of the thorax should always include inspection of the cranioverte-bral and upper/lower quarter regions as well; however, this will not be elaborated on in this chapter.

Tissue excursion, end-feel, and recoil of myofascial tissues after digital deformation should be evaluated. Firm, hard, arresting end-feels with diminished recoil often accompany collagenous restrictions with associated alteration in nonfibrous elements (i.e., glycosaminoglycan depletion, dehydration, and resulting thixotropy). These tissue characteristics are consistent with those categorized as contracture and/or cohesion-congestion (see Table 10.3).

A variety of techniques are used to assess changes in the dermis, epidermis, and superficial tissues, including general skin sliding/shearing, finger gliding, and specific-point skin sliding [29] (Figs. 10.12, 10.13, and 10.14). These three techniques allow the examiner to:

1. Identify a "general region" of fascial dysfunction (i.e., left upper posterior quadrant versus right) with general skin sliding/shearing.

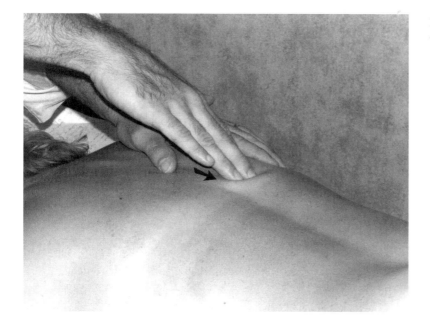

Figure 10.11. Digital contact for evaluation of superficial tissues.

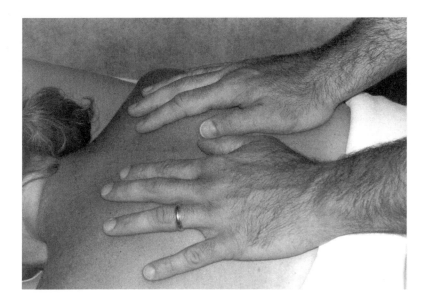

Figure 10.12. General skin slide. Used to localize a "general region," or quadrant, of myofascial dysfunction.

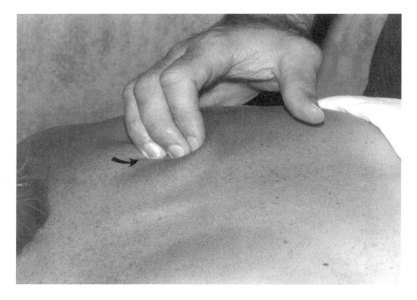

Figure 10.13. Finger glide. Used to localize a "specific site," or epicenter, of myofascial dysfunction.

2. Identify a specific spot or "epicenter" of the restriction within that region with finger gliding.
3. Identify a specific direction of fascial restriction within the restrictive barrier with specific skin sliding.

Superficial and Deep Fascia

Distinguishing between superficial and deep fascial restrictions is vital in establishing and directing ap-

propriate treatment. This is accomplished through a combination of palpatory finesse, angle of inclination of the palpating contact, and varying pressures. Palpatory experience and the skill and tacit information derived through repetition cannot be replaced with even the most eloquent of technical explanations. Determining the existence of myofascial barriers, their direction of restriction, and their exact location in the fascial planes requires much practice. The identification of "depth" is achieved via the angle of inclination the palpating digit or contact as-

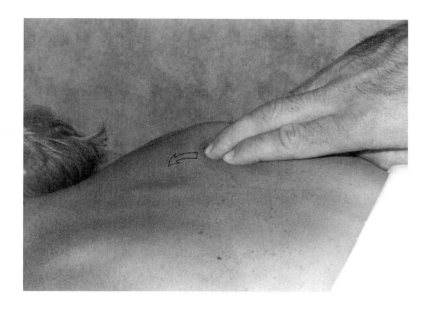

Figure 10.14. Specific skin slide. Used to localize and determine the specific depth and direction of a myofascial dysfunction.

sumes. The more horizontal the contact, the more superficial the tissue being palpated. Shearing tissues in this fashion most often identifies restrictions in the dermis and epidermis. Changing the angle of inclination to a more vertical orientation will allow for greater depth (Figs. 10.15 and 10.16).

In addition, gradually increasing the force used in palpation will provide greater depth. This option, however, should be used last, especially by a novice or inexperienced practitioner. Perceiving that additional force will provide greater proprioceptive feedback is one of the most frequent mistakes in manual medicine. Firm yet gentle compression/palpation will in fact yield the most information and give the least extraneous feedback. Force is, however, an option for depth, and is used to reach deeper fascial structures such as those existing between the septae of the muscle bellies.

Scar Tissue

Scar tissue formation results from major or minor trauma to tissues with similar histologic consequences, albeit differing in severity. Macrotrauma to myofascial tissues may include surgical incisions, traumatic lacerations, and punctures as well as intrinsic muscle and fascial tears. Microtrauma includes repetitive myofascial strain patterns and habituated postures with aberrant function. In both cases an inflammatory process or

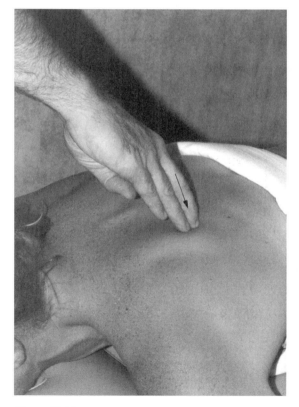

Figure 10.15. Vertical angle of inclination of the mobilizing hand to achieve greater tissue depth and treat deeper structures.

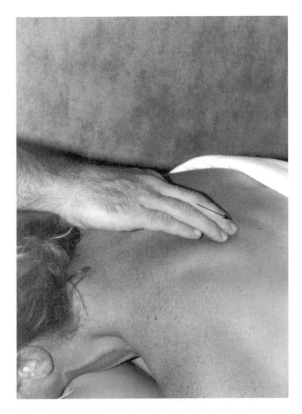

Figure 10.16. Horizontal angle of inclination of the mobilizing hand to achieve access to more superficial tissues.

phase, usually lasting 1–6 days, is followed by a postinflammatory, fibroblastic phase lasting 6–21 days [5, 63, 85]. It is during this fibroblastic phase that a proliferation of newly synthesized collagen fibers occurs with a degree of randomness. "Crosslinking" of normal collagen fibers may occur, dramatically reducing the normal "fiber glide" and therefore the mobility of the implicated tissues. Hollingshead [50] remarked that aberrance of myofascial mobility secondary to scar tissue formation ". . . may be a major factor in altering the biomechanics of the whole kinetic chain, placing strain on all related structures." This strain or altered biomechanics can have profound effects on the subtle arthrokinematics of the rib cage and thoracic vertebra and may be implicated in the primary motion restriction present in respiratory/structural lesions and type II non-neutral and type I neutral vertebral lesions. In addition, abnormal patterns of stress caused by adherent and inextensible scar tissue may contribute to chronic inflammatory disorders and perpetuate symptomatology [62–64]. Remodeling

of these newly synthesized fibers in an organized, mobile framework is critical to regaining extensibility and dynamic function at the associated motion segments as well as the entire kinetic chain.

Scar tissue is assessed by appreciating and observing:

1. Stage of healing/reactivity.
2. Intrinsic mobility of the scar (in all planes).
3. Dissociation from adjacent and underlying structures.
4. Influence of scar tissue on osteokinematic motion patterns of related articular segments.

As with skin mobility, assessment is accomplished by shearing tissues in multiplanar directions to determine barriers to movement, directions of those barriers, and quality of end-feel.

Assessment of Bony Contours

The assessment of myofascial tissues as they insert and anchor into the periosteum of the spine and extremities provides information regarding the deepest myofascial structures. The significance of these structures has been noted, since a "great deal of spinal pain may well be felt where muscle, tendon, ligament and capsule are attached to sensitive periosteum of the spine" [86].

Bony contours are evaluated via digital palpation, which proceeds along the osseous structure in a parallel or longitudinal manner. Restrictive barriers, increased tone, and adhesions between adjoining structures are noted as attention is given to the depth and direction of the tissue barrier evaluated. As with superficial tissues, increased depth is accomplished by increasing the angle of vertical inclination of the palpating digit or by increasing force. Table 10.17 identifies the key bony contours that should be evaluated in the thoracic spine and rib cage.

The assessment of bony contours also provides vital information regarding the positional dysfunction of those osseous structures. Aberrance of myofascial tissue and the related position of associated osseous structures should be correlated with motion testing (see CHARTS Method of Evaluation). This is particularly applicable in the rib cage, where structural rib dysfunction will most commonly appear with positional alterations as well as accompa-

Table 10.17. Assessment of Bony Contours

I. Supine
  A. Sternum
    1. Manubrium
    2. Body
    3. Xiphoid
    4. Sternoclavicular joints
    5. Sternorib joints
    6. Costochondral joints
    7. Anterior ribs 1–12
  B. Clavicle
    1. Superior, inferior, anterior
II. Sidelying
  A. Scapula/lateral aspect
  B. Humerus
  C. Lateral ribs
  D. Iliac crest
III. Prone
  A. Vertebral column
    1. Spinous process
    2. Posterior arch
    3. Transverse process
  B. Posterior ribs
  C. Scapula/posteromedial aspect

nying myofascial dysfunction or tissue texture abnormalities. Bony contour, myofascial abnormalities in this region commonly include the intercostal muscles circumferentially, the thoracic fibers of the iliocostalis lumborum muscle posteriorly (especially at its insertion into the rib angle) [53], and the soft-tissue attachments at the posterior costotransverse and the anterior sternocostal articulations of a dysfunctional rib or ribs (Fig. 10.17).

Laterally, the attachment of the latissimus dorsi and serratus anterior muscles become common sites of bony contour abnormalities, especially in the presence of respiratory exhalation dysfunctions. This is particularly common on the superior surface of the key rib (see Chapter 8) or with chronic laterally elevated lesions. Anteriorly, the sternum, sternal manubrial, and costochondral junctions should be carefully assessed (Fig. 10.18).

Other common areas of bony contour abnormalities include the inferior border of the clavicle (with structural or respiratory dysfunction of the first rib), the inferior border of the costochondral arch (with

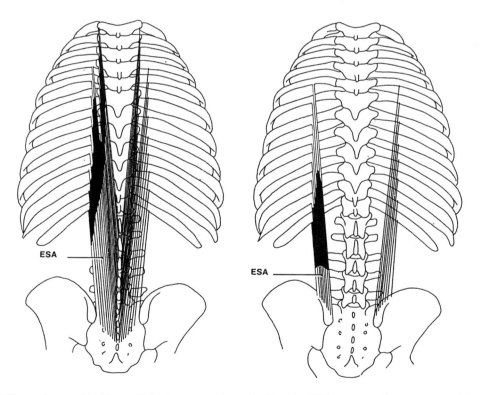

Figure 10.17. Attachment of the iliocostalis lumborum muscles to the rib angle. (ESA = erector spinae aponeurosis.) (Reprinted with permission from N Bogduk, LT Twomey. Clinical Anatomy of the Lumbar Spine. New York: Churchill Livingstone, 1987.)

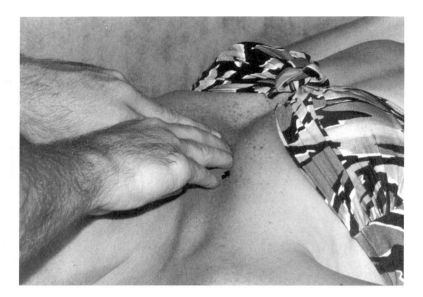

Figure 10.18. Bony contour assessment of the sternomanubrial junction.

respiratory inhalation dysfunction), and the existing groove formed between the spinous and transverse processes (i.e., the posterior arch/lamina of the thoracic spine) in the presence of type II, non-neutral vertebral dysfunction. Left untreated, this myofascial dysfunction may contribute to nonresponsive rib cage and/or vertebral dysfunction, especially when treated with an approach relying predominantly on an articulation-driven methodology (i.e., joint mobilization, manipulation techniques).

In addition, careful palpation of the bony contours will often provide vital diagnostic information, because key tissue texture abnormalities coinciding with thoracic vertebral or rib cage dysfunction are identified.

Muscular Assessment

Thorough assessment of the myofascial structures of the thorax should include evaluation of four characteristics or qualities of these structures including muscle tone, muscle play [29] or accessory mobility, functional excursion or length, and neuromuscular responsiveness and control (Table 10.18).

Muscle Tone

Muscle tone is evaluated with respect to the resting tonus of adjacent and contralateral myofascial struc-

Table 10.18. Muscle Assessment

Muscle tone
Muscle play/accessory mobility
Muscle length/functional excursion
Neuromuscular responsiveness and control

tures. Aberrance of muscle tone typically presents with increased density or hardness, tissue that is reactive or tender to touch, and often with a typical and reproducible pattern of referred pain [4, 14]. An epicenter of maximal density should be noted and will be the focal point of treatment. These epicenters are often found in myofascial tissue adjacent to and directly correlated with underlying articular dysfunction and act as diagnostic tissue texture abnormalities. This is particularly true in the case of type II non-neutral vertebral dysfunction (the multifidus and rotatores muscles) and with structural or torsional rib cage dysfunction (iliocostalis and intercostal muscles).

Muscle Play

Muscle play or accessory myofascial mobility is related to the amount of intrinsic mobility a muscle and its related noncontractile elements demonstrate in relationship to their surrounding osseous, myofascial, articular, and visceral structures. This mobility is assessed both through passive motion testing and dur-

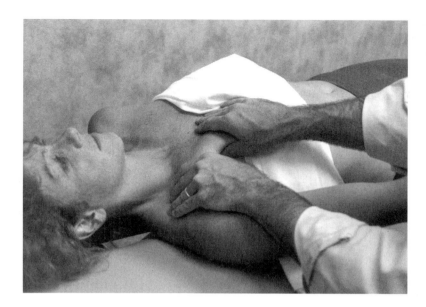

Figure 10.19. Perpendicular deformation of the pectoralis minor muscle with bilateral thumb contact to evaluate medial-lateral, lateral-medial muscle play.

ing functional movement patterns of excursion or lengthening, as well as during the shortening and broadening of fibers associated with muscle contraction. Passive motion testing is accomplished through perpendicularly directed forces (thumbs or tips of digits) described as a perpendicular/transverse deformation, and through "strumming techniques," which assess mobility in two planes [29] (Fig. 10.19).

The ability to shear muscles freely from their adjacent and underlying structures, as well as the ability to move in an uninterrupted fashion through the septae of muscle groups, is evaluated with these techniques. Specific sites, depths, directions, and degrees of restrictions should also be noted. In addition, related thoracic and costal segments and their mobility should be considered, because muscle play restrictions frequently accompany and precipitate somatic dysfunction in these regions. This is commonly seen in the rib cage between the pectoralis major, the pectoralis minor, and underlying costal segments 3, 4, and 5. Aberrant muscle play between the pectoralis major and minor muscles, or between the deeper pectoralis minor muscle and the rib cage, creates abnormal tension in the costal segments and commonly provides an environment for respiratory rib cage dysfunction. Other specific key muscle groups of the thorax that require careful assessment for muscle play abnormalities are provided in Table 10.19.

Table 10.19. Muscle of Emphasis in Muscle Play Assessment of the Thorax: Muscle Play/Accessory Mobility

Spinalis/longissimus/iliocostalis
Pectoralis major/minor complex
Rotator cuff muscles
Serratus anterior/posterior (superior/inferior)
Latissimus dorsi
Trapezius/levator scapulae
Intercostals
Respiratory diaphragm
Quadratus lumborum
Abdominals
Psoas major/minor

Functional Excursion

Functional excursion is the ability of an individual muscle to lengthen as it concomitantly narrows, as well as its ability to broaden as it simultaneously shortens. The importance of balance and symmetry with respect to excursion and length of agonist and antagonist muscle groups has been clearly identified in patients suffering from low back pain [87–89]. Tightness or diminished functional excursion in paired muscle groups (i.e., bilateral hip flexors, hamstrings, paraspinal muscle groups) are viewed as potentially contributory to aberrant static posture and

Table 10.20. Functional Excursion Axiom

With *symmetrical* muscle tightness *be aware...*
With *asymmetrical* muscle tightness *beware.*

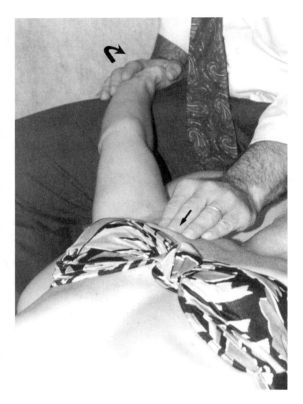

Figure 10.20. Evaluation of functional excursion with concurrent palpation of the pectoralis major muscle to identify specific dysfunctional tissue barriers.

warrant investigation. These deficiencies may result in an accentuation of sagittal plane, primary and secondary curves (i.e., cervical/lumbar lordosis, thoracic kyphosis), and the development of postural dysfunctions such as forward head posture (FHP), cervical and thoracic dowager's deformity, and thoraco-lumbar kypholordosis. Asymmetric tightness or loss of functional excursion in paired muscle groups, however, demands the utmost of evaluative scrutiny. This is chiefly because asymmetric muscle length in paired groups may create alteration in the coronal plane with rotational or torsional forces imposed on the pelvis, vertebral column, and rib cage. These forces may result in the presence of non-neutral mechanics in the vertebral column and the increased risk of myofascial and articular dysfunction. An axiom to follow when evaluating functional excursion is presented in Table 10.20.

Muscles are evaluated by taking their associated sites of origin and insertion through patterns of movement that functionally lengthen the appropriate tissues. As all osteokinematic movements in the extremities occur in curvilinear or elliptical arcs, movements should be directed with care and consideration for these pathways. Osteokinematic motions should include straight planar (i.e., sagittal, coronal) patterns of movement as well as combined patterns to create functional, diagonal patterns. In addition, movements should be performed with careful observation given to barriers of increased resistance within an overall range of excursion. Total range may belie minute yet significant restrictions in the myofascial unit and only be identified through visual and palpatory means during actual functional excursion.

Functional excursion should also be assessed through active and resisted movements where possible. Palpation of relative muscle bellies and musculotendinous and tenoperiosteal junctions should be performed throughout movements of functional excursion to identify specific points or sites of maximal restriction. These sites will frequently be the starting place for treatment (Fig. 10.20).

Neuromuscular Responsiveness and Control

Neuromuscular responsiveness consists of the initiation, control, recruitment, strength, timing, and endurance, among other qualities, of a myofascial tissue [82]. These components are critical in achieving proper function of the related articular structures and kinetic chain as a whole. This is particularly true in the case where the chronicity of somatic dysfunction has significantly affected the neuromuscular attributes of the myofascial tissues associated with articular dysfunction.

Assessment of the neuromuscular responsiveness and control of a myofascial tissue can be accomplished through the use of proprioceptive neuromuscular facilitation (PNF) patterns [38, 39, 82]. In the thoracic spine and rib cage, shoulder and pelvic girdle patterns (Table 10.21) are a valuable tool for both evaluation and treatment strategies. Guidelines for effective monitoring and administration of these patterns are also provided (Table 10.22).

Table 10.21. PNF Patterns of Assessment for Neuromuscular Responsiveness and Control

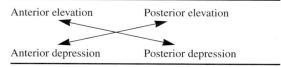

| Anterior elevation | Posterior elevation |
| Anterior depression | Posterior depression |

Source: Adapted from G Johnson, V Saliva. PNF-I: The Functional Approach to Movement Reeducation. San Anselmo, CA: The Institute of Physical Art, 1987.

Table 10.22. Guidelines for Effective Administration and Monitoring of PNF Patterns

Provide complete tension at lengthened ROM without strain to cervical or thoracic components.

Allow minimal trunk motion during pattern.

Motion should remain in a straight diagonal with an arc component.

Motion proceeds from a superior to inferior, anterior to posterior direction, or vice versa.

The head of the humerus should cross the midline.

Source: Adapted from G Johnson, V Saliva. PNF-I: The Functional Approach to Movement Reeducation. San Anselmo, CA: The Institute of Physical Art, 1987.

Principles of the Treatment Approach

Management of somatic dysfunction of the thoracic spine and rib cage requires a multifaceted, eclectic approach with careful attention paid to the objective findings enumerated in the evaluative process. In addition, several guidelines for treatment may be helpful in directing both the novice and experienced practitioner. These guidelines are provided in Table 10.23.

Be Guided by Objective Findings

Treatment must always be guided predominantly by objective findings rather than subjective presentations. Pain in the thorax is most ubiquitous and confusing, because virtually all somatic structures possess at least three spinal levels of innervation [53, 90]. In light of this, applying treatment with a palliative methodology based on subjective direction by the patient is most futile. In addition, differentiation of the various pain presentations (i.e., superficial spondylogenic, deep spondylogenic, neurogenic, radicular, viscerogenic, psychogenic), although possible and important, will provide little in the way of treatment direction. Instead,

Table 10.23. Treatment Guidelines

Be guided by objective findings rather than subjective complaints.

Treat motion dysfunction versus positional dysfunction.

Sequence treatment in order of maximal motion loss according to dysfunctional tissue end-feel or barrier.

Never barge a barrier; however, once "one has a foot in the door, never lose it."

Use the least force possible to effect the desired change.

Clear compensatory somatic dysfunction following primary dysfunctions to avoid recidivism.

Reevaluate following each procedure ("onion skin concept").

Source: JJ Ellis. LPI—Lumbo-Pelvic Integration. A Course Manual. Patchogue, NY, 1990.

the manual practitioner should trust in the observation and identification of specific and reproducible objective findings (i.e., positional and motion).

Treat Motion Dysfunction Versus Positional Dysfunction

Because function follows form and form is determined by function, it is imperative that treatment be guided toward the restoration of appropriate motion and not be guided by apparent positional findings in and of themselves. Positional findings frequently present as the end-result of aberrant myofascial function. In addition, the presentation of aberrant positional findings in the absence of motion loss may belie bony anomalies with relatively normal arthrokinematics.

Sequence Treatment in Order of Maximal Motion Loss

Although numerous axioms and strategies for treatment progression exist in the osteopathic literature [1, 35, 36], perhaps the most significant driving principle is the administration of treatment through a sequence that identifies the areas of maximal motion loss in accordance with dysfunctional tissue end-feels. This may include myofascial, articular, and, at times, visceral structures. This is particularly true in the thorax, where the rib cage provides attachment for numerous myofascial and visceral structures that often provide the primary barrier in motion restriction. Departure from a traditional progression is often warranted in this area because the costal segments and their associated myofascial structures, particularly where chronicity prevails, provide an environment for aberrant function of the thoracic vertebral segments. An example of this is the case where both a type II non-neutral ERS dysfunction and an external rib torsional dysfunction exist concomitantly. In accordance with the traditional biomechanical model, the thoracic vertebral dysfunction would be addressed first because this is seen as primary and the cause of the associated external torsion dysfunction [1, 35, 36]. This, however, may not be the most judicious approach, especially where chronicity prevails. In this example, the costal segment's chronic aberrant position is frequently associated with significant myofascial dysfunction of the related intercostal muscle groups and related connective tissue. Attempting to address the thoracic vertebral segment first may not only prove unsuccessful, but may with repeated attempts create iatrogenically induced instability in the costovertebral and costotransverse articulations. The costal segment, acting like an anchor (secondary to MFD), provides an environment where correction of the thoracic vertebral dysfunction is unattainable until an environment (of the myofascial tissues) is provided in which correction can occur and be maintained. Departure from previously learned sequences that emphasize articular technique is not only prudent in this case, but necessary if success is desired. However, a combined articular technique that addresses the costovertebral and costotransverse articulations is often effective (see Chapter 9).

Never Barge a Barrier

The application of manual therapy procedures, particularly in the myofascial tissues, demands the utmost of sensitivity and respect for patient tolerance. Aside from recognition of a tissue's reactivity and its relative stage of repair (i.e., inflammatory, fibroblastic, or remodeling stage), the patient's tolerance of treatment depth and progression must be considered. This is particularly true in the presence of increased muscle holding or tonicity. Progression of treatment must be accomplished with acute awareness of the patient's response to treatment. As the attainment of increased depth is attempted through subtle yet progressive tissue deformation, the patient's response should be carefully monitored, both verbally and somatically. Progression or depth should never substitute for pa-

tient tolerance and comfort. Once additional depth or "ground" is achieved, however, all attempts should be made to maintain that ground, keeping in mind the adage, "never pay for the same real estate twice."

Least Force Possible

The implementation of actual technique should be delivered with the least physical force possible to effect the desired somatic change. This necessitates an exacting diagnosis, enumeration of specific myofascial and articular findings, the identification of specific barriers (i.e., depth, degree, direction), and the precise localization of those barriers. Treatment should be directed at these specific barriers, with increased force being reserved as a last option. The angulation of hand contacts, use of an assisting hand, position of the body part being treated (i.e., shortened or lengthened position), and the use of associated oscillatory motions are alternative strategies that should be considered before increased force is used. Communication between the patient and practitioner will prove valuable as the patient is encouraged to assist in both the identification of the barriers and in the process of mobilizing soft tissues. In addition, patients are encouraged to report subjective changes experienced during the treatment process. This will aid them in localizing and treating these same restrictions in their own home program.

Clear Compensatory Somatic Dysfunction

Effective management of somatic dysfunction of the thoracic spine and rib cage requires thorough assessment of and amelioration of compensatory dysfunctions that exist concomitantly with the primary dysfunction. According to the biomechanical model methodology, this compensatory dysfunction may respond and correct itself concurrently with the normalization of the primary dysfunction. However, where chronicity prevails, such compensatory dysfunctions (particularly myofascial) may require specific attention. In addition, compensatory dysfunction, especially where it is associated with myofascial dysfunction, may create an environment where normalization of primary dysfunction will not occur, or where there exists a predilection for a recurrence of that dysfunction. This is seen in a patient with a chronic type II non-neutral FRS right dysfunction of T5 with a compensatory neutral type I rotoscoliosis above at T1–T4 (side-bent to the left, rotated to the right), cervical spine side-bending to the right, and subcranial sidebending back to the left. With attention focused on correction of the type II FRS dysfunction and then the thoracic type I dysfunction, the cervical and subcranial dysfunctions often are left untreated. Myofascial dysfunction of this region may provide an environment of altered posturing in the coronal plane and for non-neutral mechanics to dictate in the upper thoracic region. Although type I neutral dysfunctions are not commonly recognized as the primary dysfunction, in this case, they may provide the biomechanical prerequisites for recurrence of the type II dysfunction.

Re-Evaluate After Each Procedure

An axiom for all manual therapy procedures includes re-evaluating after each corrective procedure. Because this therapeutic intervention is "corrective versus palliative" in definition and intent, objective variables defined in the evaluative process must be continually reassessed. The normalization of myofascial dysfunction associated with vertebral and rib dysfunction frequently has profound effects on the overall presentation of that somatic dysfunction. Evaluation should focus on the positional and motion characteristics of the region being treated and include palpation of related bony landmarks and myofascial structures and the administration of one or two relative motion tests. Although re-evaluation should include the monitoring of subjective complaints, an emphasis should not be placed on this in the re-evaluation.

Principles of Myofascial Techniques

The successful administration of soft-tissue mobilization (STM) requires a keen sense of both patient and tissue response. This response is monitored through a variety of senses, including sight, palpation, and auditory feedback. Constant reassessment and adjustment of contacts, including localization, duration, and force, as well as patient positioning and assistance with the treatment technique are required for a successful outcome. In addition, a variety of soft-tissue mobilization techniques and

strategies by which to implement them contribute to the success in this endeavor.

Contacts

Numerous contacts may be used during STM and commonly include the tips of the digits, the thumb, the pisiform, the open palm, the forearm, and the elbow. Determination of which contact is used depends largely on practitioner comfort, the body part being worked on, and the dexterity and skill of the practitioner administering treatment.

Depth

Localization of the treatment contact to the dysfunctional tissue barrier is imperative for success in myofascial mobilization. Barriers must be engaged with respect to tissue depth and direction of the restriction, with localization maintained throughout the technique. Depth is obtained through the judicious use of force, contact angulation (vertical versus horizontal), and the positioning of associated myofascial tissues in a shortened position. Angulation of the contact will determine the depth of a technique and should always be used before increasing force. As with the evaluative process, the more vertical the orientation of a contact, the greater the depth achieved. Positioning adjacent soft tissues in a shortened position decreases tissue turgor and tension and will allow greater penetration. Identification and maintenance of appropriate tissue depth often proves most challenging for practitioners new to STM; however, they are critical for success. Relocalization to the new barrier must occur throughout each specific technique.

Duration

In accordance with the viscoelastic properties of connective tissue, there is a specific time dependency for the elongation of collagen and elastin fibers [48, 52]. This time may vary depending on the viability and conditions of the soft tissues being treated. Various clinicians have attempted to outline specific time frames for treating a specific myofascial restriction. These range from 10 seconds to 90

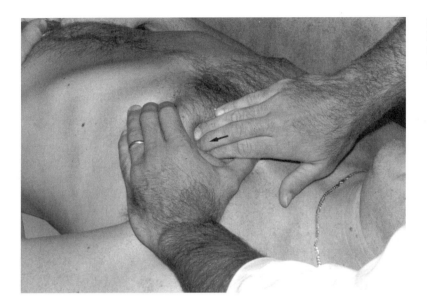

Figure 10.21. Soft-tissue mobilization of the superficial clavipectoral fascia in a shortened position.

seconds [29, 30, 79, 91]. Perhaps a more functional approach, and the one we endorse, is to apply treatment while concurrently evaluating and assessing the response of the treated and surrounding soft tissues. Instead of dogmatically assigning a time constraint on treatment, duration is based more dynamically on ongoing tissue response. Changes in tissue density (i.e., softening, elongation), turgor, tone, and elasticity (particularly with respect to endfeel) are noted as significant and warrant continued efforts. If after two to three attempts with a particular technique no noticeable change is perceived, consideration should be given to other sources as being primary or causative.

Force of Technique

As with most manual therapy procedures, force is never a substitute for accuracy or specificity of localization or for an appreciation of ductile (time dependant) properties of myofascial tissue. In STM, forces used should be only those that allow for dysfunctional tissue barriers to be engaged and corrected in accordance with their time-dependent nature of motion. Force should also be sufficient enough to maintain engagement of a barrier throughout the technique. As elongation or softening of a dysfunctional tissue barrier is perceived, the path of release should be followed.

Patient Positioning

Patient positioning should incorporate positioning the involved tissues and respective body parts in one of three static positions—resting neutral, shortened range, or lengthened range—and through various dynamic postures.

Static Postures

In the resting, prone-neutral position, the lumbopelvic girdle is in a soft lordotic position with a pillow or towel under the abdomen. The shoulders are supported to eliminate protraction, while the forehead (i.e., the table face cutout is used) and the ankles are supported. The emphasis is on attaining an environment of comfort, while reducing the cervicothoracic and thoracolumbar curves.

In the shortened position, respective tissues are placed in a slackened range by altering the surrounding tissue (at the same level) or through the positioning of a related bony or articular segment. This strategy provides an environment that dampens the feedback from surrounding myofascial structures and often allows the most efficacious palpation of the dysfunctional tissue barrier (Fig. 10.21).

Treatment with tissues in the shortened range is followed by progressing to the resting neutral position and finally into the lengthened range. In the

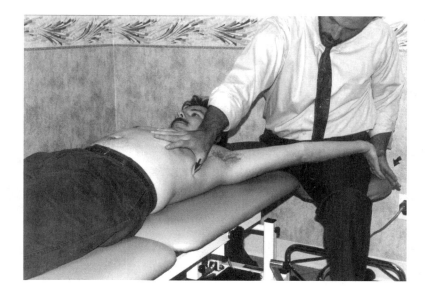

Figure 10.22. Parallel soft-tissue mobilization technique to the latissimus dorsi muscle group in a lengthened range.

lengthened range, respective tissues are placed in a position of increased tension or length by altering the surrounding tissues (at the same level) or a related bony or articular segment (Fig. 10.22).

This strategy attempts to maximize and concentrate surrounding tissue tension forces to the dysfunctional tissue barrier. Treatment progression most often concludes with the lengthened range and should be used to ascertain complete resolution of the myofascial dysfunction. These postures may be assumed through the use of such props as pillows, wedges, physio or Swiss balls, and adjustable, sectioned tables.

Dynamic Postures

Treatment of any myofascial tissue should include the use of both static and dynamic postures. As with assessment, treatment may be accomplished during dynamic movement patterns of the trunk or related extremity and should include engagement of the dysfunction tissue barrier, maintenance of localization and mobilization force throughout the movement, and a progressive increase in the tolerable amplitude of movement. These movements may include classic osteokinematic motions, or they may incorporate passive, associated oscillations of the trunk or body part. These oscillations, produced through a rhythmic rocking, most commonly at the

pelvis, shoulder, or rib cage, may be inhibitive, if slow and rhythmic, or facilitory, if fast and erratic.

Patient Assistance

When appropriate, patients should be actively involved in the treatment process. This is accomplished in several ways. The patient may be asked to contract or relax an area, provide appropriate resistance (isometric, concentric, eccentric), or to provide assistance through alternative methods such as inhalation/exhalation and coughing efforts. Each of these options provides an opportunity for greater localization of forces and more effective mobilization of dysfunctional tissue barriers. In addition, when effective, patients are encouraged to use similar strategies in their home programs.

Selected Myofascial Mobilization Techniques

During the application of STM, both hands of the practitioner participate, with one designated as the mobilizing or treating hand and the other as the assist hand. This allows for specificity of localization and the option of dynamically lengthening or shortening surrounding tissues, as well as incorporating associative oscillatory forces. A variety of specific mobilization forces are available for use with the

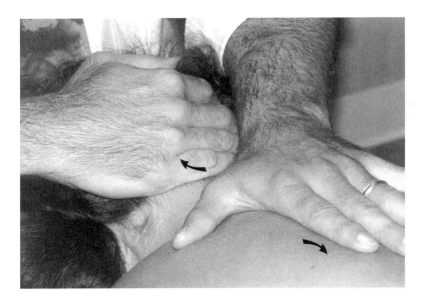

Figure 10.23. General soft-tissue mobilization technique to the superficial fascia of the posterior cervicothoracic junction.

mobilizing or treating hand, while the assisting hand controls the immediate tissue environment. The mobilizing hand is used to engage the dysfunctional tissue barrier through a pushing force (push) or a pulling/hooking force (pull). These mobilization forces are directed at the site of maximal restriction and may be delivered as sustained pressure, a perpendicular mobilization effort, end-range oscillation, a strum, or parallel mobilization technique [29].

General Junctional Release Techniques

Type II non-neutral vertebral dysfunctions and accompanying rib dysfunctions demonstrate a predilection for occurring at junctional areas of the vertebral column (i.e., occipitoatlantal, cervicothoracic, thoracolumbar, and lumbopelvic junctions). Myofascial dysfunction is also frequently encountered at these levels. General junctional release techniques provide a quick screen and clearance approach to the skin and the superficial and deep fascia of these regions before MET or mobilization efforts are used. Treatment consists of contacting the region with a bilateral, open palmar contact paravertebrally or in a cranial-to-caudal orientation, and then engaging the superficial or deep dysfunctional tissue barriers. This is accomplished through gentle compression, shearing tissues into the greatest restrictive barrier, and finally adding clockwise or counterclockwise rotation of the hands. Maximal tissue tension is maintained as both hands continue to shear in the direction of the dysfunctional tissue barrier. This approach is used posteriorly at the cervicothoracic and thoracolumbar junctions, and anteriorly at the clavipectoral tissues and the cervicothoracic/sternomanubrial junction (Figs. 10.23, 10.24, and 10.25).

Sustained Pressure

Sustained pressure involves engaging the dysfunctional tissue barrier (most commonly through the use of the distal tips of the digits) while carefully monitoring depth, direction, and degree of restriction, and maintaining a static force against the restriction until a change in density or length is perceived. This technique is primarily used for muscle tone problems; however, it is effective for myofascial play dysfunction as well. Patient participation is encouraged (especially when treating muscle tone problems) through the use of biofeedback-like techniques including controlled breathing, visual imagery, and active contraction/relaxation techniques. With the epicenter of the dysfunction tissue barrier engaged, the patient is encouraged to gradually inhale, further engaging the barrier, while pressure is maintained. During exhalation, the new barrier is engaged without provoking a localized response of pain or an increase in tone (Fig. 10.26). This is repeated until muscle tone is normalized.

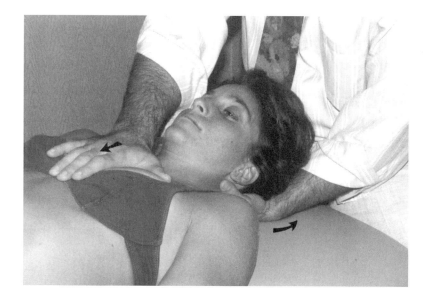

Figure 10.24. General soft-tissue mobilization technique to the superficial fascia of the anterior cervical thoracic/sternomanubrial junctions.

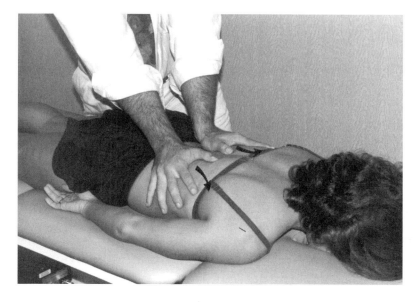

Figure 10.25. General soft-tissue mobilization technique to the superficial fascia of the posterior thoracolumbar junction.

Perpendicular Mobilization

Perpendicular mobilization efforts involve engaging the dysfunction tissue barrier and then, through a series of graded mobilization efforts of varying amplitudes, deforming the respective tissues at right angles. These amplitudes may be graded similarly to those used in the articular system (i.e., grades I–V) [92, 93]. This technique is most frequently used with muscle tissue (midbelly, tenoperiosteal) and at bony contours, and is most effective with diminution of

myofascial play, although it can be used in the presence of increased muscle tone (Fig. 10.27).

End-Range Oscillating Mobilization

The last phase of a perpendicular mobilization effort, end-range oscillating mobilization, is administered to myofascial tissue at the end-range of its available accessory motion. Applied in a perpendicular or transverse orientation, mobilization forces in

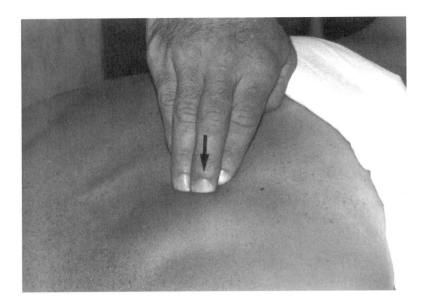

Figure 10.26. Sustained-pressure soft-tissue mobilization technique to the rhomboid muscle group.

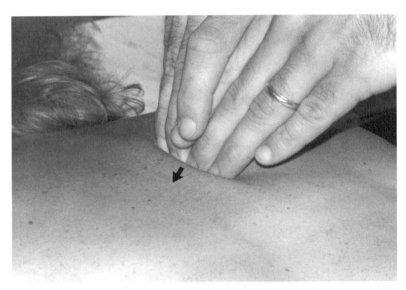

Figure 10.27. Perpendicular soft-tissue mobilization technique.

this technique are of very small amplitudes and create a transverse, end-range deformation to the site and direction of maximal tissue dysfunction. This technique is effective for both myofascial play and tonal abnormalities.

Strumming

Strumming technique incorporates a transverse mobilization effort that begins at the medial or lateral seam of a muscle belly, deforms the belly through a push or pull effort, and then strums across the belly to the opposite side without sliding over the skin. This rhythmic, synchronous movement can be used to treat both myofascial play and muscle tonal aberrations (Fig. 10.28).

Parallel Mobilization

Parallel mobilization techniques are applied between muscle belly septae, at the lateral or medial borders of a muscle, or along a bony contour. As the mobi-

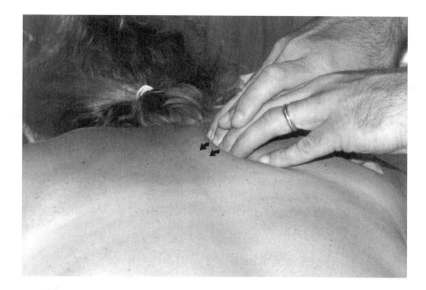

Figure 10.28. Strumming soft-tissue mobilization technique.

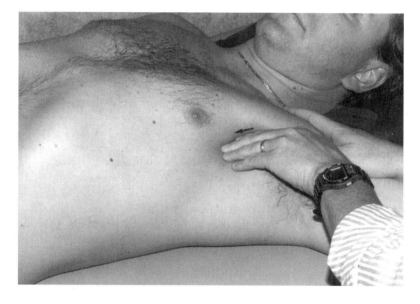

Figure 10.29. Parallel soft-tissue mobilization technique.

lizing hand or digit glides along the contour or between the septum, various angles of inclination are used to attain appropriate depth to localize and ameliorate specific dysfunctional tissue barriers. This technique is effective for both myofascial play and tonal dysfunctions (Fig. 10.29).

Functional Excursion and Muscle Length

Restoring functional excursion or length to the myofascial unit demands careful attention and cogni-

tion of that particular structure's fiber type or preponderance, orientation, relative stage of reactivity, and the osseous or articular structures to which it attaches. Myofascial structures may initially have diminished excursion in one direction. However, they may maintain a multiplanar fiber direction that, when taken through full excursion, presents multidirectional limitations. Slow, judicious, and incrementally small ranges of excursion will allow the examiner to identify and treat tissue limitations.

Specific treatment techniques for increasing excursion include static stretching [94, 95], hold-relax, contract-relax stretching [38, 82], and a combination of isotonic contractions to that particular myofascial structure (concentric, eccentric, isometric, slow reversal hold) [4, 82].

Case Studies

The following case studies illustrate the importance of identifying objective clinical findings of somatic dysfunction of the thorax. Particular attention is placed on myofascial tissues in their causal relationship of biomechanical dysfunction, as well as their potential role in promoting recalcitrant dysfunction.

Case 1

C: Chief Complaint

A 29-year-old woman reported a 6-week history of right upper quadrant and cervical pain; right greater than left episodic paresthesia in the right hand (digits 1 and 2); discomfort with all active cervical motions, most notably left side-bending; and increased symptoms on full inhalation efforts.

H: History

The patient described being injured while playing volleyball. On spiking the ball and following through, she experienced immediate cervical and right shoulder pain, which progressed to the right hand approximately 2 days later. Over a period of 1 week, the pain continued to increase in intensity and was present during examination with all inhalation efforts, with numbness in the right hand reproduced and increased with inhalation as well as left cervical side-bending efforts.

The patient denied any related family history, past mechanical or medical history, use of medications, or prior treatment for this condition. Her occupational history appeared noncontributory in the development of this dysfunction.

A: Asymmetries of Bony Landmarks

The key asymmetric findings for this patient included:

1. Elevated first rib on the right.
2. A type II non-neutral FRS left dysfunction at T1.
3. A type II non-neutral FRS right dysfunction at T2.

R: ROM/Mobility Testing

Positive findings on key motion tests for this patient included:

1. Confirmation of the type II non-neutral FRS left and FRS right dysfunctions at T1 and T2 (with diminished extension, side-bending, and rotation to the right at T1 and diminished extension, side-bending, and rotation to the left at T2).
2. Diminished caudal spring testing to the first rib on the right with firm, arresting, reactive end-feel.
3. Aberrant respiratory motion of the right upper rib cage on full exhalation.
4. Diminished active cervical range of motion, with side-bending left 75%, rotation right 50%.

T: Tissue Texture/Tension/Tonal Abnormalities

The key tissue abnormalities for this patient included:

1. Significant increase in tone of the right anterior and medial scalenes, right sternocleidomastoid, and right levator scapulae musculature.
2. Diminished mediolateral muscle play of both of the right anterior and medial scalenes at their respective musculotendinous and tenoperiosteal junctions.
3. Diminished mediolateral muscle play of the right sternocleidomastoid muscle at the mid-belly, with poor disassociation from the underlying anterior and medial scalene muscles.
4. Decreased functional excursion of the right anterior and medial scalene and right levator scapulae muscles.

S: Special Tests

Special tests for this patient revealed:

1. Positive radiologic evidence of a mildly cranially displaced first rib on the right.
2. Positive adverse neural tension signs in the right upper extremity with combined right upper ex-

tremity abduction, external rotation, and wrist and finger extension.

3. Increased subjective complaints of pain and paresthesia with concomitant cervical side-bending left and rotation right, or with full inhalation efforts.

Musculoskeletal Diagnosis

1. Elevated first rib on the right.
2. Type II non-neutral FRS left dysfunction at T1.
3. Type II non-neutral FRS right dysfunction at T2.
4. Myofascial dysfunction of the right anterior and medial scalenes (increased tone, decreased play, and functional excursion), right sternocleidomastoid (increased tone, decreased functional excursion), and levator scapulae musculature (decreased functional excursion).

Treatment

Initial treatment efforts were focused on mobilization of the type II non-neutral dysfunctions at T1 and T2 with muscle energy and high-velocity technique (see Chapter 9 for details). With vertebral correction noted with respect to positional and motion attributes, treatment efforts were directed at the first rib. Using MET, significant improvement in rib position and correlative cervical range of motion was noted (side-bending left, rotation right 90%). In addition, the patient reported a significant (75%) decrease in pain and hyperesthesia of the cervical musculature, as well as elimination of right upper extremity paresthesia (Fig. 10.30).

The patient was subsequently instructed in postural re-education, as well as self-stretching of the right anterior and medial scalene, sternocleidomastoid, and levator scapulae muscles.

On returning to the clinic for her second visit, the patient complained of a re-exacerbation of the right cervical and upper extremity symptoms (pain and paraesthesia) after self-stretching. Re-examination revealed maintained correction of the type II non-neutral dysfunctions at T1 and T2. However, the right, first rib was once again displaced cranially with associated myofascial dysfunction as initially noted.

Treatment in this session focused on normalization of myofascial dysfunction of the anterior and medial scalene, sternocleidomastoid, and levator scapulae muscles with respect to increased tone, diminished play, and functional excursion. Techniques

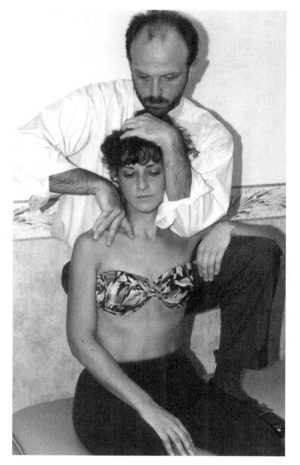

Figure 10.30. Muscle energy technique (MET) to the first rib in the seated posture to correct a superior subluxation of that rib.

used included end-range perpendicular strumming of the scalene muscles (in a shortened range), parallel technique to the sternocleidomastoid, and strumming technique to the levator scapulae (seated/lengthened position) (Figs. 10.31, 10.32, and 10.33). Muscle energy technique was then used once again with the patient in a seated position to normalize the first rib.

In addition, after the position of the first rib was restored, functional excursion of the anterior and medial scalenes was addressed with the patient in a seated position, while providing counter support and stabilization to the right first rib. This was accomplished via digital contact and through a series of hold-relax elongation techniques. The patient was then instructed in home self-stretching technique of these muscles with counter support provided

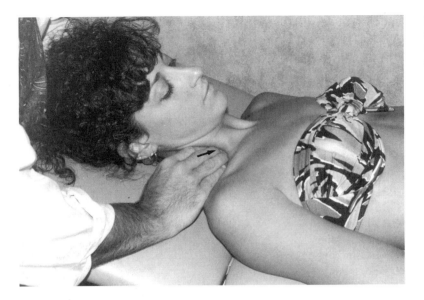

Figure 10.31. End-range perpendicular soft-tissue mobilization technique to the scalenes in a shortened position.

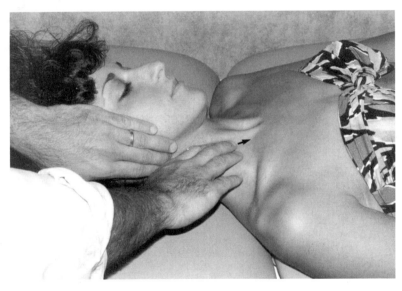

Figure 10.32. Parallel soft-tissue mobilization technique to the sternocleidomastoid.

through the use of a sheet, with a caudally directed force over the first rib (Figs. 10.34 and 10.35).

Treatment Progression and Analysis

Initial treatment efforts were directed at the correction of the type II non-neutral dysfunctions at the T1 and T2 vertebral levels. This strategy was used because position/motion dysfunction of these vertebral segments is commonly associated with and frequently causes dysfunction of the first rib, with resultant upper extremity brachialgic complaints.

These efforts were followed by successful treatment of the first rib as noted. The patient was instructed in prescriptive stretching of the involved soft tissues (anterior and medial scalenes, sternocleidomastoid, levator scapulae) for a home program. However, on returning to the clinic the patient demonstrated recurrence of the elevated first rib on the right. This reportedly occurred when the patient was performing home stretching of the anterior and medial scalenes. Treatment was redirected toward the myofascial dysfunction of the involved soft tissues with particular emphasis on normalizing the play and

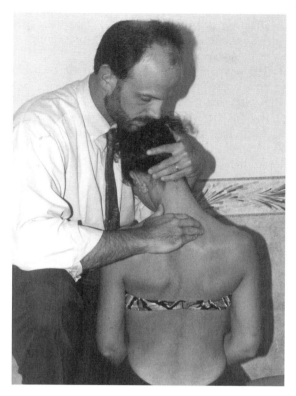

Figure 10.33. Strumming soft-tissue mobilization technique to the levator scapulae muscle.

length of the anterior and medial scalene muscles and the play of the sternocleidomastoid. In addition,

the patient was instructed in self-stretching with appropriate counter support to the first rib.

This case emphasizes the importance of clearing soft-tissue dysfunction that may be implicated in the pathogenesis of vertebral and rib cage dysfunction. It also serves to illustrate how these tissues may perpetuate or cause recurrence of these dysfunctions if left untreated.

Case 2

C: Chief Complaint

A 32-year-old right-handed man was seen with complaints of localized left anterior chest wall pain, especially on full exhalation, over a 5-week period of time. He denied any neurologic symptoms including tingling, numbness, weakness, or radiating pain into either upper extremity.

H: History

This patient described a mechanical history of injuring himself while weight training. He described performing bilateral overhead flies with a 50-pound dumbbell while in a supine position and experiencing a strain of the left pectoral muscle group, which progressed over a 3-day period to include the anterior chest wall. After approximately a 3-week rest period, with treatment including ice packs and gen-

Figure 10.34. Functional excursion/elongation of the anterior and medial scalenes with counter support provided to the first rib through the thumb and second digit.

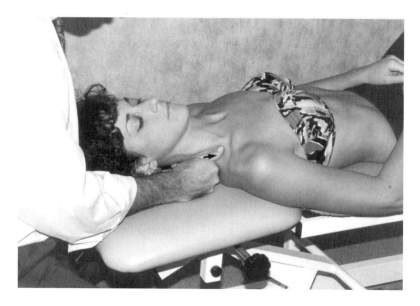

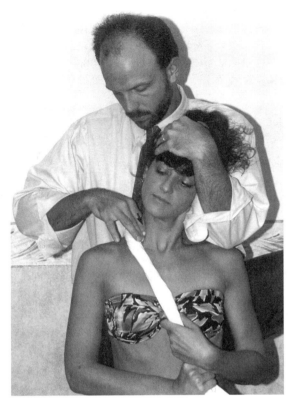

Figure 10.35. Self-stretch home program for the anterior and medial scalenes.

tle self-stretching, the patient attempted weight training once again. However, the chest wall pain increased and on examination was present with all exhalation efforts as well as overhead movements of the right upper extremity.

Other details of the history for this patient, including familial, past medical, pharmacologic, social, and occupational aspects, proved to be noncontributory.

A: Asymmetries of Bony Landmarks

The key asymmetric findings for this patient included:

1. Diminished anterior intercostal space between ribs 4 and 5 on the left with increased spacing posteriorly between ribs 4 and 5 on the left.

2. Anterior, posterior, and lateral rib contours that were unremarkable with respect to asymmetric prominence.
3. The superior margin of the fifth rib was palpable posteriorly, with a sharp border.
4. A type II non-neutral ERS left dysfunction was noted at the T4 vertebral dysfunction.
5. All other vertebral and rib segments appeared symmetric with the patient in the static seated posture.

R: ROM/Mobility Testing

Positive results of the key motion tests for this patient included:

1. Confirmation of the type II non-neutral ERS left dysfunction noted at the T4 vertebral dysfunction with diminished flexion, side-bending, and rotation to the right.
2. Aberrant respiratory motion testing on full exhalation on the left.
3. Diminished spring testing of the superior border of the left fifth anterior rib (cranial to caudal direction) with firm end-feel.
4. Diminished spring testing of the inferior border of the left fifth posterior rib (caudal to cranial direction) with firm end-feel.

T: Tissue Texture/Tension/Tonal Abnormalities

The key tissue abnormalities for this patient included:

1. Diminished caudal shear of the skin and superficial fascia in the left anterior clavipectoral region.
2. Significant decrease in mediolateral muscle play of the left pectoralis minor muscle at its proximal insertion of ribs 4 and 5.
3. Decreased functional excursion and increased tone of the left pectoralis minor muscle.
4. Increased tone of the left iliocostalis muscle at the fifth costal segment and the intercostal muscles between the fourth and fifth costal segments.

S: Special Tests

Radiologic assessment of the cervicothoracic spine produced negative findings.

Musculoskeletal Diagnosis

1. Type II non-neutral ERS left dysfunction at T4.
2. External torsion dysfunction of the left, fifth rib.
3. Exhalation respiratory dysfunction of ribs 3, 4, and 5 on the left, with rib 5 designated as the "key rib."
4. Myofascial dysfunction of the left pectoralis minor muscle (decreased muscle play, increased tone), the intercostal muscles (between costal segments 4 and 5), and the iliocostalis muscle at the fifth costal segment.

Treatment

Initial treatment efforts included MET directed at normalizing the type II non-neutral T4 ERS left dysfunction with correction noted after the first treatment session (Fig. 10.36). In addition, efforts were directed at normalizing the external torsion dysfunction of the left fifth rib with MET with the patient in both the supine and seated positions. This, however, proved resistant to treatment

During the second treatment session efforts to normalize the external torsion dysfunction with MET once again proved to be unsuccessful. Treatment efforts were redirected at the myofascial dysfunction of the superficial and deep clavipectoral fascia and the pectoralis minor and intercostal muscle groups.

The superficial fascial restrictions were ameliorated by identifying and directing treatment at the epicenter of the restrictive barrier in the fascia overlying the fifth costal segment. This was accomplished with a push technique (treating hand) and through placing the immediate surrounding tissues in a shortened range (assist hand) (Fig. 10.37).

The pectoralis minor demonstrated significant diminution in muscle play at the fourth and fifth costal segments on the left. In addition, the left pectoralis minor muscle demonstrated poor dissociation from the overlying pectoralis major muscle. These dysfunctions were treated by placing the muscle group in a shortened position and directing a perpendicular mobilization force to the respective barrier (keeping the tissue barrier level and the direction of the restriction in mind). In addition, a strum technique was used to restore muscle play while decreasing muscle tone, as well as to improve dissociation of the two muscles. A parallel technique

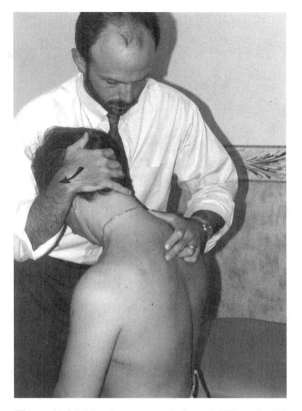

Figure 10.36. Muscle energy technique (MET) to the T4 vertebral segment in the seated position to correct a type II nonneutral ERS left dysfunction with diminished flexion, sidebending, and rotation to the right.

was also used along the lateral seam of this muscle with a significant reduction in tone and moderate gains in muscle play noted. These techniques were used while progressing from a shortened to fully lengthened position (Figs. 10.38 and 10.39).

The intercostal muscle groups between the left fourth and fifth ribs were treated with bony contour technique with the patient in a sidelying position to lengthen or increase the intercostal spacing. This technique was performed circumferentially (Fig. 10.40).

After treatment, reassessment of the external rib torsion dysfunction demonstrated improvement of approximately 75% (both objective and subjective). MET was next used to completely normalize position and motion characteristics to the structural rib dysfunction. After this correction, the respiratory movements also proved to be normalized, with absence of the previous group exhalation dysfunction noted at ribs 3, 4, and 5.

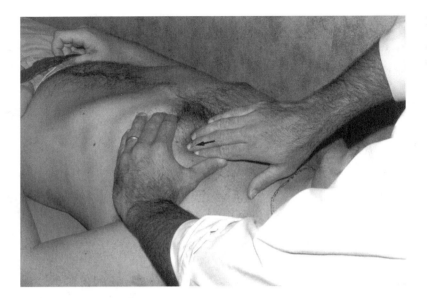

Figure 10.37. Superficial fascial soft-tissue mobilization push technique to the clavipectoral fascia over the fifth costal segment.

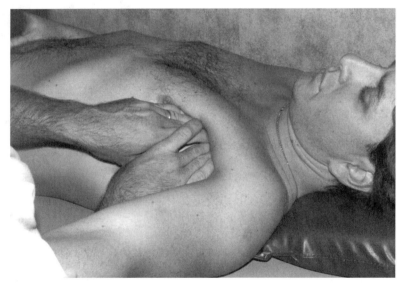

Figure 10.38. Strumming soft-tissue mobilization technique to the pectoralis major/minor complex with digital contact.

The treatment session was completed with the patient engaged in a posterior-elevation/anterior-depression proprioceptive neuromuscular facilitation (PNF) pattern with a combination of isotonics (placing, isometrics, concentrics, eccentrics, slow reversal hold) to provide neuromuscular re-education, improved functional excursion, and challenge the pectoralis minor muscle and its corresponding rib segments (Fig. 10.41 and 10.42).

The patient was instructed in a home program that included self-strumming and doorway stretch-ing to the left pectoralis minor muscles, followed by diaphragmatic, diagonal breathing patterns to maintain respiratory correction.

Treatment Progression and Analysis

Initial treatment attempts were directed at correction of the ERS T4 dysfunction because this commonly causes external torsion dysfunction of the rib cage. Correction of the vertebral dysfunction will often yield concomitant correction of the rib dysfunction.

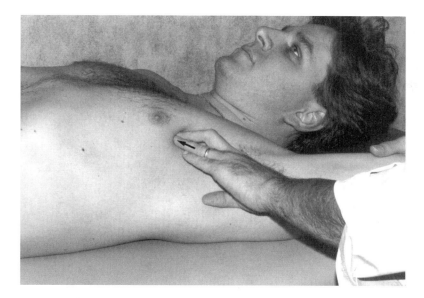

Figure 10.39. Parallel soft-tissue mobilization technique to the pectoralis major/minor complex in a lengthened position.

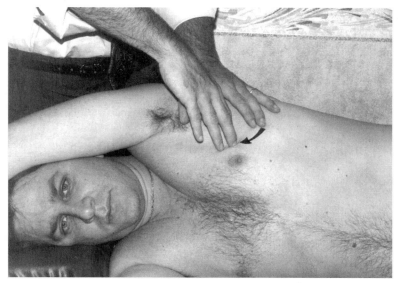

Figure 10.40. Bony contour soft-tissue mobilization technique to ribs 4 and 5. This is performed circumferentially about the entire rib cage.

This, however, is not true where chronicity and myofascial dysfunction coexist. Attempts to use MET in correcting the external rib torsion dysfunction (which was also acting as the "key rib" in the exhalation dysfunction) were unsuccessful secondary to the significant myofascial dysfunction of the pectoralis minor muscle (most notably, diminished play and increased tone). After normalization of the myofascial tissues (particularly muscle play and tone at the pectoralis minor muscle), both muscle energy and PNF techniques were carried out with success,

with the external torsion dysfunction normalized and the associated exhalation dysfunction corrected simultaneously.

This case serves to demonstrate the importance of myofascial work in combination with traditional MET as both preparative and corrective. In addition, it illustrates the importance of considering all of the attributes of soft tissues (i.e., muscle play, tone, functional excursion, and neuromuscular control) in contrast to length or functional excursion only.

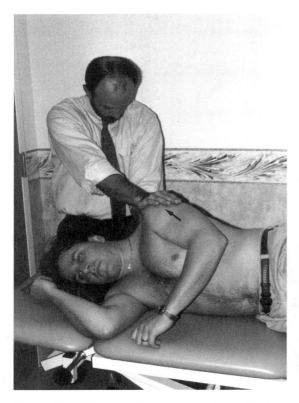

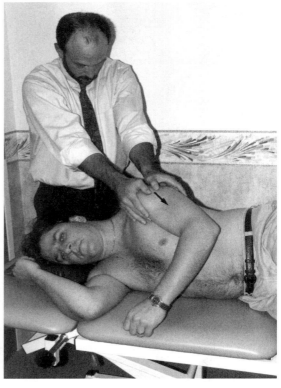

Figure 10.41. Proprioceptive neuromuscular facilitation, posterior elevation pattern to the shoulder girdle to challenge the corrected rib segment as well as improve neuromuscular control.

Figure 10.42. Proprioceptive neuromuscular facilitation, anterior depression pattern to the shoulder girdle.

Case 3

C: Chief Complaint

A 25-year-old female body-builder was seen with a 3-month history of thoracolumbar and right lower rib cage pain, especially with rotation to the left and on inhalation efforts.

H: History

This patient described injuring herself while attempting to lift a heavy object from a flexed position. She described a "catching sensation" in the lower thoracic spine and immediate discomfort in the right anterior lower rib cage. She also reported a similar injury in the same region approximately 2 years earlier.

Other details of the history for this patient, including familial, pharmacologic, social, and occupational aspects, were noncontributory.

A: Asymmetries of Bony Landmarks

The key asymmetric findings for this patient included:

1. A type II non-neutral FRS right dysfunction at T10.
2. A type I neutral, side-bent right, rotated left dysfunction at T11, T12, and L1.
3. Leg length discrepancy (short left approximately 6 mm) with an elevated right iliac crest, elevated right anterior superior iliac spine, elevated right posterior superior iliac spine, and elevated right greater trochanter and fibular head.

R: ROM/Mobility Testing

Positive findings on the key motion tests for this patient included:

1. Confirmation of a type II non-neutral FRS right dysfunction at T10 with diminished extension, side-bending, and rotation to the left.
2. Confirmation of a type I neutral, side-bent right, rotated left dysfunction at T11, T12, and L1 with diminished side-bending left and rotation right at T11, T12, and L1.
3. Aberrant respiratory motion testing on full inhalation of the right lower rib cage.

T: Tissue Texture/Tension/Tonal Abnormalities

The key tissue abnormalities for this patient included:

1. A significant increase in tone of the right iliopsoas muscle, the right respiratory diaphragm (along the inferior border of the anterior rib cage), and the right multifidus musculature (at the T10, T11, and T12 levels).
2. Diminished mediolateral muscle play of the right iliopsoas muscle at the L1, L2, and L3 levels.
3. Diminished mediolateral muscle play and functional excursion of the right quadratus lumborum musculature.

S: Special Tests

The results of special tests were all noncontributory or negative for this patient.

Musculoskeletal Diagnosis

1. Type II non-neutral FRS right dysfunction at T10.
2. Type I neutral, side-bent right, rotated left dysfunction at T11, T12, and L1.
3. Respiratory inhalation dysfunction of ribs 10, 11, and 12 on the right.
4. Leg length discrepancy, short on the left (approximately 6 mm).
5. Myofascial dysfunction of the right iliopsoas muscle (decreased muscle play, increased tone), right respiratory diaphragm (increased tone), right multifidus (increased tone), and right quadratus lumborum (decreased play and functional excursion).

Treatment

Because of the significance of this patient's myofascial dysfunction, initial treatment efforts were directed at the increased muscle tone identified along the inferior border of the rib cage (respiratory diaphragm) and the tone/muscle play problems of the right iliopsoas muscle complex. The respiratory diaphragm was initially treated with the patient seated (shortened position), followed by the supine position (lengthened position). Soft-tissue mobilization efforts included direct, sustained pressure administered to the respiratory diaphragm while the patient was encouraged to provide gentle inhalation and exhalation efforts. In addition, the bony contours of the costochondral arch were addressed with direct, end-range oscillatory mobilization technique directed at the specific restrictions encountered (Figs. 10.43 and 10.44).

The right iliopsoas muscle dysfunction was treated with a combination of perpendicular mobilization and strumming techniques. This was performed with the patient in a supine 90/90 posture (shortened position), which progressed to a lengthened position. This was followed by soft-tissue mobilization of the multifidus muscle through strumming and bony contour techniques directed along the groove between the spinous and transverse processes of the thoracolumbar spine with the patient in a quadruped, sitback position (lengthened position) (Figs. 10.45, 10.46, and 10.47).

After the correction of this MFD, MET was used to correct both the type II FRS right dysfunction at T10 (which was already approximately 50% improved) and the respiratory (inhalation) dysfunction. These efforts resulted in approximately 75% improvement with respect to vertebral and rib position/motion dysfunction, as well as specifically enumerated myofascial dysfunction. Three additional treatment sessions were required (with similar progression) to completely normalize vertebral and rib dysfunction.

On returning to the clinic for the fourth session, the patient demonstrated recurrence of the FRS right dysfunction at T10 and had complaints of pain at the thoracolumbar junction posteriorly. Treatment was redirected at the quadratus lumborum with a functional excursion/lengthening technique (treating hand), in a lengthened position over a bolster, while the assisting hand provided end-range associated oscillations (Fig. 10.48).

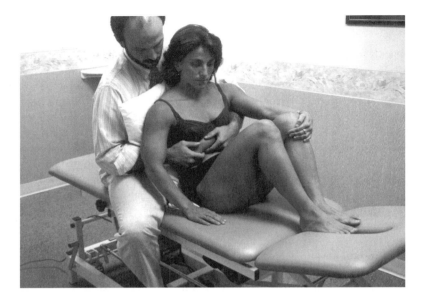

Figure 10.43. Respiratory diaphragm, bony contour, soft-tissue mobilization technique performed in a seated, shortened position.

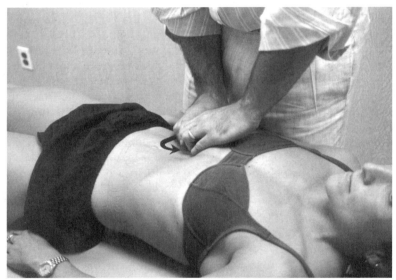

Figure 10.44. Respiratory diaphragm, bony contour, soft-tissue mobilization technique performed in a supine, lengthened position.

Once again, MET was used to correct the type II FRS right dysfunction at T10, followed by proprioceptive neuromuscular facilitation (PNF) for re-education with anterior elevation/posterior depression patterns through the pelvis (Figs. 10.49 and 10.50).

This treatment was followed by the introduction of a 6-mm heel lift to the short lower extremity to level the sacral base. No further complaints were offered and the patient was discharged.

Treatment Progression and Analysis

Treatment efforts initially directed at the myofascial dysfunction of the iliopsoas muscle and respiratory diaphragm allowed substantial progress to be realized in the normalization of the type II FRS and respiratory rib cage dysfunctions. This, however, was only temporary, and recurrence of these movement dysfunctions appeared related to the remaining my-

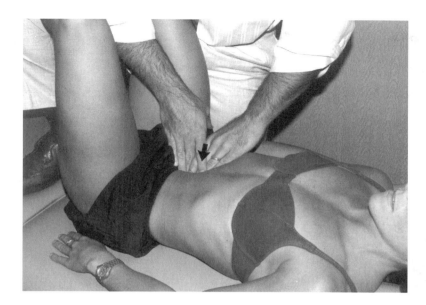

Figure 10.45. Muscle play/tone, soft-tissue mobilization technique to the iliopsoas muscle complex in a supine, shortened position.

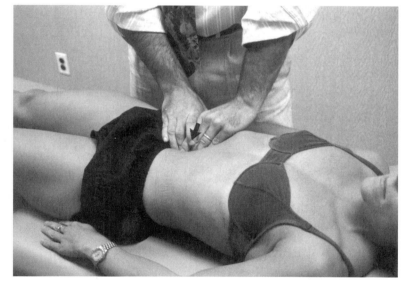

Figure 10.46. Muscle play/tone, soft-tissue mobilization technique to the iliopsoas muscle complex in a supine, lengthened position.

ofascial dysfunction and leg length discrepancy. Asymmetric muscle length and aberrant tone of the quadratus lumborum (secondary to the long right leg) provided an environment for non-neutral mechanics to exist in the thoracolumbar spine and apparently contributed to the recurrence of the type II dysfunction.

Treatment was redirected toward the quadratus lumborum and the correction of the leg length dis-crepancy. This provided an environment for the correction of the type II FRS dysfunction, accomplished through MET, to be maintained. Although type II non-neutral FRS and ERS dysfunctions are not typically recognized as being compensatory to a type I neutral dysfunction (in this case, secondary to a leg length), they are commonly seen as nonresponsive or recurrent in the presence of this static postural alteration. In addition, where chronicity prevails, related myofascial

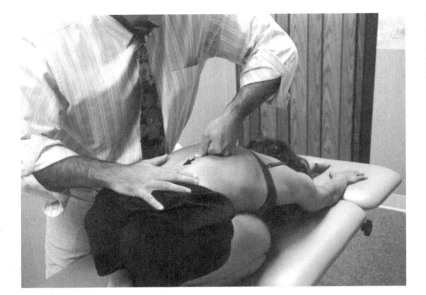

Figure 10.47. Bony contour, soft-tissue mobilization technique to the thoracic spine, paravertebral muscles and myofascial tissues in a quadruped (all fours), sit-back position.

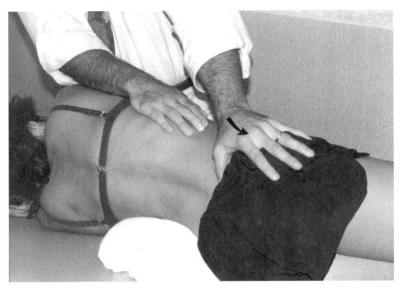

Figure 10.48. Functional excursion/lengthening technique to the quadratus lumborum with the assisting hand providing associated oscillations.

dysfunction makes correction of these articular dysfunctions more recalcitrant to treatment efforts.

This case illustrates how myofascial dysfunction accompanying static postural dysfunction (in this case, leg length dysfunction) may provide biomechanical alterations that make correction of the primary somatic dysfunction difficult, if not impossible. It also emphasizes the importance of achieving neutral mechanics in the vertebral column through the normalization of both myofascial and skeletal structures in efforts to avoid recurrence of thoracic and rib cage dysfunction.

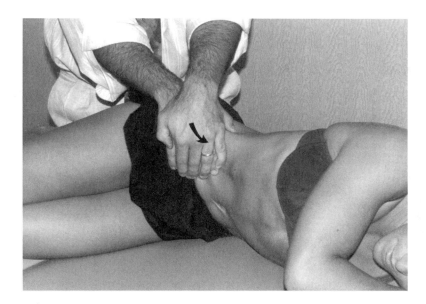

Figure 10.49. Proprioceptive neuromuscular facilitation, anterior elevation pattern to the pelvic girdle.

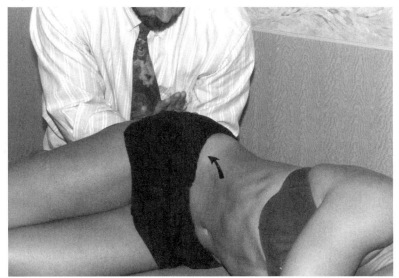

Figure 10.50. Proprioceptive neuromuscular facilitation, posterior depression pattern to the pelvic girdle.

References

1. Greenman PE. Principles of Manual Medicine. Baltimore: Williams & Wilkins, 1989.

2. Bogduk N. Anatomy of the thoracic spine: clinical article. Orthopaedic Division Newsletter 1991;November-December:5–8.

3. Lee D. Biomechanics of the thorax: a clinical model of in vivo function. J Man Manip Ther 1993;1:13–21.

4. Johnson GS. Soft Tissue Mobilization. In AH White, R Anderson (eds), Conservative Care of Low Back Pain. Baltimore: Williams & Wilkins, 1991.

5. Cantu RI. Grodin AJ. Myofascial Manipulation—Theory and Clinical Application. Gaithersburg, MD: Aspen, 1992.

6. Ellis JJ. LPI—Lumbo-Pelvic Integration, A Course Manual. Patchogue, NY, 1990.

7. Ellis JJ. The iliopsoas muscle complex as a primary motion restrictor in lumbar spine movement dysfunction. Proceedings of the International Federation of Orthopedic Manual Therapists. Vail, CO, 1992.

8. Basmajian JV. Grant's Method of Anatomy (9th ed). Baltimore: Williams & Wilkins, 1975.

9. Rolf IP. Rolfing: The Integration of Human Structures. New York: Harper & Row, 1977.

10. Cobey MC. Postural Back Pain. Springfield, IL: Thomas, 1956.

11. Kendall HO, Kendall FP, Boynton DA. Posture and Pain. Huntington, NY: Robert E. Krieger, 1977.

12. Kraus H. Clinical Treatment of Back and Neck Pain. New York: McGraw-Hill, 1970.

13. Kopell HP, Thompson WAL. Peripheral Entrapment Neuropathies. Baltimore: Williams & Wilkins, 1963.

14. Travell JG, Simons DG. Myofascial Pain and Dysfunction: The Trigger Point Manual. Baltimore: Williams & Wilkins, 1983.

15. Travell JG, Simons DG. Myofascial Pain and Dysfunction: The Trigger Point Manual. Vol. 2: The Lower Extremities. Baltimore: Williams & Wilkins, 1992.

16. Adler I. Muscular rheumatism. Med Rec 1900; 57:529–535.

17. Fassbender HG. Pathology of Rheumatic Diseases. New York: Springer-Verlag, 1975; 303–314.

18. Stockman R. Chronic Rheumatism, Chronic Muscular Rheumatism, Fibrositis. In R Stockman (ed), Rheumatism and Arthritis. Edinburgh: W. Green & Son, 1920;41–56.

19. Gutstein M. Diagnosis and treatment of muscular rheumatism. Br J Phys Med 1938;1:302–321.

20. Hunter C. Myalgia of the abdominal wall. Can Med Assoc J 1933;28:157–161.

21. Sinaki M, Merritt JL, Stillwell GK. Tension myalgia of the pelvic floor. Mayo Clin Proc 1977;52:717–722.

22. Awad EA. Interstitial myofibrositis: hypothesis of the mechanism. Arch Phys Med 1973;54:440–453.

23. Steindler A. The interpetation of sciatic radiation and the syndrome of low-back pain. J Bone Joint Surg 1940;22:28–34.

24. Albee FH. Myofascitis. A pathological explanation of many apparently dissimilar conditions. Am J Surg 1927;3:523–533.

25. Gillette HE. Office management of musculoskeletal pain. Texas State J Med 1966;62:47–53.

26. Sola AE, Kuitert JH. Quadratus lumborum myofascitis. Northwest Med 1959;53:1003–1005.

27. Steindler A, Luck JV. Differential diagnosis of pain low in the back. JAMA 1938;110:106–113.

28. Waylonis GW. Long-term followup on patients with fibrositis treated with acupuncture. Ohio State Med J 1977;73:299–302.

29. Johnson GS. FOI, Functional Orthopaedics I. San Anselmo, CA: Institute for Physical Art, 1985.

30. Johnson GS. FO-II, Functional Orthopaedics II. San Anselmo, CA: Institute for Physical Art, 1987.

31. Ellis JJ. CTI, Cervical-Thoracic Integration—A Course Manual. Patchogue, NY, 1992.

32. Korr IM. The Collected Papers of Irvin M. Korr. Colorado Springs, CO: American Academy of Osteopathy, 1979.

33. Korr IM. The facilitated segment: after injury to the body segment. American Academy of Osteopathy 1973; 11:188–190.

34. Korr IM. The Neurobiologic Mechanisms in Manipulative Therapy. New York: Plenum, 1978.

35. Mitchell FL, Moran PS, Pruzzo NA. An Evaluation and Treatment Manual of Osteopathic Muscle Energy Procedures. Valley Park, MD: Mitchell, Moran & Pruzzo, 1979.

36. Bourdillon JF, Day EA. Spinal Manipulation (4th ed). London: William Heinemann, 1987.

37. Rockwell JA. Muscle energy technique: a biomechanical approach to myofascial pain and dysfunction. J Myofascial Ther 1994;1:18–21.

38. Knott M, Voss DE. Proprioceptive Neuromuscular Facilitation: Patterns and Techniques (2nd ed). New York: Harper & Row, 1968.

39. Saliba V, Johnson G, Wardlaw C. Proprioceptive Neuromuscular Facilitation. In J Basmajian, R Nyberg (eds), Rational Manual Therapies. Baltimore: Williams & Wilkins, 1993;243.

40. Grieve GP. Common Vertebral Joint Problems (2nd ed). New York: Churchill Livingstone, 1988.

41. Kirkaldy-Willis WH, Hill RJ. A more precise diagnosis for low back pain. Spine 1979;4:102.

42. Lewit K. Manipulative Therapy in Rehabilitation of the Locomotor System (2nd ed). Boston: Butterworth, 1992.

43. Butler D. Mobilization of the Nervous System. New York: Churchill Livingstone, 1991.

44. Elvey RL. Treatment of arm pain associated with abnormal brachial plexus tension. Austral J Physiother 1986;32:224.

45. Pecina MM, Krmpotic-Nemanic J, Markiewitz AD. Tunnel Syndromes. Boca Raton, FL: CRC Press, 1991.

46. Warwick R, Williams PL (eds). Gray's Anatomy (37th ed). Edinburgh: Churchill Livingstone, 1989.

47. Ham A, Cormack D. Histology. Philadelphia: Lippincott, 1979.
48. Donatelli R, Wooden J. Orthopaedic Physical Therapy. New York: Churchill Livingstone, 1989;18.
49. Anderson JE. Gray's Atlas of Anatomy (8th ed). Baltimore: Williams & Wilkins, 1985.
50. Hollingshead WH. Functional Anatomy of the Limbs and Back: A Text for Students of the Locomotor Apparatus. Philadelphia: Saunders, 1976.
51. Hardy MA. The biology of scar formation. Phys Ther 1989;69:1014–1024.
52. Nordin M, Frankel VH. Basic Biomechanics of the Musculoskeletal System. Philadelphia: Lea & Febiger, 1989.
53. Bogduk N, Twomey LT. Clinical Anatomy of the Lumbar Spine. New York: Churchill Livingstone, 1987.
54. Frank C, Amiel D, Woo SLY et al. Pain complaint—exercise performance relationship in chronic pain. Pain 1981;10:311.
55. Bassett CA. The Effect of Force on Skeletal Tissues. In Downs, Darling (eds), Physiologic Basis of Rehabilitation Medicine. Philadelphia: Saunders, 1971.
56. Bunting CH, Eades C. Effects of mechanical tension on the polarity of growing fibroblasts. J Exp Med 1926;44:147.
57. McGaw WT. The effect of tension on collagen remodeling by fibroblasts: a stereological ultrastructural study. Connective Tissue Res 1986;14:229.
58. Arem JA, Madden WM. Effects of stress on healing wounds: intermittent noncyclical tension. J Surg Res 1976;20:93–102.
59. Brunius U, Ahren C. Healing of skin incisions during reduced tension of the wound area. Acta Chir Scand 1969;135:383–390.
60. Sussman M. Effect of increased tissue traction upon tensile strength of cutaneous incisions in rats. Proc Soc Exp Biol Med 1966;123:38–41.
61. Bland JH. Disorders of the Cervical Spine. Philadelphia: Saunders, 1994.
62. Cummings GS, Crutchfield CA, Barnes MR. Orthopaedic Physical Therapy. Vol. 1. Soft Tissue Changes in Contractures. Atlanta: Strokesville, 1983.
63. Cyriax J. Textbook of Orthopaedic Medicine: Diagnosis of Soft Tissue Lesions (8th ed). London: Baillière Tindall, 1984.
64. Palastagna N. The Use of Transverse Friction for Soft Tissue Lesions. In G Grieve (ed), Modern Manual Therapy of the Vertebral Column. London: Churchill Livingstone, 1986;819.
65. Malone TR. Muscle Injury and Rehabilitation. Vol. 1. Baltimore: Williams & Wilkins, 1988.
66. Tardieu C, Tarbary J, Tardieu G et al. Adaption of Sarcomere Numbers to the Length Imposed on Muscle. In F Gubba, G Marecahl, O Takacs (eds). Mechanics of Muscle Adaptation to Functional Requirements. Elmsford, NY: Pergamon, 1981.
67. Woo SLY, Buckwalter JA. Injury and Repair of the Musculoskeletal Soft Tissue. Park Ridge, IL: American Academy of Orthopaedic Surgery, 1988.
68. Dvorak J, Dvorak V. Manual Medicine: Diagnostics. Stuttgart: Thieme, 1984.
69. Lowenthal M, Tobias JS. Contracture in chronic neurological disease. Arch Phys Med 1951;38:640.
70. Grossman MR, Sahrmann SA, Rose SJ. Review of length associated changes in muscle. Phys Ther 1982;62:1799.
71. Miller B. Manual Therapy Treatment of Myofascial Pain and Dysfunction. In ES Rachlin (ed), Physical Therapy and Rehabilitation. St. Louis: Mosby, 1994; 415–454.
72. Adams RD. Diseases of Muscle: A Study in Pathology (3rd ed). Hagerstown, MD: Harper & Row, 1975; 280–291, 316, 317.
73. Abel Jr. O, Siebert WJ, Earp R. Fibrositis. J Mo Med Assoc 1939;36:435–437.
74. Webster's New Collegiate Dictionary. Springfield, MA: G & C Merriam Co., 1974.
75. Loring SH, Mead J. Action of the diaphragm on the rib cage inferred from a force balance analysis. J Appl Physiol 1982;53:736–760.
76. Gray H. Anatomy, Descriptive and Surgical. Philadelphia: Running Press, 1974.
77. Gratz CM. Air injection of the fascial spaces. AJR 1936;35:750.
78. Goodridge JP. Muscle energy technique: definition, explanation, methods of procedure. J Am Osteopath Assoc 1981;84:67–72.
79. Ward R. Myofascial release, course notes. East Lansing, MI: Michigan State University College of Osteopathic Medicine, April 13–15, 1984.
80. Paris S. Physical signs of instability. Spine 1985; 10:277–279.
81. Kuzmich D. The levator scapulae: making the con-Necktion. J Man Manip Ther 1994;2:43–45.
82. Johnson G, Saliva V. PNFI: The Functional Approach to Movement Reeducation. San Anselmo, CA: The Institute of Physical Art, 1987.
83. Feldenkrais M. Awareness Through Movement. New York: Harper & Row, 1977.
84. Becker RF. The meaning of fascia and fascial continuity. New York: Insight, 1975.
85. VanderMuelen JCH. Present state of knowledge on processes of healing in collagen structures. Int J Sports Med 1982;3:4.
86. Scott-Charlton W, Roebuck DJ. The significance of posterior primary divisions of spinal nerves in pain syndromes. Med J Aust 1972;2:945.
87. Magora A. Investigation of the relation between low back pain and occupation. Scand J Rehabil Med 1975; 7:146.
88. Biering-Sorensen F. Physical measurements as risk indicators for low back trouble over a one year period. Spine 1984;9:106.
89. Mayer TG, Tencer AF, Kristoferson S et al. Use of noninvasive techniques for quantification of spinal range-of-motion in normal subjects and chronic low back dysfunction patients. Spine 1984;9:588.

90. Paris SV. Anatomy as Related to Function and Pain. In Course Notes—Introduction to Spinal Evaluation and Manipulation. 1986.

91. Jones LH. Strain and Counterstrain. Ohio: The American Academy of Osteopathy, 1981.

92. Maitland GD. Vertebral Manipulation (5th ed). Boston: Butterworth, 1986.

93. Maitland GD. In R Grant (ed), Clinics in Physical Therapy: Physical Therapy of the Cervical and the Thoracic Spine. New York: Churchill Livingstone, 1988.

94. Evjenth O, Hamberg J. Muscle Stretching in Manual Therapy. A Clinical Manual: The Spinal Column and the TM Joint. Vol. 2. Sweden: Afta Rehab Forlag, 1985.

95. Johnson GS, Saliba-Johnson VL. BET—Back Education and Training: Course Outline. San Anselmo, CA: The Institute of Physical Art, 1988.

Chapter 11

Injection Techniques and Alternate Treatment Approaches

Thomas K. Szulc

Management of painful disorders of the thoracic spine and rib cage is a complex and challenging task requiring an integrated and comprehensive approach to treatment. Each patient's condition is completely unique; therefore, a program of treatment must be tailored to the individual needs of a particular patient's problem.

Regional anesthesia techniques play a very important role in treatment. The major benefits of regional anesthesia include eliminating the cause of pain, decreasing inflammation, improving mobility, and facilitating the patient's complete rehabilitation.

Depending on the individual situation, regional anesthesia may be administered alone, but in the majority of cases regional anesthesia will be administered simultaneously with other treatments including physical therapy, occupational therapy, stress management, biofeedback, relaxation, and other psychological interventions.

It is imperative that the assessment of the patient's painful condition and its treatment be done in the early and, if possible, in the acute stage of disease to prevent the development of chronicity on biological, functional, and mental levels. Therefore, the involvement of a pain specialist in the initial evaluation of a patient suffering from a painful disorder is one of the most important factors in the success of the treatment.

Emerging new innovative forms of therapy, including myeloscopy, low-reactive level laser therapy (LLLT), and pulsated electromagnetic field therapy

(PEMF) and the rediscovery of older forms of therapy such as acupuncture allow us to optimistically view the future regarding our ability to conquer the biggest enemy of humanity—pain.

Regional Anesthesia Techniques

The thoracic segment of the spine, like any other segment of the spine, is divided into ventral and dorsal compartments by a virtual frontal plane through the dorsal wall of the intervertebral foramen [1]. The ventral compartment contains the vertebral bodies, the discs, the anterior and posterior longitudinal ligaments, and the ventral dura. The dorsal compartment contains the zygopophyseal joints (facet joints), the dorsal part of the dura, and the back muscles and ligaments (Fig. 11.1).

The innervation of the thoracic spine is quite complex. The ventral compartment is supplied by interconnected neural networks in the anterior and posterior longitudinal ligaments and the plexus of the ventral dura [2–4]. The anterior longitudinal ligament plexus contains nerve branches from the thoracic sympathetic chain, the communicating rami, and the perivascular nerves. This plexus innervates the anterior part of the vertebral body, the anterior part of the annulus fibrosus, and the articulatio capitis costae (Fig. 11.2).

The posterior longitudinal ligament plexus contains nerve branches of rami communicantes, which

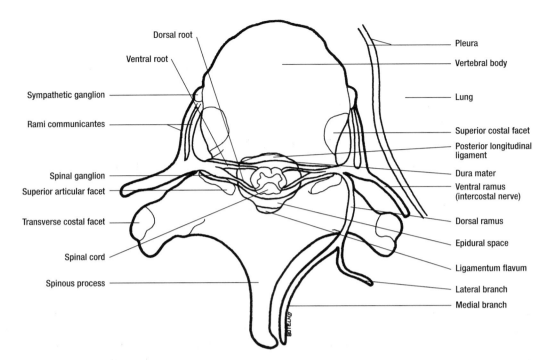

Figure 11.1. Schematic drawing of thoracic spine.

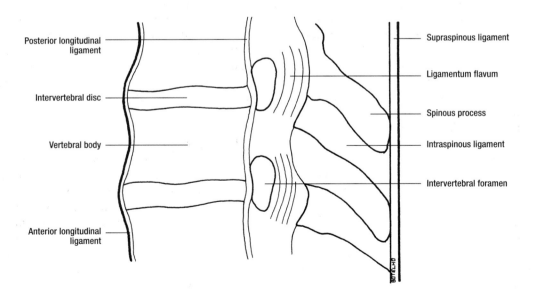

Figure 11.2. Schematic drawing of thoracic spine ligaments.

are called sinuvertebral nerves inside the spinal canal. It innervates the posterior part of the vertebral body and the posterior part of the annulus fibrosus.

The anterior and posterior longitudinal ligament plexuses are interconnected and overlap two to four levels of spinal segments.

The third neural plexus of the ventral compartment is located in ventral dura and consists of sinuvertebral nerve branches and direct branches from the posterior longitudinal ligament plexus [2]. The dorsal compartment is supplied by the dorsal rami nerves. Regional nerve blockades are performed for diagnostic, prognostic, and therapeutic purposes.

Safety precautions must be established and minimal requirements should include:

1. Intravenous cannula with fluid infusion
2. Intubation equipment
3. Ventilation equipment with an oxygen attachment
4. Medication for resuscitation and sedation

Before the procedure a careful evaluation of the patient's medical status and identification of any contraindications is a standard of care in pain management. The patient should also be adequately informed about the procedure, including possible complications and side effects, its benefit, and alternative therapies.

Thoracic Spinal Block

Indications

Indications for thoracic spinal block include [5–10]:

1. Pain control for advanced neoplastic disease.
2. Nonmalignant pain syndromes (occasionally), including postherpetic neuralgia, intercostal neuralgia, and pain from aortic aneurysm.
3. Spasticity.

To relieve intractable pain, subarachnoid injection of neurolytic agents, 5% phenol or absolute alcohol, is recommended. Intrathecal neurolysis has some advantages over narcotics or neurosurgical procedures [11], mainly the absence of nausea, vomiting, and constipation. Also, there are no personality changes and no need for prolonged hospitalization.

Contraindications

Contraindications to thoracic spinal block include:

1. Infection at the site of injection.
2. Coagulopathy.
3. Spread of the tumor within the spinal cord.
4. Widespread and poorly localized pain.
5. Inability of the patient to assume the position required for the injection.

Technique

A thoracic spinal injection [12,13] is more difficult than an injection in the cervical or lumbar spine because of the slope of spinous processes and the presence of spinal cord.

Midline Approach

The patient lies in the lateral position with the back and head flexed. The appropriate spinous processes and interspaces are identified. After the skin is anesthetized, a 22- or 25-gauge 3.5-inch spinal needle is introduced and advanced at an acute angle into the supraspinous and intraspinous ligaments. The needle is advanced deeper through ligamentum flavum into the epidural space. Finally, puncture of the dura and free flow of cerebrospinal fluid is achieved (Fig. 11.3).

Paramedian Approach

The position and the location of the interspace is the same as for the midline approach. The point of insertion of the needle is 2 cm lateral to the caudad tip of the spinous process that is immediately above the interspace to be entered. The needle is advanced until the tip of the needle hits the vertebral arch. Next the needle is walked off the arch and slowly advanced until the dura is punctured and cerebrospinal fluid appears at the needle hub (Fig. 11.4).

The injection of hyperbaric phenol requires that the patient be placed on the affected side [10]. After the needle is inserted into the subarachnoid space, the patient is tilted backward to 30–40 degrees and phenol is slowly injected. After the injection the patient remains in the oblique position for about 20 minutes [14]. The sitting position is not allowed for 1 day. The dose of 5% phenol should not exceed 1.2 ml.

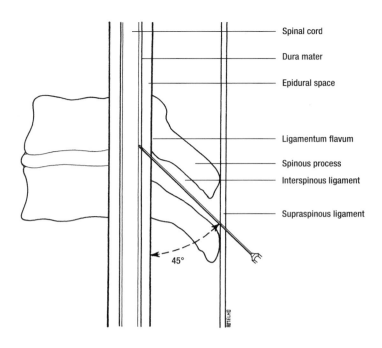

Spinal cord

Dura mater

Epidural space

Ligamentum flavum

Spinous process

Interspinous ligament

Supraspinous ligament

45°

Figure 11.3. Schematic drawing of thoracic spinal block.

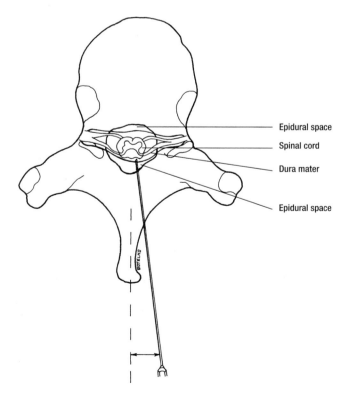

Epidural space

Spinal cord

Dura mater

Epidural space

Figure 11.4. Schematic drawing of thoracic spinal block: paramedian approach.

The injection of hypobaric alcohol (98–99.5%) requires placement of the patient in the lateral position on the side opposite the one to be blocked. The patient's body is tilted forward 45 degrees to spare the motor root from neurolysis.

The choice of puncture site depends on the level to be blocked, and the neurolytic agent should be introduced at the origin of the dorsal roots [5, 14, 15].

Complications

Complications include [9, 10, 15]:

1. Postspinal headache
2. Spinal cord damage
3. Spinal artery thrombosis [16]
4. Motor dysfunction: weakness and paralysis
5. Infection
6. Transverse myelitis, etc.

The pain may return after an apparently satisfactory block as a result of either progression of the disease or regeneration of nerve root fibers. On average, a cancer patient may obtain months of pain relief after successful neurolytic spinal block, which greatly improves the patient's quality of life.

Thoracic Epidural Block

Indications

Indications for thoracic epidural block include:

1. Ventral compartment syndrome from discopathy caused by an annular tear, or thoracic radiculopathy
2. Acute herpes zoster and postherpetic neuralgia
3. Intercostal neuralgia
4. Compression fracture
5. Postsurgical pain
6. Cancer pain

Contraindications

Contraindications include:

1. Infection at the site of injection or sepsis

2. Coagulopathy
3. Anatomic difficulties (very rare)

Technique

The patient is placed in the lateral or sitting position with the back and head flexed. The appropriate upper back area is prepared and draped in a sterile manner. The site of puncture is selected [12, 17–19].

Medial Approach

After landmarks are identified, the skin over the selected interspace is anesthetized. A Touhy or Crawford 17- or 18-gauge epidural needle then is introduced into the interspinal space in the midline at approximately a 45-degree angle. The needle is advanced slowly using the loss of resistance technique, with a 5-ml glass syringe filled with air or normal saline attached to the needle. Sudden loss of resistance on the plunger of the syringe indicates the tip of the needle is inside the epidural space. After negative aspiration, a test dose is injected to exclude dural puncture or an intravascular position of the needle.

Paramedian Approach

The skin puncture is placed 1–2 cm laterally in the desired interspinal space. After the skin and subcutaneous tissue are anesthetized, a 17- or 18-gauge epidural needle is slowly advanced at 10–15 degrees to the sagittal plane and at 45–50 degrees to the surface of the skin. If the lamina is contacted, the needle is redirected cranially and further advanced until loss of resistance is felt. The needle should enter the epidural space in the midline (Fig. 11.5).

Thoracic epidural blockade can be performed as a single injection or as a continuous block with the epidural catheter inserted through the epidural needle. Depending on the pathologic entity and the desired therapeutic effect, different medications can be administered epidurally:

1. Local anesthetic
2. Steroid
3. Opioid
4. Neurolytic agent
5. Combinations of some of these agents

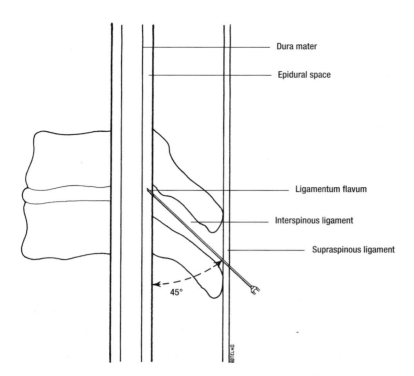

Figure 11.5. Schematic drawing of thoracic epidural block.

Labels in figure:
- Dura mater
- Epidural space
- Ligamentum flavum
- Interspinous ligament
- Supraspinous ligament
- 45°

Complications

Complications of thoracic epidural block include [18, 20]:

1. Perforation of the dura, causing headache
2. Spinal cord injury
3. Epidural hematoma
4. Infection
5. Spinal nerve injury
6. Inadvertent injection in the intrathecal space or intravascularly
7. Arachnoiditis

Case Report

A 68-year-old woman was referred to our center for treatment of severe, excruciating, constant pain across her middle back caused by a compression fracture of T7 and osteoporosis. Her symptoms had started over 3 months before after a minor fall. She underwent conservative treatment with anti-inflammatory and analgesic medications, transcutaneous electrical nerve stimulation (TENS), and a physical therapy program with no improvement.

During the initial consultation, the patient described her pain as 8 on a scale of 0–10. Because of evident symptoms of thoracic radiculopathy, an established plan of treatment included a thoracic epidural block with a steroid. The procedure was performed with the patient in a sitting position, and the epidural needle was inserted into the epidural space at the level T6–T7. Ten milliliters of 0.125% bupivacaine mixed with 80 mg of methylprednisolone acetate (Depo-Medrol) was slowly injected into the thoracic epidural space. The patient responded to this treatment very well with a decrease in pain of over 60%. After the second thoracic epidural block, which was performed 2 weeks later, an improvement of almost 80% was achieved and the patient returned to her routine lifestyle.

Continuous Epidural Neurolysis

Epidural adhesions may occur after spinal surgery or can follow any intraspinal pathologic condition associated with a chronic inflammatory process. In animal studies, epidural fibrosis was demonstrated after leakage of proteoglycans from nucleus pulposus into the epidural space [21, 22], which is evidence that epidural adhesions may develop without previous surgery. The recent development of epidural endoscopy [19a] may be helpful in accurately diagnosing the intraspinal pathologic entities responsible for painful disorders.

Indications

Indications for continuous epidural neurolysis include:

1. Pain caused by epidural adhesions and scarring
2. Thoracic radiculopathy
3. Compression fracture of a vertebral body
4. Discopathy
5. Degenerative joint disease of the thoracic spine

Contraindications

The contraindications for continuous epidural neurolysis are the same as for epidural injection.

Technique

The patient is positioned in the lateral decubitus or prone position [23]. The appropriate area of the upper back is prepared with sterile technique. A 16-gauge RK epidural needle is inserted into the epidural space under fluoroscopic guidance at the intervertebral space closest to the site of pain using the previously described technique.

The RK needle has some advantages over regular epidural needles. Mainly it decreases the risk of shearing the catheter and allows multiple passes of the epidural catheter [24]. After the RK needle is placed into the epidural space, an epidurogram is performed by injecting 7–10 ml of water-soluble contrast (Omnipaque 240) to outline defects caused by epidural scarring and to locate compression and inflammation of spinal nerve roots. Next, the spring-tipped polytetrafluororethylene (Teflon)-coated epidural catheter is inserted into the epidural space and its tip is placed as close as possible to the site of epidural scarring. The catheter is aspirated for blood or cerebrospinal fluid (CSF) and a test dose of short-acting local anesthetic is injected. It is followed by an injection of 10 ml 0.25% bupivacaine mixed with 40–80 mg Depo-Medrol or 40 mg triamcinolone. Thirty minutes later, after sensory block is achieved, 6–8 ml 10% NaCl is slowly injected. Injection of local anesthetic and hypertonic saline is repeated on the next two consecutive days to complete the course of treatment.

To improve the effectiveness of epidural neurolysis, 1,500 units of hyaluronidase was used together with or instead of hypertonic saline [25]. Hyaluronidase is known for breaking down hyaluronic acid, which is a major component of mucopolysaccharides.

Complications

Complications include:

1. Intrathecal injection with nerve damage
2. Neural deficits
3. Intravenous injection
4. Infection
5. Catheter shearing

Case Report

A 74-year-old bedridden woman was in severe, constant, sharp pain in the middle and lower back. The pain in her back was associated with any movement of her body and was not relieved by analgesics or weak opioids. She required moderate doses of morphine to control her pain.

Her past medical history included a status post hysterectomy 40 years earlier and long-standing osteoporosis complicated by multiple compression fractures of the thoracic spine. The patient was hospitalized with a diagnosis of chronic intractable back pain caused by compression fractures of the vertebral bodies of the thoracic spine from T7 to T12 and osteoporosis. Orthopedic evaluation excluded surgical intervention and referred the patient to pain services.

After careful evaluation of the patient's condition, a program of treatment was established in which continuous epidural neurolysis played the most important role. Under local anesthesia and fluoroscopic guidance an RK epidural needle was inserted into the epidural space at the level of T12–L1 and an injection of 8 ml of water-soluble dye revealed bilateral patchy defects at levels T9–T10 and T10–T11 suggesting epidural scarring. Next, a special epidural

Racz-type catheter was inserted into the epidural space and the tip of the catheter was placed at the level T9–T10, where resistance was met. Then 10 ml of 0.25% bupivacaine with 40 mg Depo-Medrol and, 20 minutes later, 5 ml of 10% NaCl was injected through the catheter into the epidural space. Daily injections of local anesthetic and hypertonic saline for the next two consecutive days were carried out. On the third day the epidural catheter was removed, and at that time the patient noted over 50% pain relief. She also began ambulation with the help of a therapist and a walker. Soon after, the patient was discharged home completely pain free with the ability to ambulate and to perform her basic daily activities. At last follow-up she had been pain free for 3 years.

Thoracic Sympathetic Block

Blockade of the sympathetic nervous system eliminates vasomotor, sudomotor, and visceromotor activities. The thoracic ganglia are positioned more posterior than in the lumbar and cervical spine. The first thoracic ganglion is usually fused with the lower cervical ganglia creating a stellate ganglion. The second thoracic ganglion is located anterior to the neck of the second rib. The T3–T6 ganglia lie in front of the head of the rib and the T7–T10 ganglia are located below the ribs along the posterosuperior aspect of the vertebral bodies [26].

Indications

Indications for thoracic sympathetic block include [26, 30]:

1. Reflex sympathetic dystrophy and causalgia of the upper extremity and chest wall
2. Postamputation pain
3. Herpes zoster infection
4. Thoracic visceral pain from acute myocardial infarction, angina pectoris, aortic pain, pulmonary embolism, or intractable asthma

Contraindications

Contraindications to thoracic sympathetic block include:

1. Infection at the site of injection
2. Coagulopathy
3. Pneumothorax

Technique [13, 26, 30]

The patient is positioned prone on the x-ray table. After sterile preparation of the upper back, the skin is anesthetized 3–4 cm lateral to the midline at the level of the transverse process. A 22-gauge 3.5-inch spinal needle is introduced paravertebrally and advanced until the transverse process is contacted. The needle is repositioned inferiorly and medially, and advanced another 4–5 cm to the lateral aspect of the vertebral body. The position of the needle is confirmed by anteroposterior and lateral fluoroscopic imaging. After negative aspiration, 2–3 ml local anesthetic is injected in each ganglion. A neurolytic blockade is performed with 2–3 ml 6% phenol in normal saline. It is advisable to inject contrast to ensure proper placement of the needle before any neurolytic block (Fig. 11.6).

Complications

Generally, there is a greater incidence of complications from thoracic sympathetic block than from any other sympathetic block.

Complications includes pneumothorax, intraspinal injection, and intravascular injection.

Case Report

A 14-year-old girl sustained a pulling injury to her right wrist and her right shoulder. Her injury was diagnosed as a wrist sprain by an orthopedic surgeon, and she underwent conservative treatment with no success. Four months later she was seen in our center with symptoms of the second stage of reflex sympathetic dystrophy, which included:

Constant severe burning and aching pain in the right upper limb
Vascular dysfunction with swelling and cyanotic discoloration
Temperature changes
Hyperhidrosis

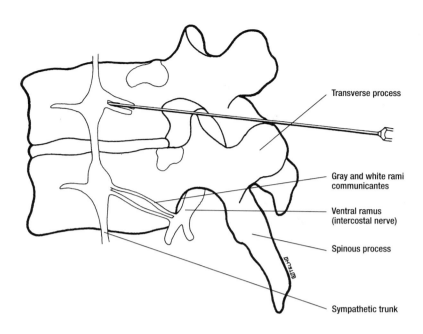

Figure 11.6. Schematic drawing of thoracic sympathetic block.

Transverse process

Gray and white rami communicantes

Ventral ramus (intercostal nerve)

Spinous process

Sympathetic trunk

Allodynia

Motor dysfunction and weakness in her right upper extremity.

The program of treatment included sympathetic blockades and physical therapy with a stress loading program, psychological support with biofeedback, and relaxation training. The patient underwent multiple sympathetic and somatic blocks by means of stellate ganglion blocks, intravenous regional sympathetic blocks with guanethidine, a continuous brachial plexus block, and a continuous cervical epidural block with good but temporary relief of symptoms.

Finally a thoracic sympathetic blockade was performed to the right sympathetic chain at the T3 and T4 levels. The patient noted excellent analgesia and marked improvement of circulation and motor function lasting for a prolonged time (7–10 days). A radiofrequency lesion of the thoracic sympathetic chain was discussed with the patient and her family.

Facet Joint Block

Thoracic zygopophyseal joint pain syndrome has received little attention in the medical literature. The thoracic facet joints are paired synovial joints located between the superior and inferior pillars from C7–T1 to T12–L1. The articular surface is inclined 60 degrees from the horizontal to the frontal plane and rotated 20 degrees from the frontal to the sagittal plane in a medial direction (see Chapter 1) [27]. The thoracic facet joints are innervated from posterior rami branches. Because the dissection of human thoracic facet joints has never been done, it is assumed that articular branches originate from the medial branch of the dorsal rami.

Weight bearing in a forward flexed position increases the stress on joints. The neck, shoulders, abdominal muscles, and quadratum lumborum muscles exert large forces on the thoracic spine [28].

Indications

Indications for facet joint block include:

1. Thoracic facet joint syndrome.
2. Thoracic sprain.
3. Compression fracture.

Contraindications

Infection at the site of injection is a contraindication to facet joint block (Fig. 11.7).

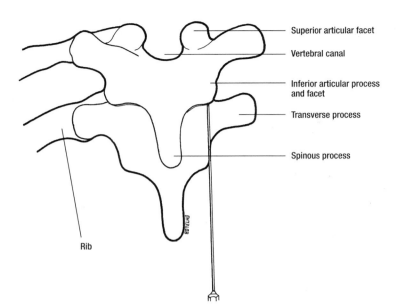

Superior articular facet

Vertebral canal

Inferior articular process and facet

Transverse process

Spinous process

Rib

Figure 11.7. Schematic drawing of facet joint block.

Technique

The patient is placed in the prone position on the x-ray table. The appropriate area of the back is prepared and draped in a sterile manner. The procedure is performed under fluoroscopic control. Skin over the inferior margin of the pedicle below the joint to be blocked is anesthetized. Under x-ray imaging, a 22- or 25-gauge 3.5-inch spinal needle is introduced at an angle of approximately 60–70 degrees to the skin toward the target facet joint. The needle is advanced cephalad until it is positioned into the joint. Proper placement of the needle is confirmed from a C-arm image intensified through injection of a small amount of dye. Next, medication is injected, but the amount should not exceed 0.5 ml to prevent rupturing the joint capsule.

In my experience, more successful results were achieved when an intra-articular injection was combined with medial branch blocks on two or three levels. Although there is no clear anatomic study of the innervation of the thoracic zygopophyseal joints and medial branch block techniques in the thoracic spine have not yet been described, I believe it is similar to the cervical and lumbar spine. Therefore a 22- or 25-gauge 3.5-inch needle is placed in the superior, medial aspect of thoracic transverse process and 1–3 ml of local anesthetic is injected.

Injection of a facet joint can be performed as a diagnostic procedure using a short-acting local anes-

thetic or as a therapeutic procedure using mixture of local anesthetic and steroid (methylprednisolone [Depo-Medrol] or triamcinolone [Aristocort]).

If the patient receives good but short-term relief of pain after two to three injections, radiofrequency denervation of the joint may be the next rational choice of treatment [29].

Complications

Complications include intraspinal or intravascular injection and infection.

Case Report

A 22-year-old college student had sustained an injury to his upper back during weight lifting over 2 years before being examined in our pain clinic. Despite intensive chiropractic treatment for 2 years twice a week, the pain in his upper back, which radiated to his left shoulder blade, persisted. During the examination the only positive clinical findings were tenderness and pain to palpation over the left facet joints T3–T4 and T4–T5.

A diagnostic facet joint block at the T3–T4 and T4–T5 levels was performed with complete pain relief. The patient required an additional two facet joint blocks with a local anesthetic and cortico-steroid to eliminate his symptoms totally.

Two months later he returned with minimal pain in the upper back that recurred after strenuous exercises. Treatment with low-level energy laser therapy and a work loading exercise program was used with excellent results. The patient returned to his regular, active daily schedule, including weight lifting, with no restrictions.

Intercostal Block

Indications

The indications for intercostal block include:

1. Acute pain [12]:
   Postoperative pain relief
   Posttraumatic pain control
   Acute herpes zoster infection
2. Chronic pain [13]:
   Postherpetic neuralgia
   Intercostal neuralgia
   Pain in distribution of thoracic nerve roots
   Metastases to ribs

Contraindications

Contraindications to intercostal block include skin infection at site of injection, and pneumothorax.

Technique

The thoracic spinal nerve is formed by the fusion of dorsal and ventral roots distal to the spinal root ganglion (see Fig. 2.3). The thoracic spinal nerve communicates with the sympathetic system through rami communicantes and sends back to the spinal canal a small recurrent meningeal branch to innervate the meninges. Distal to the rami communicantes, the spinal nerve divides into dorsal and ventral branches. The dorsal branch innervates skin, muscles, and vertebrae. The ventral branch follows a rib and, at the level of the midaxillary line, the lateral branch rises. It divides into posterior and anterior divisions supplying the skin over the back and the anterior chest wall, respectively. The lateral cutaneous branches of the seventh to twelfth intercostal nerves supply sensory and motor innervation to the anterior abdominal wall.

The following techniques [13] can be used to administer an intercostal block: (1) paravertebral, (2) dorsolateral, or (3) anterolateral.

Paravertebral Block

The patient is placed in the prone position and the skin is prepared and draped in sterile manner. The point of entry for the block of the thoracic spinal nerve is 3 cm lateral and 3 cm caudal to the upper edge of the spinous process. The skin over the point of entry is anesthetized and a 22- or 25-gauge 3.5-inch short bevel needle is advanced vertically until the transverse process is felt. The needle then is repositioned caudally and advanced another 3 cm beyond the transverse process. After negative aspiration, medication is injected: for temporary blockade 5 ml of local anesthetic; for prolonged blockade 2–3 ml of 95–98% ethyl alcohol or 6–8% phenol in normal saline (Fig. 11.8).

Dorsolateral Intercostal Block

Dorsolateral intercostal block is a blockade of the ventral branch in the posterior axillary line. The patient is placed in the supine position and tilted 30 degrees to the contralateral side. The arm on the blocked side is abducted and the hand is placed under the neck. The area is prepared and draped using sterile technique. The site of entry is at the intersection of the posterior axillary line with the inferior margin of the rib. After placement of a skin wheal a 25- or 22-gauge short bevel needle is inserted in the direction of the palpated rib until bone contact is made. The needle then is "walked off" the rib caudally and advanced another 2–3 mm below the inferior margin of the rib. After negative aspiration, injection is performed: for temporary block 3 ml of local anesthetic; for prolonged blockade 2–3 ml absolute alcohol.

Anterolateral Intercostal Block

Anterolateral intercostal block is a blockade of the ventral branch in the anterior axillary line. The patient is placed in the supine position. After the skin is sterilized, landmarks are identified and a skin wheal is made at the intersection of the anterior axillary line and the inferior margin of the rib.

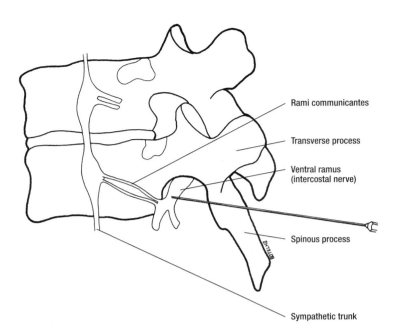

Figure 11.8. Schematic drawing of paravertebral thoracic block.

Rami communicantes

Transverse process

Ventral ramus
(intercostal nerve)

Spinous process

Sympathetic trunk

The same technique is used as for a posterolateral intercostal block, but the tip of the needle is advanced more caudally to the middle of the intercostal space (Fig. 11.9).

Complications

Possible complications include:

1. Pneumothorax
2. Hemothorax
3. Toxicity of anesthetic agent
4. Neuritis in neurolytic block

Case Study

A 40-year-old physician who fractured two ribs while playing football one week earlier was admitted to pain services because of a severe, sharp, constant pain in the right anterior chest wall that was aggravated by any movement as well as breathing, sneezing, or coughing. The pain was not relieved well enough with strong analgesics.

Chest x-ray films confirmed fractures of the T7 and T8 ribs without any other pathologic conditions. The patient's condition was diagnosed as intercostal neuralgia caused by the rib fractures, and an inter-

costal nerve block was performed at the T7 and T8 level using local anesthetic with complete pain relief and restoration of the mechanics of respiration. Relief from pain lasted over 24 hours and a second intercostal block was administered with excellent results. In the next few days he experienced only minimal tolerable discomfort that disappeared without any sequelae.

Intrapleural Analgesia

Injection of local anesthetic into the pleural cavity produces analgesia and sympathetic blockade in the chest wall and cavity, the shoulder, the upper limb, and in the upper abdomen [31]. To date there is no clear understanding of the mechanism of interpleural block. Spread of local anesthetic through the pleural cavity and surrounding nerve structures such as the intercostal nerves, sympathetic chain, splanchnic nerves, and celiac ganglion and the intrathoracic plexuses (aortic, pulmonary, and esophageal) may be responsible for interpleural analgesia.

The use of interpleural analgesia for postoperative pain relief was first reported by Reisted and Kvalheim [32] in 1984, and it was discovered as a complication of continuous intercostal nerve block. The use of interpleural analgesia has not been common practice in the management of pain, but in se-

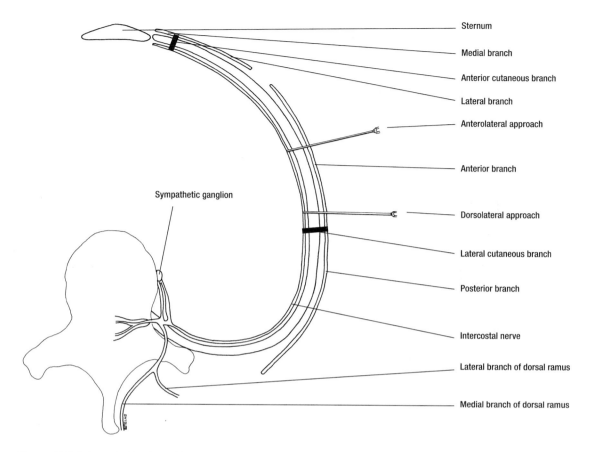

Figure 11.9. Schematic drawing of intercostal block.

lected cases direct interpleural infusion of local anesthetic can be very successful treatment for many painful conditions of the thorax and upper abdomen. Despite excellent results, the use of interpleural analgesia has declined because of the increase in popularity of the epidural local anesthetic/opioid technique and patient-controlled anesthesia (PCA) administration in the control of postoperative pain (Fig. 11.10).

Indications

Unilateral or bilateral interpleural analgesia has been used in the management of postoperative (acute), chronic, and cancer pain [33].

Acute Pain

Indications for the management of acute pain include:

    Postsurgical
        Postthoracotomy
        Unilateral breast surgery
        Minor chest wall procedures (e.g., chest tube insertion)
        Cholecystectomy
        Kidney surgery: nephrectomy, lithotripsy, percutaneous nephrostomy, nephrolithotomy
    Radiologic percutaneous procedure
    Rib fracture and blunt trauma to the chest

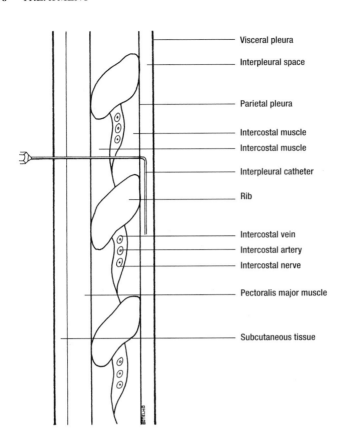

Visceral pleura

Interpleural space

Parietal pleura

Intercostal muscle
Intercostal muscle

Interpleural catheter

Rib

Intercostal vein
Intercostal artery
Intercostal nerve

Pectoralis major muscle

Subcutaneous tissue

Figure 11.10. Schematic drawing of interpleural block.

Injection of pleurodesis substances for recurrent pneumothorax and pleural effusion [34].

Chronic Pain

Indications for the control of chronic pain include:

Reflex sympathetic dystrophy and causalgia of the upper extremity and chest wall [35]
Postherpetic neuralgia and acute herpes zoster infection [36]
Phantom pain [33]
Intercostal neuralgia
Other chronic chest wall pain syndromes

Cancer Pain

Indications for the control of cancer pain include:

Intrathoracic carcinoma
Intra-abdominal cancers (e.g., pancreatic carcinoma) [37]

Advantages of Interpleural Analgesia Over Other Methods

No respiratory depression and no suppression of cough reflex
Good hemodynamic stability
Contralateral side of the body cannot be affected

Contraindications

Contraindications to the use of intrapleural anesthesia include [33]:

1. Local infection
2. Coagulopathies
3. Pneumonia or bronchitis with persistent cough
4. Bronchopleural fistula
5. Multiple emphysematous bullae
6. Respiratory failure
7. Extensive pleural fibrosis

Technique

The interpleural space should be approached at intercostal space 3–8 at the angle of the rib approximately 7–10 cm from the midline posteriorly [38]. The needle is introduced at the superior border of the inferior rib in the intercostal space.

The patient is placed in the lateral decubitus position with the affected side uppermost. The skin is prepared and draped in a sterile manner. The skin wheal is raised in the appropriate intercostal space over the superior border of the rib 7–10 cm from the posterior midline. A 17-gauge Huber-point Touhy epidural needle is introduced at the superior border of the rib and advanced toward the midline at an angle of about 60 degrees to the skin. The bevel of the needle is directed cephalad and against the chest wall. After walking off the edge of the rib, the stylet is removed and a 5-ml glass syringe is attached to the Touhy needle. The needle is slowly advanced; when it enters the pleural space a loss of resistance is felt on the plunger of the glass syringe. The syringe is removed, and a catheter is quickly introduced into the interpleural space to prevent entry of air. A hanging-drop method instead of the loss of resistance technique can be used. An interpleural catheter can be tunneled subcutaneously to decrease the possibility of infection, especially for long-term use.

Injection of local anesthetic is followed up. Bupivacaine is widely used because of its prolonged pain relief; 20 ml 0.25–0.50% bupivacaine lasts 4–12 hours. The addition of epinephrine, 1:200,000, to bupivacaine does not drastically change the duration of the block. The recommended dose is 0.3 ml/kg of 0.5% bupivacaine with epinephrine, not to exceed 10 mg/kg/24 hours. Continuous infusion can be used by infusing 5–10 ml/hour.

The patient should be kept supine for 20–30 minutes after the injection. In thoracic sympathetic block for upper extremity pain, the interpleural catheter is placed at the third or fourth intercostal space with the patient in 30 degrees of Trendelenburg.

Complications

There are a number of possible complications of intrapleural anesthesia [33]:

1. Pneumothorax
2. Hemothorax
3. Infection
4. Chylous thorax
5. Bronchospasm
6. Pleural effusion
7. Local anesthetic toxicity
8. Phrenic nerve paralysis (right intrapleural analgesia)
9. Rare complications: Fibrous thorax, pyothorax, etc.

Case Report

A 57-year-old building inspector suffering from inoperable metastatic adenocarcinoma of the upper lobe of the left lung and symptoms of a superior pulmonary sulcus syndrome was seen for pain control in our facility. At that time the patient was placed on oxycodone and acetaminophen (Percocet), 2 tablets every 3 hours. He could not tolerate stronger opioids such as morphine, dilaudid, or fentanyl patches because of undesirable side effects including nausea, vomiting, and drowsiness. The patient complained of severe constant pain in the left shoulder and left upper back associated with symptoms of brachial plexopathy; extensive left upper extremity weakness; Horner's syndrome; and swelling and changes of temperature in his left hand. An MRI study of the cervical spine revealed a neoplastic process involving the vertebral bodies of C5 and C6.

Because of the advanced stage of the disease, pain control was the medical priority. A trial epidural infusion of opioids was performed with some relief of pain but was unacceptable to the patient because of side effects. The patient also refused a cervical epidural neurolytic block. Therefore, an interpleural block was instituted, which almost completely controlled the patient's pain. The implanted interpleural catheter was connected to the external pump and 0.5% bupivacaine was continuously delivered into the interpleural space. The patient, relieved of pain, was sent home, where he died 3 weeks later.

Advanced Invasive Therapies

Spinal Cord Stimulation

Spinal cord stimulation was introduced by Shealy in 1967 as a nondestructive modality for controlling chronic, intractable pain [39]. Since that time, significant technical improvements in the device have been made, which markedly improved clinical results [40].

There are two techniques for the placement of spinal cord stimulator electrodes: surgically, through a thoracic laminectomy, and percutaneously, through a special 15-gauge epidural needle.

During placement of the electrodes, trial stimulation is applied, so the patient has to be awake to confirm the most optimal localization of electrodes. The mechanism of action of the spinal cord stimulator is still unclear, but it appears to block or reduce transmission of painful stimuli to the brain by electrical stimulation of the dorsal columns. Spinal cord stimulation produces paresthesia in the affected painful area.

Indications

Indications for spinal cord stimulation for control of pain in the thoracic spine include:

1. Chronic intractable neuropathic thoracic pain from reflex sympathetic dystrophy or postherpetic neuralgia.
2. Thoracic dorsal root injury.
3. Postcordotomy pain.

Contraindications

The contraindications for spinal cord stimulation are the same as those for epidural block.

Technique

The patient is placed in the prone position on an x-ray table in the operating room [41]. Under local anesthesia and with fluoroscopic guidance, using meticulous sterile technique, a special 15-gauge epidural needle is placed at the desired level into the epidural space using the loss of resistance technique.

Spinal cord stimulator electrodes are inserted through the epidural needle into the posterior epidural space, dorsally to the spinal cord and in the midline or slightly lateral to the midline if unilateral pain is present. Trial stimulation is then performed to find the optimal placement for the electrodes. After successful positioning of the electrode, the epidural needle is withdrawn and the electrode is an-

chored to the interspinous ligament. Subcutaneous implantation of the receiver or generator of the spinal cord stimulator and its connection with the electrode is the final step of operation.

Complications

Complications include:

1. Infection
2. Technical problems—e.g., fracture of the electrode wire, electrode migration
3. Puncture of the dura
4. Epidural hematoma
5. Postoperative allodynia
6. Neurologic sensory and motor deficit

Case Report

A 58-year-old retired businessman had a 30-year history of intractable, constant pain in the upper back radiating to the right infrascapular area associated with muscular spasm in the lower back and weakness of the right leg. Thirty years earlier while in military service he was involved in a fall from an armored vehicle and sustained a fracture of the T4 vertebral body with spinal cord contusion. The injuries required surgical decompression and because of the development of severe upper back pain he subsequently underwent another thoracic laminectomy and later a cordotomy at that level. Alleviation of pain lasted about 1 year and since that time he had "learned to live" with his pain and had also used TENS, analgesics, and anti-inflammatory medications for its control.

Because of the progressive deterioration of his condition and the failure of all other therapies, a spinal cord stimulator was implanted using a Resume electrode system (Medtronic) through an open laminectomy. Percutaneous implantation was unsuccessful because of calcification of the interspinal ligaments. Resume electrodes were positioned dorsally between T1 and T3 slightly to the right of the midline.

During the trial stimulation, complete relief of pain was achieved and therefore permanent implantation of a generator was performed under local anesthesia. At follow-up 6 months after the implantation of the spinal cord stimulator, the patient had been pain free with no restrictions in his active life.

Intraspinal Opioid Infusion System

Spinally administered narcotics when injected epidurally or intrathecally produce profound analgesia as a result of blocking of opiate receptors in the substantia gelatinosa of the spinal cord [42]. Control of cancer or chronic intractable pain can be achieved by the infusion of opioid intraspinally through the use of a totally implanted drug delivery system. Selection criteria for cancer patients [43] include poor pain relief with high, escalating doses of oral or subcutaneous narcotics; intolerable side-effects from systemic opioids; a life expectancy of more than 3 months.

There are many advantages of spinal infusion therapy for cancer patients, among them continuous delivery of small amounts of opioid directly to spinal opiate receptors, which produces profound analgesia; a decreased need for systemic medications; good improvement in the quality of life; no requirement for hospitalization after implantation; a lower risk of infection than with external systems.

Indications

Indications include chronic malignant pain and chronic intractable nonmalignant pain not responding to any other modality of treatment. Trial infusion therapy must be successful before implantation.

Contraindications

Contraindications include:

1. Infection or decubitus ulcer at the site of implantation
2. Coagulopathy
3. Predicted survival less than 3 months
4. Severe lung disease with hypoxemia
5. Poor general health

Technique

The surgical implantation of the intraspinal catheter and pump can be done under local and general anesthesia. The intraspinal catheter is placed percutaneously through a 14- or 15-gauge epidural needle and can be placed epidurally or intrathecally using routine techniques described previously [44, 45]. The spinal catheter is tunneled subcutaneously and connected to the pump implanted subcutaneously and suprafascially in the lower or upper quadrant of the abdomen. The pump is refilled with morphine every 30–60 days.

Complications

Complications include:

1. Infection
2. Postsurgical bleeding
3. CSF leakage
4. Postspinal headache
5. Catheter obstruction

Prolotherapy

Prolotherapy, also known as sclerotherapy or reconstructive therapy, is the therapeutic process of injecting a proliferative agent into connective tissues, mostly into ligaments, tendons, and fascia, to create a controlled, localized inflammatory reaction. Inflammation triggers a healing reaction, including proliferation of fibroblasts and new collagen production [46]. This process significantly increases the mass of the connective tissue, which, by becoming stronger and more elastic, normalizes the biomechanics of the spinal segments.

The term *prolotherapy* was popularized by Hackett [47], a physician from Canton, Ohio, in the mid-1950s. Hackett had observed tissue contracture after the use of sclerosant agents in the treatment of inguinal hernias. He demonstrated good results with injection of sclerosants into ligaments of the lower back, with a cure rate of 82% in 1600 patients. The positive effects of prolotherapy were reported by Liu in 1983 [48], Ongley in 1987 [46], and Klein in 1989 [49] with documentation of strengthened ligaments, decreased pain, and objective increases in range of motion.

Indications

Indications for prolotherapy include:

1. Thoracic facet joint instability associated with

scoliosis, osteoarthritis, compression fracture, or spondylolisthesis
2. Discopathy
3. Laxity of ligaments of the thoracic spine
4. Chronic persistent pain associated with stiffness and an inability to maintain any posture for a prolonged time that is aggravated by bending and twisting movements, with no neurologic deficit suggesting ligament injury.

Contraindications

Contraindications to prolotherapy include infection at the site of injection and sensitivity to the proliferative agent.

Agents

1. 12.5% Dextrose: a mixture of 2.5 ml 50% dextrose with 7.5 ml 0.5% lidocaine. Twenty to 30 ml of this solution can be safely used.
2. Ongley's solution or P25G solution [46]: a mixture of 2.5% phenol, 25% glucose, and 25% glycerine. The solution is diluted half and half with 0.5% lidocaine.

Some other proliferative agents, not used in my practice, include sodium morrhuate, PQU solution, zinc sulfate solution, and pumice suspension [50].

Technique

The patient is placed in a prone position. The thoracic spine is examined and all tender areas, especially those located over the facet joints, are identified. Under sterile conditions and after the skin is anesthetized, a 22- or 25-gauge 3.5-inch needle is advanced into the facet joint capsules and also in the midline into corresponding segments of the interspinous ligaments. Approximately 0.2–0.5 ml of the proliferative solution is deposited at each site. Occasionally, additional injections are made in the periosteum of the transverse processes.

After the prolotherapy treatment, patients are encouraged to perform simple stretching exercises to diminish postinjection pain and improve spreading of the proliferative agent.

Most patients experience soreness and discomfort at the injection sites for 24–48 hours after the treatment.

Complications

Complications of prolotherapy include:

1. Infection
2. Allergic reaction
3. Neuritis
4. Periostitis
5. Headache from inadvertent dural puncture
6. Intravascular injection

Case Report

A 40-year-old travel agent had a 3-year history of aching and occasionally sharp pain in the left side of the upper and lower back associated with muscular spasms and difficulty in bending and rotation of her trunk. This otherwise relatively healthy woman underwent multiple conservative treatments including chiropractic manipulations, physical therapy programs, pharmacologic treatment, and psychological evaluation with no success. During the physical examination of the initial consultation the only positive findings found were pain and tenderness to palpation of the facet joints and intercostal spaces in the left paramedial line at the T8–T12 level.

A magnetic resonance imaging (MRI) study of the thoracolumbar spine was interpreted as negative. Prolotherapy to the spinal ligaments and facet joint capsules at the T8–T12 level was performed under fluoroscopic control by using 12.5% dextrose in 0.5% lidocaine as a proliferant. The patient underwent a series of four treatments of prolotherapy, once every 2 weeks. At the same time she participated in a physical therapy program. Results of the treatment were successful, with complete relief of pain and improvement of mobility.

Acupuncture

Traditional Chinese medicine considers movement of energy as a source of life. This vital life energy circulates through the human body and also through all living organisms. The energy, called Qi (Chi), can flow because of polarity between two different states: Yin and Yang, where Yang is active and positive, and Yin is passive and negative [70]. The same principle governs the cyclic changes of the seasons, the change of day and night, and change of the function of every living cell, from the resting to the active state.

Vital energy, Qi, contains many different forms of energy; hereditary, cosmic, nutritional, protective, and so forth. This energy flows through very specific, unchangeable pathways called meridians. There are 12 paired symmetric meridians, each corresponding to a major body organ. Energy flows through the meridians in a characteristic order at a specific time of the day. It runs from the lung meridian to the large intestine, to the stomach, spleen, heart, small intestine, urinary bladder, kidney, pericardium, triple heater, gallbladder, liver, and back to the lung meridian [71]. Any disturbances in the flow of the Qi, either a deficiency or an excess, will disrupt the cycle and create a disease process. In traditional Chinese medicine the human body is considered as a whole system, and the role of the physician is to optimize the movement of Qi forces, working with them to achieve perfect balance and harmony. The physician should not only treat any pathologic state of the body but should also take an active role in the maintenance of health.

In addition to 12 principal meridians, there are tendomuscular meridians, distinct meridians, curious meridians, and other systems of transmitting energy between meridians or directly to the organs [71]. In every meridian there are multiple acupuncture points that can be stimulated to achieve balance in the flow of Qi through the body. Interestingly, at acupuncture points considerably lower electrical resistance was found, and stimulation of these points produced strong physiologic effects [70], including changes in the levels of most neurotransmitters, changes in white and red blood counts, increases in levels of endorphins, and changes in immunoglobulin levels.

Traditional acupuncture is a technique involving the insertion of special needles into acupuncture points at specific meridians to balance the disturbed energy system. Acupuncture can be practiced with any kind of needle, but the needle has to work as a conductor of electrons. Usually the needle is made of stainless steel, silver, or gold.

Indications

All illnesses of whatever nature can be successfully treated with acupuncture treatment.

Contraindications

Contraindications to acupuncture include:

1. Local infection
2. Pregnancy
3. Alcohol intoxication
4. Emotional disturbances
5. Patient fatigue

Depending on the medical condition, the nature of the energy flow disturbance, the patient's personality, and the results of careful medical examination, acupuncture points are chosen. Two different techniques of point stimulation can be administered: tonification or dispersion. During tonification, local excitation produces a local depolarization. Tonification of the distal point of the meridian will create a wave of depolarization-repolarization along the meridian. During dispersion a needle placed into an acupuncture point will move ions and electrolytes along the meridian, acting like microbattery.

There are very few complications of acupuncture practice, including infection, which is very rare, and vertigo or fainting during the treatment. In spite of many years of research and generalized acceptance of acupuncture across the world as an effective and safe treatment, to date the American Medical Association and the Food and Drug Administration consider acupuncture an experimental form of therapy.

Acupuncture and traditional Chinese medicine are not merely a technical skill, but a profound philosophy and science requiring extensive knowledge and many years of practice and study.

Newest Noninvasive Therapies

Low-Reactive Level Laser Therapy (LLLT)

The laser (light amplification by stimulated emission of radiation) was first developed by Maiman in 1960 [51]. It rapidly found application in the medical field, especially in ophthalmology, surgery, and dermatology. During the use of surgical lasers additional effects were noted, mainly decreases in pain and tissue inflammation. The importance of this biological phenomenon was recognized by researchers and low-power and low-energy density systems were developed.

The first experimental and clinical applications of low-reactive level laser therapy (LLLT) were reported in 1968 by Mester in Hungary for the treatment of vascular ulcers [52, 53]. Since that time therapeutic lasers have been widely used in most European and Asiatic countries. In the United States, the Food and Drug Administration has yet to approve LLLT devices for a single application in medicine.

Low-level energy laser biostimulation has nonthermic effects in tissues and most LLLT lasers can be separated into two groups according to wavelength: visible light lasers (e.g., He Ne: 632.8 nm), and infrared lasers (e.g., Ga Al As: 820 or 904 nm). Most generate 5–200 mW of power and are classified as class 3b medical devices (International Standards System). This means that the LLLT lasers are considered to present a potential hazard to the eyes, and protective goggles must be used by a therapist and a patient during the treatment [54].

The mechanism of action of LLLT is still not completely known. Many published theories suggest that LLLT of visible red light activates the enzymatic system in the cell, mostly in the mitochondria, increasing the level of the ATP and starting cell proliferation [54–56]. In infrared laser irradiation, the energy is absorbed in the cell membrane, affecting membrane permeability and ion transfer and increasing Na-K-ATPase activity [55, 56]. The LLLT photobioactivation follows the principle of the biologic Arndt-Schultz law.

General Indications

General indications for LLLT include [54, 55]:

1. Wound healing [57]
2. Acute soft- and hard-tissue injuries
3. Acute inflammatory conditions
4. Chronic inflammatory conditions (e.g., arthritis) [58, 59]
5. Musculoskeletal disorders
6. Neuralgias and neuropathies
7. Temporomandibular joint dysfunction
8. Chronic pain disorders

The use of LLLT offers many therapeutic advantages in irradiated areas, including pain attenuation, anti-inflammatory action, increased blood flow, and decreased edema.

Contraindications

Contraindications to LLLT include:

1. Conditions in which direct application to the eye is necessary
2. Pregnancy
3. Neoplasm at the site of the irradiation
4. Skin photosensitivity

Technique

The LLLT beam can be applied to the affected area using a contact or noncontact technique with an initial dosage of 1–4 J/cm^2 depending on the type of the tissue involved in the disease process. For noncontact technique, scanning devices or manual scanning is recommended [55].

In the early stages of therapy, daily treatments are advised. A regimen with a minimum of two treatments per week regimen showed successful therapeutic effects in the published literature [54].

Complications

Complications of LLLT include occasional transient nausea, dizziness, or headache.

Pulsated Electromagnetic Field Therapy

Low-frequency, low-energy pulsated electromagnetic field therapy (PEMF) has been used for a few decades for wound healing and bone regeneration [60]. Recently, magnetic therapy has gained interest because of the latest scientific explanation for its biological effects on human cells [62, 63]. The magnetic fields completely permeate the body and therefore may reach every single cell. A pulsated electromagnetic wave is able to reactivate the transport of ions through the cell membrane by normalizing the membrane potentials [63, 64]. It also influences the activity of enzymes and coenzymes by stimulating the paramagnetic ions such as iron, chromium, copper, molybdenum, etc. [65, 66]. In experimental studies, PEMF showed an influence on liquid crystals, which are part of many biologic structures [64, 66, 67]. Additional positive effects of PEMF have been observed [63], including:

Increases in regeneration processes
Antispasmodic and anti-inflammatory effects
Improvements in oxygen utilization
Vasodilatation
Acceleration of callus formation
Alleviation of pain

Pulsated electromagnetic field therapy uses pulsated sinusoidal or rectangular electromagnetic waves, with a field density of 10–100 Gauss and a frequency of 1–50 Hz. It is a completely painless, non-invasive, office-based treatment.

Indications

Indications for PEMF include [63]:

1. Wound healing.
2. Nonunion of fracture [60, 61].
3. Delayed bone healing and failed arthrodeses [68].
4. Osteoporosis [69].
5. Avascular necrosis of the hip.
6. Legg-Calvé-Perthes disease.
7. Degenerative spine disease.
8. Osteoarthritis and rheumatoid arthritis.
9. Soft-tissue injuries.
10. Chronic pain conditions.

There are no known complications of PEMF and the only contraindication is pacemaker usage.

References

1. Bogduk N. The innervation of lumbar spine. Spine 1983;8:286–293.
2. Groen G, Baljet B, Drukker J. Nerves and nerve plexuses of the human vertebral column. Am J Anat 1990; 188:282–296.
3. Groen G, Baljet B, Drukker J. The innervation of the spinal dura mater: anatomy and clinical implications. Acta Neurochir (Wien) 1988;92:39–46.
4. Groen G, Baljet B, Boekelaar A et al. Branches of the thoracic sympathetic trunk in the human fetus. Anat Embryol 1987;176:401–411.
5. Stern E. Relief of intractable pain by intraspinal subarachnoid injection of alcohol. Am J Surg 1934;25: 217–227.
6. Bonica J. Subarachnoid Alcohol Block. In J Bonica (ed), The Management of Pain. Philadelphia: Lea & Febiger, 1953.
7. Swerdlow M. Subarachnoid and Extradural Neurolytic Block. In Advances in Pain Research and Therapy. Vol. 2. New York: Raven, 1979;325–337.
8. Perese D. Subarachnoid alcohol block in the management of pain of malignant disease. AMA Arch Surg 1958;76:347–354.
9. Blanchard J, Ramamurhty S. Subarachnoid Alcohol Block. In G Racz (ed), Techniques of Neurolysis. Boston: Kulwer Academic, 1989.
10. Lloyd J. Subarachnoid and Other Clinical Uses of Phenol. In G Racz (ed), Techniques of Neurolysis. Boston: Kulwer Academic, 1989.
11. Bonica J. The management of pain of malignant disease with nerve blocks. Anesthesiology 1954;15:134–145.
12. Katz J, Renck H. Handbook of Thoraco-Abdominal Nerve Block. Orlando, FL: Grune & Stratton, 1987.
13. Bonica J, Buckley P. Regional Analgesia with Local Anesthetics. In J Bonica (ed), The Management of Pain. Philadelphia: Lea & Febiger, 1990.
14. Swerdlow M. Intrathecal neurolysis. Anesthesia 1978;33:733–740.
15. Swerdlow M. Intrathecal and Extradural Block in Pain Relief. In M Swerdlow (ed), Relief of Intractable Pain. New York: Elsevier, 1983;174–211.
16. Hughes J. Thrombosis of the posterior spinal artery. Neurology 1970;20:659.
17. Wagner F. Thoracic Epidural Anesthesia. In Regional Anesthesia. Chicago: Year Book, 1985;117–125.
18. Cousins M, Brindenbaugh P. Neural Blockade in Clinical Anesthesia and Management of Pain. Philadelphia: Lippincott, 1988.
19. Scott D. Techniques of Regional Anesthesia. Norwalk, CT: Appleton & Lange, 1989.
19a. Blomberg R. A method for epiduroscopy and spinalscopy, presentation of preliminary results. Acta Anesth Scand 1985;29:113–116.
20. Zenz M, Panhans C, Niesel H. Regional Anesthesia. Chicago: Year Book, 1988.
21. McCarron R. Epidural Fibrosis: Experimental Models and Therapeutic Alternatives. In G Racz (ed), Techniques of Neurolysis. Boston: Kluwer, 1989.
22. McCarron R, Wimpee M, Hudkins P et al. The inflammatory effect of nucleus pulposus: a possible element in the pathogenesis of low back pain. Spine 1987;12: 760–764.
23. Racz G, Holubec J. Lysis of Adhesions in the Epidural Space. In G Racz (ed), Techniques of Neurolysis. Boston: Kulwer Academic, 1989.
24. Racz G, Sabonghy M, Gintautas J et al. Intractable pain therapy using a new epidural catheter. JAMA 1982; 248:646–647.

25. Stolker R, Vervest A. Percutaneous Epidural Adhesiolysis in "Failed Back Syndrome." In Proceedings of the Third European Congress on Back Pain, Glasgow, 1990.

26. Bonica J. Sympathetic Nerve Blocks for Pain Diagnosis and Therapy. New York: Breon Laboratories, 1980.

27. Dvorak J, Dvorak V. Manual of Medicine Diagnostics. New York: Thieme, 1990.

28. Grieve G. Common Vertebral Joint Problems. Edinburgh: Churchill Livingstone, 1988.

29. Stolker R, Vervest A, Groen G. Percutaneous facet denervation in chronic thoracic spinal pain. Acta Neurochir (Wien) 1993;122:82–90.

30. Stanton-Hicks M. Blocks of the Sympathetic Nervous System. In M Stanton-Hicks (ed), Pain and the Sympathetic Nervous Syndrome. Boston: Kulwer, 1989.

31. Rosenberg P. Interpleural analgesia. Pain Digest 1992;2:1–2.

32. Kvalheim L, Reiestad F. Intrapleural catheter in the management of postoperative pain. Anesthesiology 1984; 61:A231.

33. Stromskag K. Interpleural regional analgesia: clinical and experimental aspects. Tapir Forlag 1991;1:37.

34. Shanta T. Interpleural analgesia to relieve pain induced by tetracycline pleurodesis. Pain Digest 1992;2:28–29.

35. Shanta T. Causalgia induced by telephone mediated lightning electrical injury and treated by interpleural block. Anesth Analg 1991;73:502–503.

36. Reiestad F, McIlvaine W, Barnes M. Interpleural analgesia in the treatment of severe postherpetic neuralgia. Reg Anesth 1990;15:113–117.

37. Durrani Z, Winnie A, Ikuta P. Interpleural catheter analgesia for pancreatic pain. Anesth Analg 1988;67: 479–481.

38. Reiestad F, Stromskag K. Interpleural catheter in the management of postoperative pain, a preliminary study. Reg Anesth 1986;11:89–91.

39. Shealy N, Mortimer J, Reswick J. Electrical inhibition of pain by stimulation of the dorsal columns: a preliminary report. Anesth Analg 1967;46:489–491.

40. North R, Kidd D, Zahurak M et al. Spinal cord stimulation for chronic intractable pain: experience over two decades. Neurosurgery 1993;32:384–394.

41. North R. Spinal Cord Stimulation for Intractable Pain: Indication and Technique. In Current Therapy in Neurological Surgery. Toronto: BC Decker, 1988.

42. Duggan A, Hall J, Headley P. Suppression of transmission of nociceptive impulses by morphine: selective effects of morphine administered in the region of substantia gelatinosa. Br J Pharmacol 1977;61:65–67.

43. Penn R, Paice J. Chronic intrathecal morphine for intractable pain. J Neurosurg 1987;67:182–186.

44. Krames F, Gershow J, Glassberg A et al. Continuous infusion of spinally administered narcotics for the relief of pain due to malignant disorders. Cancer 1985;56:3.

45. Penn R, Paice J et al. Cancer pain relief using chronic morphine infusion early experience with programmable implanted drug pump. J Neurosurg 1984;61:302–306.

46. Ongley M, Klein R, Dorman T et al. A new approach to the treatment of chronic back pain. Lancet 1987;2: 143–146.

47. Hackett G. Ligament and Tendon Relaxation Treated by Prolotherapy. Springfield, IL: Thomas, 1958.

48. Liu Y, Tipton C, Matthews R et al. An in situ study of the influence of sclerosing solution in rabbit medial collateral ligaments and its junction strength. Conn. Tissue Res 1983;11:95–102.

49. Klein R, Dorman T, Johnson C. Proliferant injection for low back pain: histological changes of injected ligaments and objective measurements of lumbar spine mobility before and after treatment. J Neuro Orthop Med Surg 1989;10:123–126.

50. Dorman T, Ravin T. Diagnosis and Injection Techniques in Orthopedic Medicine. Baltimore: Williams & Wilkins, 1991.

51. Maiman T. Stimulated optical radiation in ruby. Nature 1960;187:493.

52. Mester E, Szende B, Tota J. Effect of laser on hair growth of mice. (In Hungarian.) Kiserl Oversud 1967;19:628–631.

53. Mester E, Juhasz J, Varga P et al. Lasers in clinical practice. Acta Chir Acad Hung 1968;9:349–357.

54. Baxter D. Therapeutic Lasers: Theory and Practice. New York: Churchill Livingstone, 1994.

55. Ohshiro T, Calderhead R. Progress in Laser Therapy. New York: Wiley, 1991.

56. Kudoh C, Inomata K, Okajima K et al. Effects of 830-nm GaAlAs diode laser radiation on rat saphenous nerve sodium-potassium-adenosine triphosphatase activity: a possible pain attenuation mechanism examined. Laser Ther 1989;2:63–67.

57. Mester A, Mester A. Wound healing. Laser Ther 1989;1:7–15.

58. Goldman J, Chiapella J, Casey H et al. Laser therapy of rheumatoid arthritis. Lasers Surg Med 1980;1:93–101.

59. Gartner C. Low reactive level laser therapy (LLLT) in rheumatology: a review of clinical experience in the author's laboratory. Laser Ther 1992;4:107–115.

60. Bassett C, Mitchell S, Gaston S. Treatment of ununited tibial diaphyseal fractures with pulsing electromagnetic fields. J Bone Joint Surg 1981;63:511–523.

61. Bassett C, Pawluk R, Pilla A. Acceleration of fracture repair by electromagnetic fields. Ann N Y Acad Sci 1974;238:242–262.

62. McCaig C, Rajnicek A. Electrical fields, nerve growth and nerve regeneration. Exp Physiol 1991;76:473–494.

63. Sieron A, Cieslak G, Adamek M. Low energy magnetic therapy and laser therapy. (In Polish.) Silesia Medical School, Katowice, 1993.

64. Becker A. A theory of interaction between DC and ELF electromagnetic fields and living organisms. J Bioelect 1985;11:133–140.

65. Cook E, Smith M. Biological Effects of Magnetic Fields. New York: Plenum, 1964.

66. Villa M et al. Biological effects of magnetic fields. Life Sci 1991;49:85–92.

67. Tenforde T. Biological interactions of extremely low frequency electric and magnetic fields. Bioelectrochem Bioenerg 1991;25:1–17.

68. Bassett C, Mitchell S, Gaston S. Pulsing electromagnetic field treatment in non united fractures and failed arthrodeses. JAMA 1982;247:623–628.

69. Tabrah F, Hoffmeier M, Gilbert F Jr et al. Bone density changes in osteoporosis-prone women exposed to pulsed electromagnetic fields (PEMF). J Bone Miner Res 1990;5:437–442.

70. Stux G, Pomeranz B. Acupuncture. New York: Springer, 1987.

71. Wu Pei Ping. Chinese Acupuncture. Paris: Health Science Press, 1962.

Chapter 12

Therapeutic Exercise and Self-Correction Programs

Beate Carrière

Role and Function of the Body Segment Thorax

The body segment thorax acts as the stabilizing "center" of the body and is greatly influenced by posture and movement. Klein-Vogelbach stated that movement impulses coming from the legs via the pelvis, from the arms via the shoulder girdle, and from the head via the neck have to be stabilized and coordinated [1]. Dynamic stability (one or several joints stabilized through muscular activity) of the thoracic spine is required when leaning the neutral spine forward, backward, or sideways or during rotation. The definition of a neutral spine is when the pelvis, thorax, and head are aligned in the longitudinal axis of the body. The body weight should be evenly distributed over the base of support while sitting or standing. Muscle activity is then economized, thus preventing wear and tear of joint and ligamentous structures. To prevent injuries to the spine, this dynamic stability must be maintained regardless of the speed of movement of the trunk, head, or arms and any additional load they may be carrying.

Adequate mobility of the spine is necessary to enable the spinal canal to elongate between 5 and 9 cm from spinal extension to spinal flexion [2]. Butler stated that humans are capable of highly skilled movements with the nervous system stretched, slack, stationary, or mobile [3]. Loss of flexibility of the thoracic spine is therefore clinically important. An inflexible person may no longer move eco-

nomically, thus requiring greater energy expenditure and abnormal muscle substitution to complete even simple tasks.

Therapeutic exercises of the thoracic spine should support gains achieved by the techniques described in previous chapters. The global treatment goals may include improving mobility of the entire spine, achieving dynamic stability of the thoracic spine through progressive strengthening exercises, and obtaining normal abdominal breathing. A mobile spine allows for postural adjustments. A dynamically stable trunk in neutral position is required to facilitate normal breathing, to maintain good posture, and to provide a solid base for the shoulder girdle, upper extremities, neck, and head. This dynamic stability allows the arms to move freely in an open kinetic chain.

Functional Abdominal Breathing

Functional abdominal breathing decreases the load on the auxiliary breathing muscles, such as the scalene. It allows the thoracic spine to maintain dynamic stability during respiration. Inspiration (elevation of the ribs) causes a movement impulse that, if allowed to continue, would extend the thoracic spine past neutral. This extension of the spine should be prevented by the stabilizing muscle activity of the antagonists. The term *active buttressing* describes this stabilizing activity of the trunk flexors during inspiration [1]. This is reversed during expiration where the trunk extensors, through active buttressing, maintain a neutral spine. Breathing exercises that only encourage expiration with flexion and inspiration with extension of the thoracic spine promote faulty movement patterns and should be avoided [4].

All patients with thoracic spine or rib cage dysfunction should be instructed in functional abdominal breathing. During the initial instruction, the patient should be in a supine position with both hands placed on the upper abdomen and the lower rib cage. The patient should be instructed to feel the abdomen lift with inspiration and lower with expiration. The length of the trunk must remain stable. This training may require verbal cues such as "don't arch your back." After mastering abdominal breathing in the supine position, the patient should progress to sitting and standing while applying the same breathing technique. The practitioner can then progress to manual resistance to the abdomen or rib cage during inspiration [5].

Postural Balance

Posture is a physiologic and psychological phenomenon. It is not only an expression of personality, it is also a complex reaction to a multitude of influences from the environment [6]. Both have to be considered when treating a patient. Faulty movement patterns often appear "normal" to a patient. These patterns can only be altered when the patient is ready to change the perception of movement. For example, a depressed or grieving person may have greater difficulties changing posture. Behavioral responses usually include withdrawal and decreased postural adaption. Umphred emphasized that the practitioner should know about the limbic system and its connection to the motor system. Sensitivity to the emotional state of a patient is a key factor in understanding the motor responses observed during therapy. Cooperation and follow through with postural changes are dependent on the patient's motivation, concentration, and alertness [7].

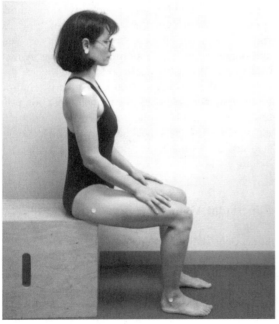 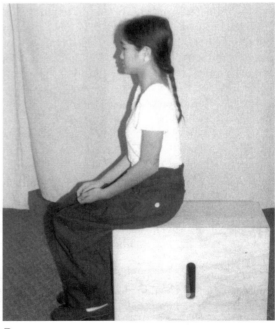

A   B

Figure 12.1. A. In correct upright posture while sitting (healthy subject), a plumb line in the mid-frontal plane bisects the ear, the middle of the acromion, and the trochanter. B. An optimal compromised upright sitting posture in a 13-year-old girl after T12 and L1 compression fractures, a right acetabulum fracture, and a right femur fracture. There is maximal hip flexion of 90 degrees in this patient.

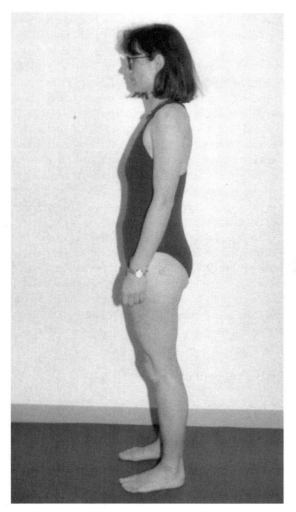

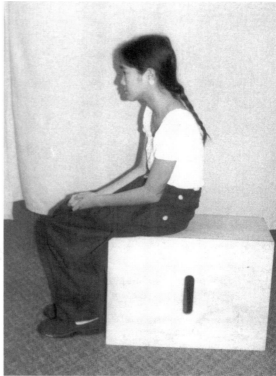

Figure 12.3. Faulty sitting posture secondary to loss of hip flexion after multiple fractures of the spine, acetabulum, and femur.

Figure 12.2. In good upright standing posture (healthy subject), a plumb line passes through the ear, the middle of the acromion, the greater trochanter, and anterior to the lateral malleolus.

Postural balance should be evaluated with the patient sitting and standing. In the sitting position, the pelvis, trunk, and head should be aligned such that a vertical plumb line would bisect the ear, the middle of the acromion, and the greater trochanter (Fig. 12.1). In the standing position, the plumb line should also bisect the lateral femoral condyle and pass just anterior to the lateral malleolus (Fig. 12.2). A common mistake in correcting standing posture is to have the patient perform a chin tuck. Even with poor postural alignment, in the standing position the head is positioned over the feet. When correcting posture, the practitioner should consider the relative position

of the head and feet. For example, moving the thorax forward and upward will move the neck toward its normal neutral position if the head is still above the feet.

Good mobility of the pelvis in all directions is of paramount importance for the thoracic spine. If while sitting the pelvis is locked in a posterior tilt (possibly caused by short proximal hamstrings or decreased active hip flexion), the result is flexion of the lumbar and thoracic spine and a forward head posture (Fig. 12.3). In attempting to counteract gravity, a reactive hypertonus of the upper trapezius and other posterior neck muscles occurs. Flexion of the

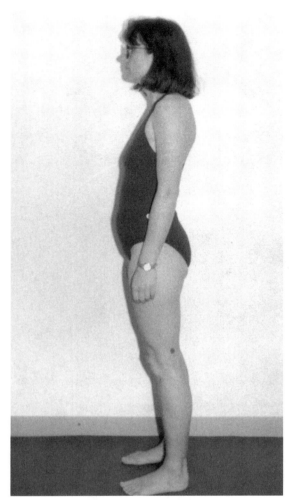

Figure 12.4. Faulty standing posture (healthy subject). Note the increased anterior pelvic tilt, the trunk leaning backward, and the forward head position.

thoracic spine results in protraction of the shoulders and shortening of the pectoral muscles. The back extensor muscles become overstretched, the rectus abdominis muscle becomes shortened, and the oblique abdominal muscles become weakened. Abdominal breathing may be compromised. This, in turn, may result in using auxiliary muscles such as the scalene for breathing. This example of a deviation of sitting posture demonstrates that when treating thoracic spine problems the practitioner should not limit the exercises to the thoracic spine but may include hamstring stretches, hip flexion strengthening exercises, and abdominal breathing in the treatment program.

Another example of postural imbalance is when shortened hip flexor muscles (both the rectus femoris and the iliopsoas muscles) cause an anterior tilt of the pelvis while standing (Fig. 12.4). This results in a postural imbalance, where the trunk leans backward, resulting in an overstretched rectus abdominis, the shoulders and head being "pulled" forward, and the pectoral muscles being shortened. There is also a shortening of the posterior neck muscles and increased extension at the atlanto-occipital joint. Therefore, stretching the hip flexor muscles is necessary to allow the patient to achieve a neutral spine and correct this cascade of compensatory changes.

Other possible causes of postural deviations are a difference in leg length or pelvic asymmetries. With prolonged sitting or when performing exercises, it may be necessary for the patient to sit on a pad that accommodates the asymmetry of the pelvis. Heel lifts or orthotics may be indicated for leg length discrepancies [8].

Body Proportions

Body proportions [1,9] (Fig. 12.5) should be considered when planning exercises for the thoracic spine. Body segments or body parts constitute body weights. For example, when doing a sit-up, a patient with a long trunk will be required to generate a greater abdominal force (or hip flexion substitution) than an individual with a short trunk. This exercise should be designed differently depending on the patient's proportions so that each patient performs the task correctly. Thus, the long-trunked patient could be asked to start the exercise in a sitting position, leaning the stable trunk backward as far as possible without giving up stability and then returning to a neutral sitting posture (Fig. 12.6).

On the other hand, a patient with long legs and a short trunk should not be asked to train the lower abdominal muscles in a supine position with straight leg raises. Instead, the knees should be flexed, thus decreasing the length of the resistance lever. Hip flexion then is initiated, thereby avoiding undue strain to the low back (Fig. 12.7).

Depending on the patient's proportions, external adjustments such as raising or lowering the chair or table may be necessary for the patient to be able to maintain a neutral spine in sitting. Special attention

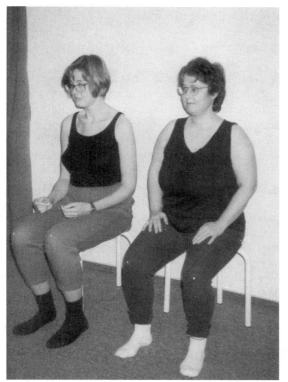

A

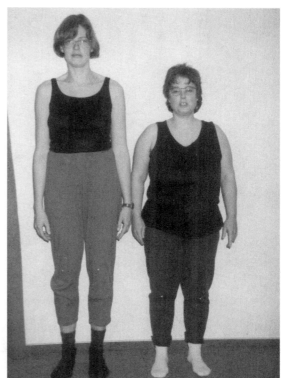

B

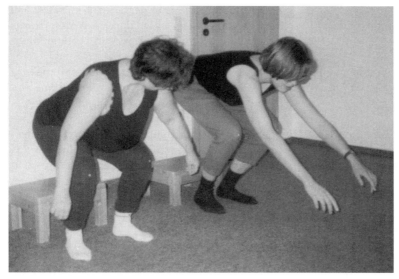

C

Figure 12.5. Body proportions. A. Note similar size while sitting. B. Note the difference in the length of the arms and legs when standing. C. Note the effect when trying to stand from sitting. The person with long thighs has to lean farther forward and use her arms to counterbalance the weight of the trunk.

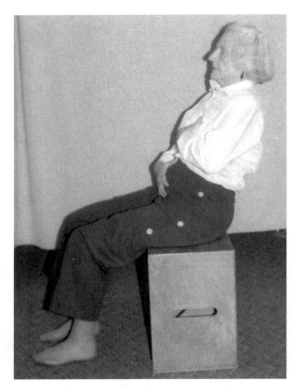

Figure 12.6. Leaning backward with the trunk aligned to strengthen the abdominal muscles.

should be paid to the length of the patient's upper arm. Short upper arms can cause a destabilization of the thorax if the armrests or the table are too low [1, 8, 9].

The practitioner should also consider the patient's bone structure when designing exercises. Heavy bone structure means greater constitutional weight than light or normal bone structure. A patient's constitution cannot be altered and usually does not cause pain if it is a variant within the norm [1]. Although excessive muscle mass of the shoulder girdle, arms, or neck in weightlifters may produce pain and dysfunction in the thoracic spine, this constitutes a distal weight, which has to be stabilized by the thoracic spine when leaning forward. This can be avoided by a weight training regimen that includes posterior shoulder and trunk extensor exercises. Obesity can also be considered an added resistance to the maintenance of a neutral posture and must be addressed in any thoracic exercise program.

Principles of Exercises

"Imbalance of Length and Strength"

A tight muscle loses its elasticity and shortens at rest. The consequences can be altered joint mechanics with a resultant uneven distribution of pressure, changed proprioceptive input, and altered programming of movement patterns. Janda, in describing muscles that have a tendency to develop tightness and affect the function of the thoracic spine, reported that tightness of the iliopsoas, rectus femoris, and the hamstring muscles can prevent mobility of the pelvis and hip joints [10]. Good mobility of the pelvis and the hips is necessary to align the thoracic spine in the sagittal plane of the body. In the trunk and neck, the quadratus lumborum, spinal erectors, pectoralis, upper trapezius, levator scapulae, and sternocleidomastoid are muscles that routinely develop tightness and produce malalignment of the thoracic spine in the sagittal plane. Unilateral tightness of a muscle group can result in asymmetries in all body planes. Janda also described that muscles such as the rectus abdominus, the lower stabilizers of the scapula (rhomboids, middle and lower trapezius, and serratus anterior), the deep neck flexor muscles, and the extensor muscles of the upper extremity have a tendency to acquire weakness and become inhibited and hypotonic.

The combination of tightness and weakness of muscles in one region affects posture and can contribute to thoracic spine problems. Janda [11] described a "crossed syndrome" in the pelvic area as an imbalance of tight and weak muscles causing a forward pelvic tilt, an increased lumbar lordosis, and an increased hip flexion. The "proximal crossed syndrome" typically has tightness and weakness in the neck and shoulder/scapula area causing postural changes such as protraction and elevation of the shoulders, a forward head, winging scapulae, and hypermobility of the C4–C5 and the T4 segments. This should be recognized and addressed when exercising the patient. Both tight and overstretched muscles develop weakness. Stretching a tight muscle to its normal length enables the antagonist to shorten to its normal length and to contract efficiently. Tight muscles should only be strengthened when they reach a reasonable flexibility.

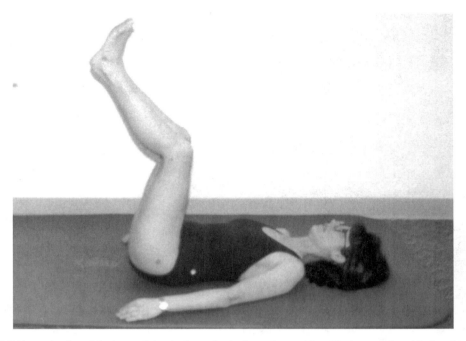

Figure 12.7. Strengthening of the lower abdominal muscles in the supine position. The legs are flexed before they are raised.

White and Sahrmann agreed with Janda on the significance of precise analysis of faulty movement patterns and that the restoration of the proper muscle length is necessary to achieve a movement system balance. Faulty muscle dominance can increase the disuse of the synergistic muscles, causing a greater muscular imbalance. The possible effect on joints is increased wear and tear because of the deviation of the kinesiologic standard of movement for each axis of motion. White and Sahrmann emphasized shortening muscles and connective tissue structures that are too long by employing specific strengthening exercises in an attempt to correct the faulty movement [12].

Exercises in general should not cause pain, since pain is a poor motivator. Discomfort from stretching a tight muscle is temporary and acceptable. Patients with good body awareness have less difficulty changing faulty movement patterns. Improving body awareness should be part of the treatment when teaching exercises. Feldenkrais's treatment approach emphasizes restoration of function through body awareness training [13].

Functional Muscle Training

The goal of all treatment strategies should be to regain maximum pain-free function. After evaluation, the practitioner should have specific short-term goals that will assist in this endeavor. For example, a goal of maintaining a neutral spine in walking may require the stretching of shortened hamstring and hip flexor muscles while strengthening the back extensor and abdominal muscles. Even though weak back extensor muscles can be trained in a prone position, it may be more beneficial to exercise them in an upright position, which more readily translates into the functional task of walking.

A patient whose goal is to maintain an upright posture when working at a desk should benefit from learning to maintain a neutral spine while leaning forward and back. For example, to keep the trunk and pelvis in alignment, the patient palpates the distance between the symphysis pubis and the navel with the thumb and middle finger of one hand while sitting in an upright neutral posture. With the other hand the distance between the navel and xiphoid

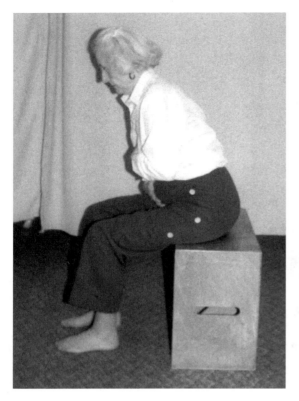

Figure 12.8. Functional muscle training leaning forward, using body awareness to maintain stability of the trunk.

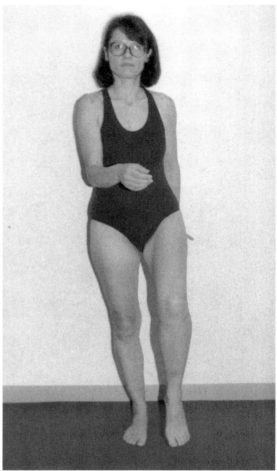

Figure 12.9. Diagonal arm swing, facilitating shortness of the pectoral muscles.

process is palpated and the patient learns to lean the trunk forward and back, maintaining the same distances between points (see Fig. 12.6) (Fig. 12.8). Only the distance between the anterior superior iliac spine and the thigh will change if the movement is done correctly. The patient also can palpate the abdominal muscles with one hand, the back extensor muscles with the other hand, and "feel" the muscle tonus alternate when leaning forward and back.

Finally, a goal of maintaining a stable trunk with neutral head and shoulder alignment during walking is often appropriate. The arm swing of a patient who walks with a unstable trunk and forward shoulders is often diagonal, which may contribute to shortened pectoral muscles and a kyphotic thoracic spine (Fig. 12.9). Functional muscle training would be achieved if the patient learns to align the pelvis, trunk, and head while swinging the arms in a forward direction (sagittal plane) when walking

(Fig. 12.10). Such a correction, during the walking cycle, would encourage neutral posture by gently stretching the pectoral muscles and strengthening the antagonistic thoracic extensor muscles and scapula stabilizers.

Reactive Muscle Training

When a patient is given a task such as swinging the arms forward instead of diagonally while walking, a subconscious activity is taking place in the shoulder-scapulae muscles as a reaction. The patient is not being told to tighten the rhomboid and the mid-

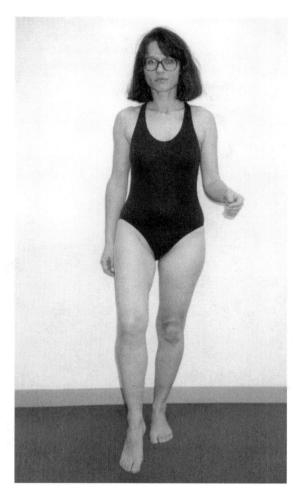

Figure 12.10. Arm swing in the sagittal plane, promoting stretching of shortened pectoral muscles and rhomboid strengthening.

dle trapezius muscles, yet it happens automatically if the instructions were followed correctly. The advantage of incorporating reactive exercises into the treatment is the automatic correction of a faulty movement. Often, balance or equilibrium reactions are provoked, which can assist the practitioner in guiding the patient through correct movement patterns. It may be necessary to give precise instructions to elicit the desired reaction. Instructions may include maintaining or altering body distances, dictating movement direc- tion, or modifying movement speed—for example, "stand on your right leg, move your left hand in a straight line as far forward as you can without falling or taking a step." The

patient response most likely would be a reactive hip extension on the left side (Fig. 12.11) [6].

Treatment Regimens

Any exercise that promotes the economical use of muscles, ligaments, and joints and restores good mobility, strength, coordination, and skill to the thoracic spine should improve the patient's level of function. However, to have a lasting treatment effect the practitioner has to observe what is happening below and above the "problem area," how the movement continues, and what avoidance mechanisms may be present. The practitioner must identify movement limitations, which joints and soft tissues are involved, and if there is sympathetic nervous system involvement (e.g., unusual perspiration, itching, mottled skin). During the examination the practitioner should determine if there is weakness, tightness, lack of coordination, faulty recruitment patterning (e.g., patient side-bends the trunk immediately when abducting an arm) or, perhaps, an avoidance of end range. In addition, the practitioner should determine the patient's body awareness and the readiness for change. The practitioner can then choose from a variety of treatment concepts as long as a healthy, normal movement or the best possible compromise will be the result.

It is important for the practitioner to develop keen observational and listening skills. Exercises can only be "custom tailored" if the practitioner pieces together what he or she sees and hears. Handout sheets should be used only as models and must be adapted to the patient's abilities and needs rather than the opposite.

A careful analysis of the patient's constitution, physical condition, postural alignment, and mobility gives the practitioner an indication of what goals to set for the treatment. The practitioner has to know about precautions arising from the diagnosis before planning the exercises. The patient has to be able to do the exercises correctly and without substitution. Joint or muscle pain arising from exercises is a contraindication to continuing. However, mild postexercise muscle soreness is acceptable. When exercises are executed incorrectly and cause joint or muscle pain, a correction is indicated. On the other hand, when the exercises are not appropriate for the patient's present condition, the practitioner then has to find more appropriate exercises.

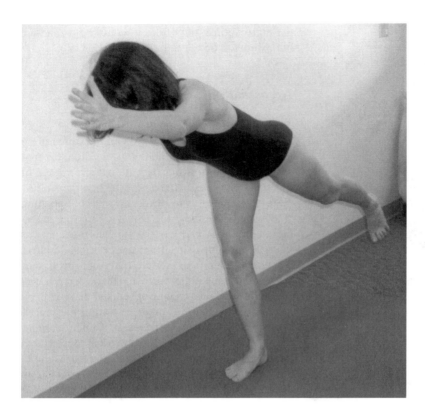

Figure 12.11. Reactive muscle training. When balancing on the right leg and moving the left hand as far forward as possible, the reaction will be to extend the left leg.

Selective Muscle Training

The practitioner has many more specific exercise prescription possibilities than just eccentric (the muscle lengthens and acts as a brake), concentric (the muscle shortens), or isometric (the muscle maintains the same length while contracting). For example, to increase the muscle activity, the practitioner can decrease the patient's base of support. The practitioner can also decide to use a long or a short body segment lever for resistance. An example of this is having a patient kneel on all fours on a wooden box. The patient now has a decreased base of support because the lower legs are not touching the ground (at home the patient can kneel on all fours at the side of the bed with the legs over the edge, kneel on a stool, or simply lift the lower legs when kneeling on hands and knees on the floor) (Fig. 12.12). To make this more challenging, the patient can be asked to flex the right arm in the mid-frontal plane. This will further reduce the base of support. The patient's triangular support base now is determined by one hand and both knees supporting the weight of the body. This exercise may be indicated for patients with weakness of the back

extensors and an overstretched middle trapezius muscle as often seen in scoliosis, nonfixated kyphosis, and osteoporosis. When only one knee and one hand must support the body weight, a further reduction of the base of support is taking place. The same exercise of lifting the flexed right upper arm into the mid-frontal plane becomes increasingly difficult when the opposite leg is extended as well. The weight of the right arm has to be held by the upper back muscles in an open kinetic chain, with the left arm supporting the weight of the trunk, head, and right arm.

When the right elbow is extended in the mid-frontal plane, the length of its lever increases, adding additional body weight, which must be stabilized. A further progression would consist of adding a small dumbbell (free weight) held in the right hand (Fig. 12.13). In this kneeling position on the box, when maintaining a neutral spine in a horizontal position, the abdominal muscles support the "arch of the bridge" against the force of gravity. The rotator muscles of the thoracic spine together with the back extensor muscles must prevent the fall of the right side of the thorax, thus stabilizing the weight of the thorax, the right arm, and the head. A lateral flexion

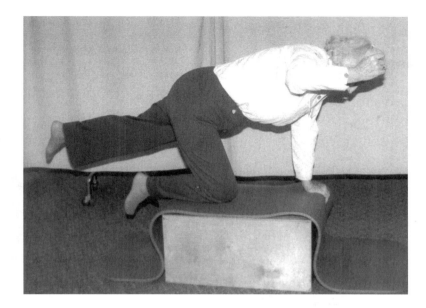

Figure 12.12. Exercise on a wooden box, which decreases the patient's base of support.

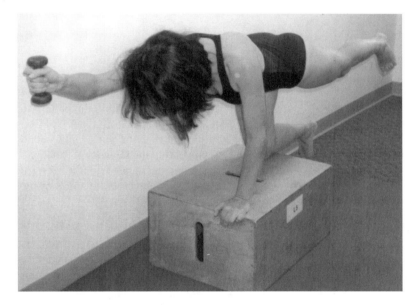

Figure 12.13. Kneeling on the box with the opposite hand on the box, free arm extended, holding a free weight.

movement can be facilitated in this position, since the longitudinal axis of the body is horizontal in space, the lateral flexors (side benders) can work with "gravity eliminated." When the practitioner wants to limit the continuation of the movement impulse, the instruction, "do not move the pelvis any direction," can be given. Active buttressing will result, since muscle activity prevents the movement impulse from continuing into the lumbar spine and pelvis.

A final possibility on the box exercise would be the initiation of a countermovement. The practitioner instructs the patient to move the tip of the left elbow in the mid-frontal plane laterally and caudally. At the same time the patient is asked to turn the left knee medially, which results in lateral flexion (side-bending) of the pelvis and the lumbar spine (Fig. 12.14). This exercise would be beneficial in improving restricted lateral flexion (side-bending) of the thoracic spine.

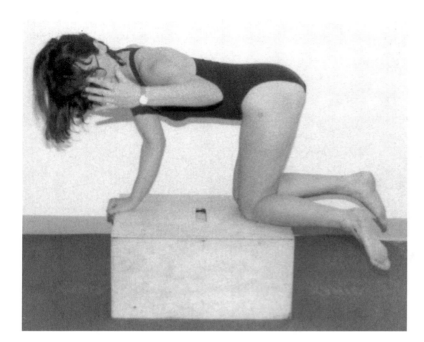

Figure 12.14. Kneeling on the box. Lateral flexion of the left side of the spine through counter-movement of the left arm and the left leg.

Another selective muscle training exercise uses the concept of two movement impulses going in the opposite directions to maximize a selected movement. The exercise "Turn again Whittington" serves as an example [6]. During this exercise the patient is positioned supine with both arms elevated in a transverse plane at about 90 degrees of shoulder flexion with the hips and knees flexed (Fig. 12.15A). The patient is then instructed to lift the head off the floor and turn it to the right while straightening the right arm and bending the left arm. While rolling onto the right side the left leg flexes and the right leg extends (Fig. 12.15B). This exercise requires the patient to coordinate five simultaneous movement impulses of the head and all extremities. The result is clockwise rotation of the pelvis and head, counterclockwise rotation of the trunk, flexion of the left hip, extension of the right hip, horizontal abduction of the left and right shoulder with the left elbow flexed and the right elbow extended.

This complicated exercise can improve the strength, coordination, and postural awareness of the thoracic spine, but it demands concentration, motivation, and good mobility for proper execution.

Finally, selective muscle training of agonists and antagonists can be elicited by asking the patient to imagine a certain movement taking place. For example, "sit upright and imagine you want to bend your trunk." By preventing the movement "an invisible wall will not allow you to bend your trunk even if you try," the patient elicits co-contraction of the trunk flexors and extensors.

Swiss Ball Exercises

The Swiss ball [14–16] has become a valuable inexpensive exercise tool for managing patients with thoracic spine dysfunction. It can be used by the practitioner to assist in the training of mobility, stability, strength, motor skill, and coordination. Because of the ball's labile base of support, balance and equilibrium reactions are required during use. The proprioceptive and vestibular systems can be stimulated by sitting upright on the ball and bouncing. Continuous postural adjustments are required, thus facilitating the smooth coordination of posture and movement. The patient's reward for exercising with the Swiss ball is to easily recognize the pro-

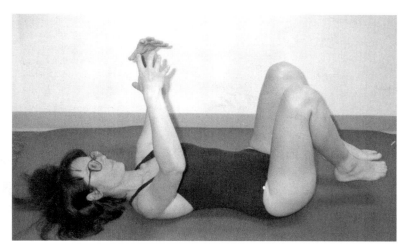

A

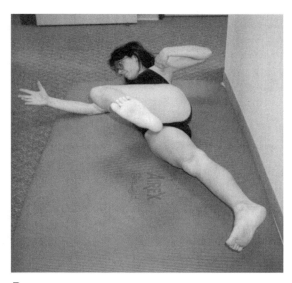

B

gression from initial learning to mastering the task required [17, 18]. All Swiss ball exercises must be performed correctly and should not cause joint or muscle pain. The ball should be firm and roll easily. Exercises should be selected carefully and progressed as the patient masters simple exercises.

"The cowboy" exercise stimulates good vertical alignment and gentle compression and decompression of the spine similar to weight acceptance during gait. It is performed by sitting upright on a Swiss ball with the hips at least the same distance from the floor as the knees or greater (if the pelvis, thorax, and head cannot be put in alignment otherwise).

Bouncing the ball is then initiated with either the trunk, the shoulder girdle, or the extremities.

The "Indian fakir" is an exercise that stimulates muscle activity by changing the base of support (Fig. 12.16). Starting from the cowboy position, the patient takes small forward steps while leaning the stable trunk backward into a horizontal position. This exercise promotes stabilization of the trunk by strengthening the abdominal muscles on both the way down to the horizontal position and the way back up. In the horizontal position, the back extensor muscles are activated in a bridge activity. Patients with poor posture, weakness of either the trunk flexor or extensor muscles, or alignment problems from scoliosis should do well with this exercise.

The goal of "the scissors" exercise is smooth coordinated thoracic spine rotation under a stable shoulder girdle (Figure 12.17). The weight of the legs must be held and stabilized by the trunk. This exercise challenges the patient's balance and coordination while improving thoracic spine rotary range of motion and strengthening the back extensor and rotator muscles against gravity. This exercise can be useful in patients with postural insufficiency and ankylosing spondylitis.

Maximum flexion of the spine, hips, and knees is achieved in the end position of the "sea urchin" (Fig. 12.18). This is useful in patients with recurrent restrictions of flexion and rotation and side-bending to the ipsilateral side (ERS dysfunction).

The "figurehead" exercise assists in strengthening and mobilization of the thoracic spine into extension against gravity (Fig. 12.19). In the end

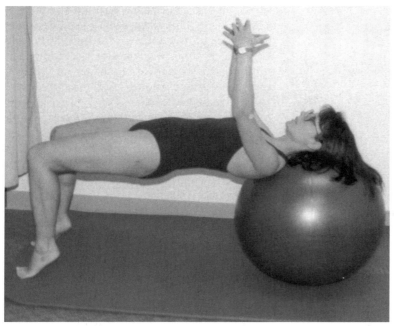

A

B

Figure 12.16. "Indian fakir." A. Leaning the stable trunk backward to horizontal position. B. Bridge activity of the back and hip extensors in the end position.

position, stabilization of the spine is the goal. This exercise is helpful in strengthening the middle trapezius, the suboccipital muscles, and the back extensor musculature.

The Swiss ball is also useful in the management of patients with kyphoscoliosis or a neutral group dysfunction. An example adapted from Klapp [19] starts by resting the trunk on a ball 45 or 55 cm in diameter (Fig. 12.20). The right arm is then flexed at the elbow, which serves as a body segment weight to strengthen and shorten the overstretched right midthoracic spine muscles. The left arm is extended to stretch and elongate the shortened left midthoracic spine.

Finally, the ball can be used to support the head and arms while the thoracic spine is gently extended (Fig. 12.21). This exercise is useful in the management of patients with osteoporosis who need to maintain back extension mobility.

The double ball or PhysioRoll (Ball Dynamics International, Inc., Denver, CO) is used for patients who require more stability. The PhysioRoll has a groove and only rolls forward and back, not side-

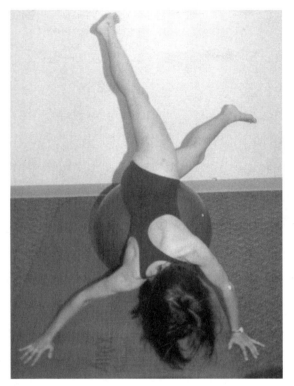

Figure 12.17. "Scissors." The thoracic spine rotates under the shoulder girdle. The weight of the legs has to be stabilized by the trunk.

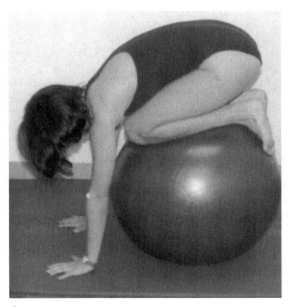

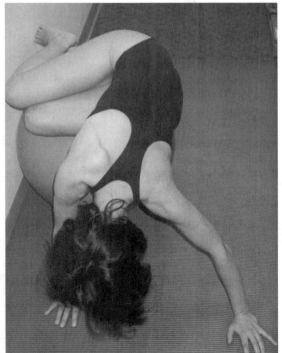

A

B

Figure 12.18. "Sea urchin." A. Total flexion of spine and hips. B. Flexion and rotation of the spine.

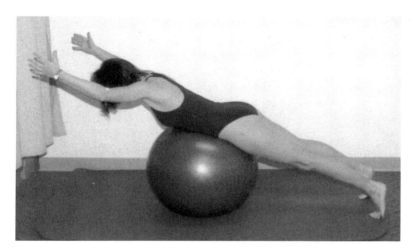

Figure 12.19. "Figurehead." End position with arms extended in the frontal plane.

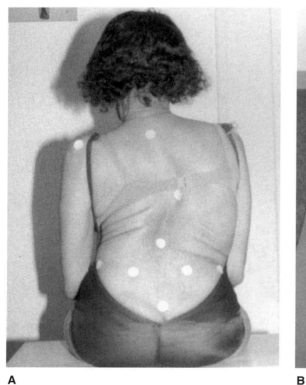

A

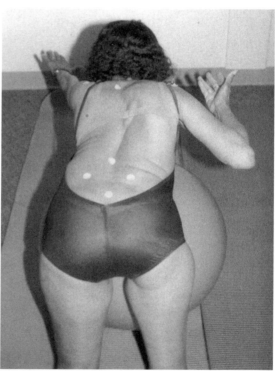

B

Figure 12.20. A. A 47-year-old woman with severe scoliosis. B. Same patient as in A, demonstrating activation of the midthoracic spinal muscles with scoliotic correction while supporting the abdomen on the Swiss ball (adapted from Klapp exercises).

ways (Fig. 12.22). The groove provides guidance when maintenance of spinal alignment is a problem. The greater base of support helps patients prepare for exercises with the more challenging Swiss ball.

The PhysioRoll is especially useful for mobilization and stretching into lateral flexion of the thoracic spine, especially for those patients with tightness of the rib cage, scoliosis, or neutral group dysfunction.

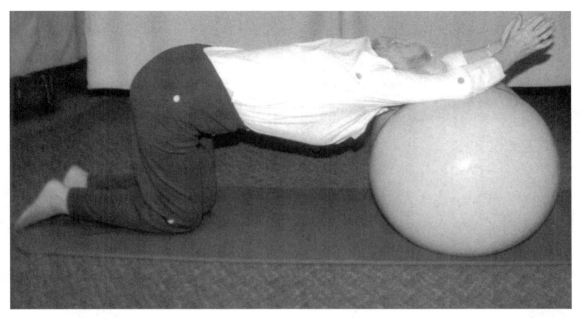

Figure 12.21. A patient with osteoporosis using a Swiss ball to support the head and arms while gently extending the spine.

The author has found this exercise useful for self-mobilization of the rib cage in the management of a patient after multiple healed rib fractures (Fig. 12.23). Soft-tissue and joint mobilization can precede this exercise.

The Foam Roll

The "foam roll" exercises were developed by Parker, a physical therapist who trained with Feldenkrais [20, 21]. The rolls can be used for destabilization of the base of support when kneeling on two rolls, thus stimulating increased muscle firing (Fig. 12.24).

Exercises for abdominal training adapted from Sahrmann can be done on one foam roll. To do this, the patient lies with the entire spine and head in a supine position on the roll with hips and knees flexed. By instructing the patient to lift one leg the abdominal muscles and hip flexor muscles will be activated (Fig. 12.25). The weight of the leg must then be stabilized by co-contraction of the extensor muscles. Performing this exercise demands balance, coordination, and skill. Feeling the roll under the spine increases the body's awareness of the trunk alignment while providing sen-

sory and proprioceptive feedback. The amount of upper trunk muscular stabilization depends on the arm position, whether or not the hands touch the floor, and on the size of the roll (1–6 inches in diameter).

Another use of the foam roll is for self-mobilization. This can be accomplished by rolling back and forth over the foam roll (Figure 12.26). Flexion and extension of hypomobile segments of the thoracic spine are mobilized by actively flexing a segment of the spine against gravity and passively extending the segment with gravity assistance.

Thera-Band

The use of a Thera-Band (North Coast Medical, Inc., San José, CA) [22, 23] in patients with weakness of trunk or extremity muscles has been popular for some time. Thera-Bands are color coded according to stiffness and can be used to provide resistance to muscles. The practitioner must ensure that the patient learns to perform Thera-Band exercises in a position of correct postural alignment and while using the appropriate amount of resistance. The resistance is correct when the patient can execute the exercises

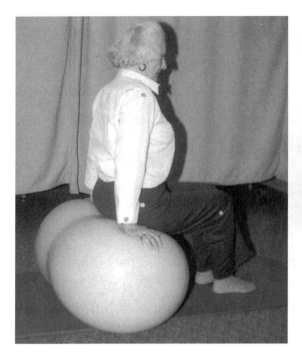

Figure 12.22. Double ball (PhysioRoll) used for increased support by a patient with osteoporosis.

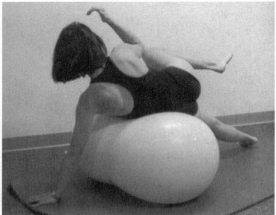

A

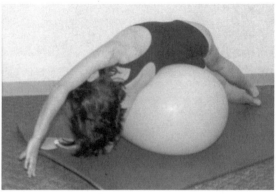

B

Figure 12.23. Lateral stretching and mobilization. A. Lateral flexion again gravity. B. Lateral extension with gravity over the PhysioRoll.

without substitution through the full range of motion and in good postural alignment.

The Thera-Band can be used by patients to promote stability of the thoracic spine while introducing a vertical loading activity. An example of this is a patient suffering from osteoporosis (Fig. 12.27). Gently bouncing on a trampoline while firing the extensor muscles of the thoracic spine and shoulder girdle should promote spinal stability and slow osteoporotic activity. To train muscles concentrically and eccentrically the patient should decelerate the movement when returning the tension of the Thera-Band to the start position.

Free Weights

It is important for any practitioner to use free weights only when the patient is capable of holding and moving his or her own body segment weights. An arm, the head, or a leg are body segment weights that the patient must be able to move in space without difficulty or substitution before free weights are added. A substitution is often noticeable by monitoring a change of pressure over the patient's base of support. For example, a patient with weak trunk extensor muscles may lean the thorax backward during active arm flexion. To prevent this, ask the patient to feel the pressure under his or her feet and not allow it to change when lifting the arms. Active buttressing of the abdominal muscles will prevent this backward leaning (Fig. 12.28). Before adding weight to this activity, the practitioner should introduce manually quick chopping movements of the patient's arms into shoulder flexion and extension while observing the stability of the trunk. If the patient can maintain a neutral spine, weight can be introduced.

When using free weights it is important to begin with small amounts of weight, such as small

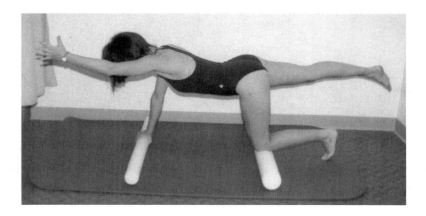

Figure 12.24. Foam roll exercise. Kneeling on two rolls to destabilize the base of support.

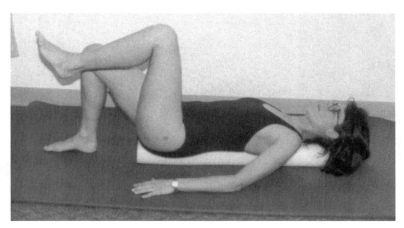

Figure 12.25. Abdominal training while supine on foam roll.

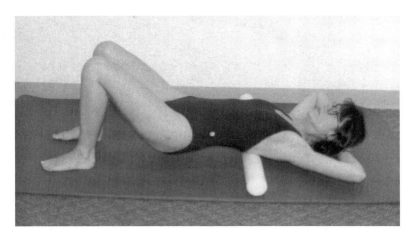

Figure 12.26. Self-mobilization of the thoracic spine into extension with the foam roll.

food cans, before increasing the amount. The number of repetitions depends on the correct execution of the exercise. The patient must be able to recognize the point at which substitution begins to limit the development of these faulty movement patterns. Pain beyond the normal delayed onset muscle soreness from weightlifting is a contraindication to continuation.

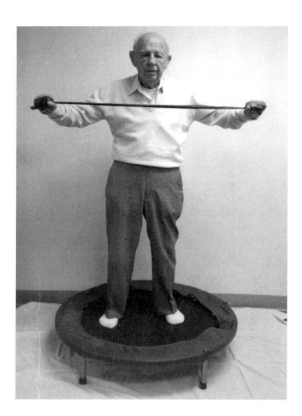

Figure 12.27. Thera-Band used by patient with osteoporosis while bouncing on trampoline.

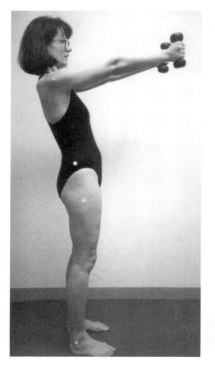

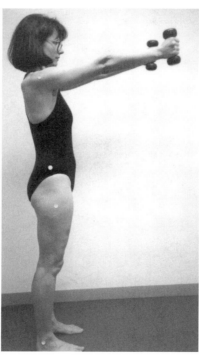

Figure 12.28. Raising arms into forward flexion. A. Without instructions. B. With instruction not to alter the pressure under the feet. Observe the backward leaning in A as a normal balance reaction to lifting the weight of the arms. This reaction is increased when dumbbells are held in the hands.

A

B

Frequency of Exercises

The patient who has been made aware of optimal posture and movement will ideally exercise many times throughout the day by finding occasions to stretch or adjust posture or to perform breathing exercises. If a patient does better when given instructions to do certain exercises three times a day, the practitioner should then develop such a program. Some patients require extensive explanations while others require only a few drawings. A change in movement pattern, a decrease of pain, or an increase in mobility should occur after three to four treatment sessions.

Summary

In the treatment of thoracic spine dysfunction there are numerous exercises from which to choose: PNF [5], Sahrmann [24], Janda [10], Butler [3], and Klein-Vogelbach [6, 14] serve as examples, but the basic principles remain the same. The goal is to retrain function and to restore normal movement or the best possible compromise. The amount and the types of exercises that the practitioner has in his or her repertoire are not as important as the precise application of the exercise and the patient's compliance in regularly performing them.

References

1. Klein-Vogelbach S. Functional Kinetics. New York: Springer, 1990;76, 110–121, 219–221.
2. Louis R. Vertebroradicular and vertebromedullar dynamics. Anat Clin 1981;3:1–11.
3. Butler DS. Mobilisation of the Nervous System. Melbourne: Churchill Livingstone, 1991;38.
4. Klein-Vogelbach S. Die Stabilisation der Körpermitte und die aktive Widerlagerbildung als Ausgangspunkt einer Bewegungserziehung. Krankengymnastik 1963; 5:1–9.
5. Voss DE, Ionta MK, Myers BJ. Proprioceptive Neuromuscular Facilitation. Philadelphia: Harper & Row, 1985;315–319.
6. Klein-Vogelbach S. Therapeutic Exercises in Functional Kinetics. New York: Springer, 1991;2–3, 371.
7. Umphred DA. Limbic Complex. In DA Umphred (ed), Neurological Rehabilitation (3rd ed). St. Louis: Mosby, 1995;4:93–101.
8. Travell JG, Simons DG. Myofacial Pain and Dysfunction. Baltimore: Williams & Wilkins, 1992;42–54.
9. Carrière B, Felix L. In consideration of proportions. PT: Magazine of Physical Therapy 1993;4:56–61.
10. Janda V. Muscle Weakness and Inhibition (Pseudoparesis) in Back Pain Syndromes. In GP Grieve (ed), Modern Manual Therapy of the Vertebral Column. New York: Churchill Livingstone, 1986;19:197–201.
11. Janda V. Workshop: Assessment and Treatment of Impaired Movement Pattern. Los Angeles, March 1993, handout January 1993.
12. White SG, Sahrmann S. A Movement System Balance Approach to Management of Musculoskeletal Pain. In R Grant (ed), Physiotherapy of the Cervical and Thoracic Spine (2nd ed). New York: Churchill Livingstone, 1994.
13. Feldenkrais M. Awareness Through Movement. New York: Harper & Row, 1972.
14. Klein-Vogelbach S. Functional Kinetics: Swiss Ball Exercises. Videotape. New York: Springer, 1992.
15. Klein-Vogelbach S. Ball Exercises in Functional Kinetics. New York: Springer, (English translation in preparation).
16. Carrière B. Swiss ball exercises. PT: Magazine of Physical Therapy 1993;9:92–100.
17. Frank JS, Earl M. Coordination of posture and movement. Phys Ther 1990;70:855–863.
18. Winstein CJ. Knowledge of results and motor learning implications for physical therapy. Phys Ther 1991; 71:140–149.
19. Klapp B. Das Klapp'sche Kriechverfahren. Stuttgart: Thieme, 1990.
20. Parker I. Beyond conventional exercises. Physical Therapy Forum 1992;7:4–7.
21. Parker I. Functional exercise program. Vol.1, part 1. Balance. Video. San Francisco: Ilana Parker Physical Therapy Service, 1993.
22. Mayer JA, Zappalla L. Fit Ball. Video. Boulder, CO: FitBall USA, 1993.
23. Placht W. Therafit Rückenschule. Schöngeising: Joachim Heymans, 1990.
24. Sahrmann S. Exercise Video, Series I. St. Louis: Videoscope, 1991.

PART IV
Clinical Perspectives and Concerns

Chapter 13

Clinical Presentations and Examples: An Osteopathic Perspective

Edward G. Stiles

Basic Principles

Providing manual therapy is an art based on science. Many factors enable the practitioner to design the most advantageous approach for each individual patient, irrespective of the presenting problems. Specific principles for assisting the practitioner in developing a management strategy will be discussed in this chapter. This conceptual approach is supported by the career and writings of A. T. Still, the founder of osteopathy. Interestingly, Still wrote several books, all dealing with osteopathic philosophy, but none could be described as a technique manual. It appears Still concluded that if a physician understood the role of the musculoskeletal system in health and disease, he or she would examine patients searching for evidence of mechanical dysfunction (somatic dysfunction) and develop a specific manipulative strategy for alleviating any discovered dysfunction. Viewed in this context, the techniques are not the key issue; they are only of secondary importance to the application of osteopathic philosophy within the practice of medicine.

Although not the sole reason for the development of the profession, manipulative approaches can be viewed as a cornerstone of osteopathic medicine. Still's stated purpose, in the late 1800s, was to improve the practice of medicine. Manipulative techniques therefore exist as a tool for providing osteopathic care for patients with a multitude of clinical problems. Naturally, beneficial effects will result only if mechanical dysfunction plays a contributing role in the clinical condition. Many il-

lustrations related to the clinical specialties will be discussed later in this chapter, once a few basic principles concerning the development of an "osteopathic prescription" or clinical strategy are examined.

The famous Canadian, American, and British physician Sir William Osler is quoted as saying, "It is more important to know the patient who has a disease than the disease that has the patient." It is crucial to paraphrase this statement in terms of osteopathic principles by stating, "It is more important to know the patient who has somatic dysfunction than it is to know the somatic dysfunction that has the patient." This is a crucial concept for providing quality manual care because each patient owns a unique history. The history of injuries, life-style patterns, and occupational and personal stress factors ensure the somatic dysfunction pattern will be unique for each patient. An individualized manipulative approach must be designed to take into account these particular factors.

Goals of Manual Medicine in Reference to Somatic Dysfunction

The two basic goals of manual medicine are:

1. To attempt to restore normal range of motion in the dysfunctional joints (somatic dysfunction) rather than "putting a structure back in place."
2. To integrate the movement and function of the joints and soft tissues throughout the body. In

terms of a computer metaphor, this would be equivalent to reprogramming the "software" of the system or central nervous system component. The improved musculoskeletal function can then have widespread physiologic responses, which will be further discussed later in the chapter.

Manual medicine techniques, although primarily addressing the musculoskeletal system, must be viewed and appreciated in terms of their widespread physiologic responses affecting other systems of the body. It is helpful to view the patient with a health problem as representing an illness that is the net result of a disease process occurring within the host or patient: Host + Disease = Illness. This explains why patients with the same medical or surgical diagnosis will each have a unique clinical picture. This occurs because the host's homeostatic mechanisms respond differently and uniquely to the same disease process. It is important for an accurate medical and surgical diagnosis of the disease process to be established and properly managed. The manipulative management is directed at the host component of the illness, not at the disease component! If the mechanical dysfunction within the body is playing a role in the patient's clinical picture, manipulative approaches, by alleviating the mechanical dysfunction, may have a beneficial impact in assisting the patient to realize his or her health potential. Thus, patients with a wide variety of medical and surgical problems can frequently benefit from an evaluation and proper management of any somatic/mechanical dysfunction within the musculoskeletal system of the host.

As with any medical or surgical procedure, both indications and contraindications must be considered and discussed. In my opinion, there is a single indication for manipulative medicine: the presence of somatic dysfunction. The HICDA-9 defines somatic dysfunction as impaired or altered function of related components of the somatic (body framework) system—skeletal, arthrodial, and myofascial structures—and the related vascular, lymphatic, and neural elements. In this context, pain is not an indication for manipulative care. If pain, or other visceral symptomatology, is associated with mechanical dysfunction, then manipulative care may be indicated and beneficial. In terms of contraindications, these can only be discussed once the general health of the patient is assessed, the somatic dysfunction

has been specifically diagnosed, a specific technique has been selected, and the skill of the practitioner has been determined. After considering these four components, one can then discuss whether a specific technique may or may not be indicated or contraindicated.

The barrier concept has been previously introduced in Chapter 8. However, some elaboration on the barrier concept and its relationship to mechanical dysfunction in related areas will be addressed now. In the spinal region, the segments above and below a restricted vertebra (somatic dysfunction) will frequently become neurophysiologically hypermobile, attempting to compensate for the lost range of motion at the restricted vertebral segment. If a specific mechanical diagnosis is not established and a nonspecific technique is used, a "pop" may occur in the hypermobile joints, whereas the hypomobile segment may never be properly released. In this situation, the patient may, at best, experience temporary relief and assume the vertebra "keeps going out" when in reality the restricted segment has never been properly treated and mobilized.

With the conceptual model of somatic dysfunction just discussed, somatic dysfunction can be understood to be an altered range of motion or function rather than a problem of something being "out of place" and needing to be "put back in place" with a manipulative procedure. An excellent analogy is to compare somatic dysfunction to a door that is not off its hinges, but is unable to properly and completely open and close.

With these thoughts in mind, consider some of the common ways in which somatic dysfunction can develop or be produced. This understanding is important, since it can be helpful in designing a specific manual medicine strategy for each patient. Some common mechanisms could be:

1. Major trauma
2. Minor trauma
3. Positional or occupational strains resulting in fatigue and muscle spasm
4. Viscerosomatic reflex phenomena
5. Emotional stress resulting in the patient's becoming an "uptight" patient
6. Nutritional deficiencies that may result in altered metabolic activity secondary to a vitamin or mineral imbalance or deficiency
7. Destructive lifestyles

Each of these factors could contribute to the development of somatic dysfunction. In most patients, several of these factors play a role and must be specifically addressed if the patient is to realize his or her health potential.

Management of Somatic Dysfunction: Direct and Indirect Technique

How does one manage mechanical dysfunction? There are several different general or generic strategies that the clinician can use in the management of somatic dysfunction. The previous chapters have outlined direct treatment techniques of the restrictive barrier including muscle energy, high velocity thrust, myofascial, and selected exercise techniques. Another generic group of techniques are classified as indirect or functional techniques. With these techniques, the practitioner passively takes the restricted segment away from the restrictive barrier toward the normal physiologic barrier. There will be a point in this continuum, somewhere between the restrictive and the normal physiologic barrier, at which the surrounding soft tissues of the restricted segment will be in a state of maximal relaxation. This point should be simultaneously reached within several ranges of motion (flexion-extension, side-bending right and left, rotation right and left, anterior-posterior translation, right-left translation, and cephalad-caudad translation). This point of maximal soft-tissue relaxation is also the point of maximal movement potential and is called the dynamic balance point (DBP). Once the DBP is attained by simultaneously stacking the DBP of each of the six ranges of motion, the practitioner has several treatment options: (1) holding the segment in that position (position/hold) while using a maximally held respiratory inspiration or expiration, which provides further soft-tissue relaxation; (2) allowing the treated segment to passively unwind to the point of mechanical release (indirect/passive); or (3) actively and gently taking the restricted segment through the soft tissue maze by following the path of least resistance through the restrictive barrier to the point of mechanical release (indirect/active). With each of these indirect technique approaches, the end-point is attained when the tissues relax, the restrictive barrier releases, and normal physiologic motion is restored to the dysfunctional joint.

In addition, the various aspects of the direct and indirect approaches can be combined. For example, once the restricted segment is gently positioned directly against the "feather edge" of the restrictive barrier, "fine-tuning" can be attained by slightly altering the flexion-extension, side-bending, and rotational position to attain maximal tissue relaxation while the treated segment is maintained against the restrictive barrier. Thus, the segment is positioned directly against the restrictive barrier according to muscle energy principles but is "fine-tuned" using functional palpatory skills to attain maximal parasegmental tissue relaxation. This example illustrates the goal of specifically positioning the restricted segment in such a way that the dysfunctional segment is "made an offer it can't refuse." Another way of conceptualizing this "fine-tuned" position is to imagine the segment as "floated" against the restrictive barrier. In this position, a minimal muscle effort by the patient will initiate a maximal mechanical response at the dysfunctional joint.

The Structural Goals for Manual Medicine

The structural goals for manual medicine are, first, to establish a normal range of physiologic motion, in terms of both quality and quantity of movement, for each dysfunctional joint. Second, one hopes to integrate the movements of each joint into an overall pattern of movement. Attention to the overall movement pattern is particularly important after the clinician has treated the various dysfunctional areas but the patient's clinical condition demonstrates little objective or subjective change. As an example, a patient may have acute low back pain, but on performing a screening examination with the patient in the standing position, the practitioner finds that the area of greatest restriction is in the cervical region. This could be significant since, embryologically, the large superficial muscles of the low back originate or develop in the cervical area but migrate down the back as the fetus develops. In this example, once the cervical area is properly treated, the secondary symptoms of low back pain may be alleviated. If there should be remaining low back mechanical dysfunction, it must now be treated, provided this is the next area of greatest restriction. An analogy may be helpful. Once an injury has occurred, the body begins to compensate and attempts to alleviate the detrimental effects of the mechanical dysfunction. If this adaptive process has developed over several months or years, reversing the process with manual procedures is like "peeling the layers off an onion." As each layer of dysfunction is removed, a new underlying layer or pattern of mechanical dysfunction will appear and must be appropriately treated.

Another goal of manual medicine merits discussion. Manipulative care will completely alleviate the mechanical dysfunction and integrate multiple joint functions of some patients and enable the patient to become asymptomatic. Other patients, who have developed chronic patterns of dysfunction and compensation secondary to an anomalous situation, may never become asymptomatic. The goal for managing their care is to assist the patient in realizing his or her specific and unique health potential. The phrase "Don't give up if you get a lemon, you can always make lemonade" illustrates the management philosophy for these patients.

An additional benefit of treating any mechanical dysfunction is that it may assist the host in realizing his or her health potential, especially if the mechanical dysfunction is contributing to symptoms mimicking or complicating a visceral pathologic state. Once effective manual therapy is initiated, the patient may experience an alleviation of symptoms and signs mimicking visceral dysfunction.

This perspective is best illustrated with a case history. The patient, in his 40s, contracted tuberculosis 20 years earlier and developed an unresolved atelectasis. As a result, the patient experienced marked fatigue while performing his duties as an accountant. Because of fatigue, the patient participated in few family activities and frequently missed work because of secondary pulmonary infections. Marked somatic dysfunction was diagnosed in the cervical and thoracic spine, rib cage, and upper extremity regions. After 6 months of manual therapy, the following pulmonary data were obtained.

	11/9/76	4/8/77
FEVC	54%	54%
PEF	18%	16%
FEV 0.5	13%	13%
FEV 1.0	17%	16%
FEF 2–12	4%	3%
FEF 25–75%	5%	4%

FEVC = forced expiratory vital capactiy; PEF = peak expiratory flow; FEV = forced expiratory volume; FEF = forced expiratory flow.

These data demonstrated marked and permanent pulmonary changes and damage. I, as treating physician, was amazed by the unchanged pulmonary data, because the patient experienced many life-style benefits once manipulative care was combined with the care provided by his medical internist. For the first time he was able to go through the winter months in his home state of Maine without the need for an antibiotic. Previously, antibiotics had been necessary on a yearly basis for several consecutive winters. He reported no loss of work and once again participated in family activities. This became more understandable when the pulmonary data were further analyzed.

	11/9/76	4/8/77
TV	204%	114%
MV	177%	69%
IC	50%	64%
IRC	14%	53%
VC	49%	51%

TV = tidal volume; MV = minute volume; IC = inspiratory capacity; IRC = inspiratory reserve capacity; VC = vital capactiy

Although the patient developed marked and permanent pulmonary damage, improvement of the mechanics of the dysfunctional regions with manual therapy resulted in positive clinical benefits and assisted the patient in realizing his health potential. The patient continued manual therapy on a once-a-month basis and went through the next three winters without developing a secondary pulmonary infection.

As previously mentioned, once the somatic/mechanical dysfunction is appropriately addressed, systemic benefits may be observed because the adverse impact of the somatic dysfunction is removed. The following benefits may be observed and be of assistance in understanding and appreciating the possible mechanisms operating in both the previously discussed pulmonary patient and the clinical discussions in the remaining portion of the chapter.

System Energy Demands

Inman and Saunders have demonstrated how gait dysfunctions can markedly increase the energy demands on the total musculoskeletal system. Since the musculoskeletal system makes up two-thirds of the total body mass, mechanical dysfunction in the lower extremities may have a marked impact on the viscera of the body by increasing the energy and metabolic demands on every system. For example, gait dysfunctions have been reported to increase the energy demands on the body by up to 300% while the subject is walking on a level plane. There must be an appropriate increase in visceral functions to meet these increased physiologic demands imposed by the altered musculoskeletal function. If the patient has an impaired cardiovascular or respiratory system, the superimposed energy demands of the mechanical dysfunction might cause the "weak link" system—i.e., the cardiovascular or respiratory system—to decompensate or fail to realize its potential. The treatment plan should therefore include medical management of the cardiovascular or respiratory problems. Simultaneously, appropriate management of the musculoskeletal component should be initiated, thus decreasing the energy demands on the compromised visceral system.

Arterial Supply

The sympathetic nervous system (SNS) is recognized as the vasomotor regulating system of the body, controlling both vasoconstriction and vasodilation. Conceptually, this may be significant when one considers the anatomic relationship of the sympathetic ganglia. In the cervical and lumbar regions of the spine, the SNS ganglia are positionally maintained against the vertebrae by the surrounding fascias. In the thoracic region of the spine, the SNS ganglia again are positionally maintained by the fascias in an intimate relationship with the costovertebral regions. It is suggested that mechanical dysfunction might be associated with the typical inflammatory reaction of pain, edema, and restriction of motion. Furthermore, the resulting edema may be associated with a localized entrapment phenomenon involving the unyielding fascia on the SNS ganglia. Experimental stimulation of SNS ganglia in animals has been shown to be associated with both vasomotor and vascular changes in the viscera innervated by the chronically stimulated SNS ganglia. It is suggested that thoracic somatic/mechanical dysfunction might be associated with vasomotor changes in the tissues innervated by the involved SNS ganglia. This might impair tissue perfusion and the tissue blood level of both endogenous and medical substances.

Neurologic: Impulses

Mechanical dysfunction has been shown to have a facilitation effect on the segmentally related areas of the spinal cord. The resulting facilitation may have either a stimulatory or an inhibitory impact; it is impossible to predict the clinical effect. For example, mechanical dysfunction in the midthoracic region might facilitate the sympathetic innervation to the segmentally related viscera. If this should be an inhibitory effect, the physician may observe a sympathetic/parasympathetic imbalance on the stomach resulting in hyperacidity and increased peristalsis. If the sympathetic innervation from the dysfunctional area is stimulatory in nature, changes in vasomotor control to the stomach, hypoacidity, and a decrease in peristalsis might be observed. It is impossible to predict whether the mechanical dysfunction will have a stimulatory or inhibitory impact. Clinical examples are presented later in this chapter to further explore these potential clinical patterns.

Neurologic: Trophic Factors

Basic science research demonstrates that protein and lipid trophic substances, which originate in the nuclear region of the nerve, actually flow along the axon and ultimately cross the neuromuscular junction. These trophic substances are crucial for the normal function and health of the innervated end-organ. Mechanical dysfunction, with the resulting fascial tension and muscular guarding, might produce an axon entrapment phenomena that impedes the flow of trophic substances to the end-organ. This could have an adverse impact on the functional potential of that end-organ. This might lower tissue resistance and increase the susceptibility of the related viscera to develop a wide variety of pathologic conditions.

Ventilation, Venous, and Lymphatic Circulation

Functional anatomists have demonstrated that normal rib cage mechanics, during the inspiratory phase, are associated with expansion of the thoracic cage as well as the descent of the thoracoabdominal diaphragm toward the abdominal cavity. As a result, a decrease of intrathoracic pressure develops. This pressure change during inspiration is also associated with a decrease in both central venous and lymphatic pressure, which assists in both venous and lymphatic circulation. Thus, normal rib cage mechanics may play a crucial role in ventilation, venous, and lymphatic circulation and one might expect that somatic dysfunction of the thoracic spine or rib cage regions might have an adverse impact on any one, two, or all three of these functions.

Afferent Sensory and Trophic Flow to the Spinal Cord from the End-Organ

Mechanical dysfunction could also have a detrimental impact on both of these functions via facilitation mechanisms, fascial entrapment, or by impeding axon trophic flow as previously mentioned.

Therefore, it is postulated that mechanical dysfunction may have a detrimental impact on energy demands; vasomotor/arterial circulation; neurologic aspects of impulse and trophic flow; ventilation, venous, or lymphatic circulation; and afferent impulse patterns or trophic flow. This dysfunction might have a detrimental impact on any one of these functions, all of them, or any of the possible combinations. A myriad of symptoms and altered functions might be associated with somatic/mechanical dysfunction and be secondarily resolved once the related somatic dysfunction is properly diagnosed and effectively managed.

It is also widely recognized that the body manufactures a myriad of endogenous substances, which could be characterized as the "body manufacturing its own medicines." Mechanical dysfunction might have a detrimental impact on arterial/vasomotor supply, innervation and trophic functions, ventilation/oxygenation of tissues, and venous and lymphatic circulation, and that these alterations could adversely affect the manufacture, metabolic breakdown, and circulation of these endogenous substances. The net affect could further alter normal homeostatic function and balance. Widespread pathophysiologic and clinical changes might result. Alteration in the production, circulation, and metabolism of the body's own "medicines" along with the possible detrimental effects of mechanical dysfunction on energy demands; on vasomotor tone; on neurologic impulse patterns; on neurotrophic flow; on ventilation and venous and lymphatic circulation; and on afferent sensory and trophic flow

might enable one to begin to appreciate the potential widespread and detrimental affects that might occur clinically when somatic/mechanical dysfunction is present.

Somatic dysfunction may or may not represent a direct etiologic factor and might be better viewed as a risk factor. Bernard is quoted as saying, "Systems do not exist in nature but only in the minds of men." Thus, dysfunction in the musculoskeletal system, which makes up two thirds of the total body mass, may have a marked and detrimental impact on the other systems of this complexly integrated body. Again, the somatic dysfunction may not represent a direct etiologic factor, but rather a risk factor. This might render the patient more vulnerable if other risk factors associated with the disease process are also present. Somatic dysfunction with the resulting pathophysiologic mechanisms may be a determining factor as to which organ will eventually become the target organ.

It must be emphasized that managing the somatic component of the patient's health problems merely addresses the host aspect of the illness. Appropriate medical and surgical diagnostic and therapeutic measures must also be used in the management plan of the patient. These somatic aspects will be discussed in the following section.

Clinical Illustrations

In this section, clinical diagnoses will be used to discuss the various potential sites of somatic dysfunction and the possible clinical significance of these findings. This understanding comes from 7 years of in-hospital practice, where I served as a manual medicine specialist for internists, surgeons, and other specialists. The emphasis of treatment is placed on the host, or the somatic component of the illness, while appropriate medical and surgical care is concurrently directed at the disease process.

Cardiovascular System

In a patient with congestive heart failure, a specific manual medicine approach can be developed. It is common to find somatic dysfunction in the cervical area of the spine that may facilitate the parasympathetic input to the cardiac plexus. If the somatic dysfunction stimulates the vagal input, a decrease in cardiac rate and lower blood pressure might be expected because of the predominance of parasympathetic input. If somatic dysfunction in the cervical and thoracic areas of the spine stimulates the sympathetic innervation to the cardiac plexus, an increase in cardiac rate and blood pressure might be observed. Dysfunction in these areas may also affect sympathetic vasomotor function and be associated with anginal symptomatology secondary to coronary artery vasoconstriction. If the upper thoracic dysfunction inhibits the sympathetic motor input to the cardiac plexus, a slowing of the heart rate and a decrease in blood pressure might be expected. Somatic dysfunction involving the thoracic spinal region and rib cage might impair the patient's ventilation, venous, and lymphatic circulation potentials, producing a secondary impact on fluids and electrolyte balances, which could further contribute to arrhythmias, shock, or congestive failure. Somatic dysfunction of the lower extremities, low back, or pelvis might increase the energy demands of the body and further compromise the impaired cardiovascular system, contributing to the congestive failure.

While the patient is in the intensive care unit, functional techniques can be used to specifically treat any somatic dysfunction. Once the patient stabilizes and gains strength, muscle energy techniques may be used to effectively alleviate any remaining somatic dysfunction.

It should be noted that a similar strategy may be used and somatic dysfunction findings may be present with a patient who has experienced a myocardial infarction or angina. Again, functional techniques can be used in the early stages of clinical management along with appropriate medical care. Both the disease process and the host/somatic components can, and should, be managed in an effort to assist the patient in realizing his or her unique health potential.

Another interesting clinical phenomenon is a condition I classify as "pseudo-angina." Mechanical dysfunction involving the third, fourth, or fifth left ribs might have an impact on the pectoralis minor, which takes its origin from these ribs. The neurovascular bundle to the arm courses under the pectoralis minor muscle. With rib dysfunction in this region, the patient can be asymptomatic at rest. With exertion the increased ventilatory efforts of the dysfunctional rib cage may cause the patient to experience chest pain in the area of the third, fourth, and fifth ribs. This may be associated with increased tone of the pectoralis minor muscle and pain radiating into the left shoulder. The associated entrapment phenomenon involving the neurovascular bundle, as occurs in the hyperabduction syndrome, may result in pain radiating down the left arm. Naturally, the symptomatology would subside with rest. From my clinical experience, it is not uncommon for this pattern of mechanical dysfunction to also be present in patients with myocardial pathologic states. In this instance the patient, and frequently the physician, concludes the chest pain being experienced is of myocardial origin, when in reality it is of mechanical origin. Once the mechanical dysfunction is alleviated in these cases, there will be a significant decrease in the frequency, and often the severity, of the chest pain. Now only the true anginal pain is experienced and the development of a cardiac cripple has been prevented.

While at Waterville Osteopathic Hospital (Maine), patients admitted with a chief complaint of chest pain and referred to the Service of Osteopathic Medicine were followed to analyze the discharge diagnosis. In 36% of the patients, the attending physicians listed the discharge diagnosis as chest pain caused by somatic dysfunction. It is suspected that in institutions where the musculoskeletal system is not examined for somatic dysfunction, the discharge diagnosis would have included such medical diagnoses such as Tietze's syndrome, costochondritis, or anterior chest wall syndrome. I suspect these diagnoses would occur with approximately the same frequency as somatic dysfunction was detected at Waterville Osteopathic Hospital.

Another interesting entity, from a manual medicine vantage point, is essential hypertension. By definition, the cause is unknown. If the patients are evaluated mechanically, somatic dysfunction in the cervical area is frequently found, which may inhibit the parasympathetic input and result in a predominant sympathetic input to the cardiac plexus. Somatic dysfunction in the upper thoracic area may stimulate the sympathetic motor innervation from this area, increase cardiac output, and contribute to the essential hypertension. Somatic dysfunction in the lower extremities might secondarily increase the energy demands on the cardiovascular system, increase the cardiac workload, and be expressed clinically as essential hypertension.

The somatic dysfunction findings may be of benefit in assisting the physician in initially selecting an appropriate medical strategy. For example, in a patient with congestive heart failure, somatic dysfunction in the upper thoracic area may inhibit the sympathetic innervation to the cardiac plexus, resulting in bradycardia and poor cardiac output. In these patients, a sympathomimetic medication might be of benefit. If the patient's major area of somatic dysfunction is in the cervical area, it may stimulate the parasympathetic-vagal input to the cardiac plexus and also contribute to the bradycardia or decreased cardiac output. Theoretically a greater amount of sympathomimetic drug would be required to overcome the predominance of vagal/parasympathetic input, potentially increasing the incidence of side effects. With cervical somatic dysfunction, a parasympatholytic drug might be considered. If the major area of somatic dysfunction is in the thoracic region and rib cage, this could conceivably impair both diaphragmatic and rib cage excursion and secondarily impair both the venous and lymphatic circulation or return, resulting in peripheral edema. When peripheral edema exists in our theoretical patient, the patient might initially respond well to a diuretic. This could especially be true if the cervical and thoracic areas display little somatic dysfunction, which might suggest an innervation imbalance to the myocardium and edema secondary to low cardiac output. Thus, the mechanical findings might provide an additional clue for assisting the clinician in the initial development of the most advantageous therapeutic program for that patient.

Respiratory System

A multitude of somatic dysfunction patterns may be present in a patient with pneumonia. Somatic dysfunction in the upper thoracic and cervical areas of the spine may have an adverse impact on the sympathetic ganglia and affect the vasomotor supply to the pulmonary tissues. This might impair the arterial supply to the pulmonary system, lower the resistance of these tissues, and render them more susceptible to an infectious process. Somatic dysfunction involving the thoracic spine and rib cage area may impair the patient's ability to ventilate and realize maximal venous or lymphatic circulation. Venous and lymphatic stasis may also adversely affect tissue resistance and increase the susceptibility to an infectious process.

My clinical experience suggests that it is not uncommon for a patient to be placed on an appropriate antibiotic, selected on the basis of the sputum culture, yet clinically respond poorly. Once the associated mechanical dysfunctions are effectively managed, it is not unusual to observe, within an hour or two, a drop in the temperature and white blood cell count, suggesting that the somatic dysfunction may have had an detrimental impact on the sympathetic vasomotor system. This dysfunction may have altered the circulation to the site of infection, secondarily lowering the tissue level of antibiotic in spite of an appropriate systemic blood level of antibiotic. Once the vasomotor control was improved, a clinically effective amount of antibiotic was delivered to the infected tissues and the patient began to clinically demonstrate improvement.

With a patient suffering from chronic obstructive pulmonary disease (COPD) or asthma, a similar pattern of dysfunction can be observed. Cervical somatic dysfunction may have a stimulatory impact on the vagal-parasympathetic supply to the bronchial tree and contribute to the bronchial constriction. Somatic dysfunction in the upper thoracic and cervical region may affect the related sympathetic ganglia, inhibit the sympathetic motor innervation to the bronchial tree, and impair bronchial dilation. Somatic dysfunction in the upper thoracic and cervical regions of the spine might also adversely affect the sympathetic-vasomotor supply to the pulmonary region and decrease the tissue level of any medications or endogenous substances necessary for proper pulmonary function. Thoracic and rib cage somatic dysfunction might impair the patient's ability to ventilate and maintain optimal venous and lymphatic circulation, further contributing to pulmonary congestion. Somatic dysfunction of the lower extremities increases the energy demands on the already compromised respiratory system. It becomes obvious that a total musculoskeletal evaluation is indicated and any diagnosed somatic dysfunction should be appropriately managed.

With an acutely ill pulmonary patient, functional techniques are frequently very effective and can be used in the intensive care unit, even with a patient on a ventilator. If the patient is less acute, muscle energy techniques can also be used in the intensive care unit. Once the patient is stabilized, high-velocity thrust techniques may be effective in treating any fibrotic restrictive barriers.

Two case histories are of value in illustrating these principles.

Case 1. A 20-year-old woman was admitted to Waterville Osteopathic Hospital with complaints of chest pain and shortness of breath of 1 month's duration. There was no history of previous respiratory or cardiac problems. Three years earlier, she had broken her left arm. After the initial examination in the emergency room, pulmonary function tests were performed by the attending internist and were repeated after a bronchial dilator was administered. She was admitted and a consultation was requested with the Osteopathic Medicine service. Marked somatic dysfunction was found in the cervical and thoracic spine, the rib cage, and the left upper extremity. The somatic dysfunction was treated with manipulation. Manual therapy was used on a daily basis for 3 days. Other than the bronchial dilator used in the initial pulmonary function testing procedures in the emergency room, no other medications were used during the hospitalization.

	10/17[a]	10/17[b]	10/20	3/15
FEVC	62%	65%	83%	84%
PEF	42%	46%	73%	69%
FEV0.5	51%	46%	87%	73%
FEV1.0	69%	67%	92%	92%
FEF 2–12%	44%	43%	77%	73%
FEF 25–75%	69%	66%	105%	100%

[a]Prebronchial dilator.
[b]Postbronchial dilator.
FEVC = forced expiratory vital capacity; PEF = peak expiratory flow; FEV = forced expiratory volume; FEF = forced expiratory flow.

Thus, a healthy woman sustained trauma to the musculoskeletal system, and this apparently had an adverse impact on pulmonary function. The symptoms of chest pain and shortness of breath cleared and pulmonary function improved once the somatic dysfunction was alleviated. This improvement persisted at the 5-month follow-up examination.

Case 2. A 62-year-old woman was being treated in the intensive care unit. She was known to have COPD, congestive heart failure, and Parkinson's disease. When admitted on October 23 she was in un-

compensated congestive heart failure. The initial treatment regime consisted of adjusting the dosage of her medications. Because no new medications were introduced, the internist felt that within 3 days the maximal clinical benefit should have been realized. On the third day (October 26) after hospitalization, consultation with the addition of manipulative management was added to the medical regime. Three days after manipulative care was initiated, marked improvement was noted in the pulmonary function data.

	10/23	10/26	10/29
FEVC	27%	31.4%	71%
PEF	50.4%	38.7%	59%
FEV0.5	24.8%	31.1%	78%
FEV1.0	24.3%	34.8%	80%
FEF 2–12%	—	34.9%	83%
FEF 25–75%	30.9%	—	61%

FEVC = forced expiratory vital capacity; PEF = peak expiratory flow; FEV = forced expiratory volume; FEF = forced expiratory flow.

This case illustrates the value of simultaneously providing patients with quality medical and surgical care along with comprehensive manipulative care to manage both the disease process and the host/mechanical component of the illness.

With a patient suffering from asthma or COPD, the somatic dysfunction findings might be of value in suggesting the initial medical strategy. If the major somatic dysfunction is in the upper thoracic area, one might observe an inhibiting effect on the sympathetic motor input that could impair the patient's ability to obtain maximal bronchial dilation. With this patient, one might expect the best response to a sympathomimetic medication. When the major area of somatic dysfunction is in the cervical area of the spine, it might have a stimulatory impact on the parasympathetic-vagal input and contribute to bronchial constriction. With this patient, it would be conceptually advantageous to use a parasympatholytic medication, providing it would not dry out the bronchial mucosa. In the case of facilitation of the parasympathetic supply secondary to cervical dysfunction, one might expect a larger dose of sympathomimetic drug being required to override the stimulated parasympathetic system. Therefore, an increased incidence of side effects to the sympathomimetic medication might be noted.

Somatic dysfunction in the cervical and thoracic spine, rib cage, and upper extremity regions may have an adverse impact on sympathetic vasomotor control, sympathetic and parasympathetic motor innervation, trophic flow, ventilation, and energy demands, as well as on venous and lymphatic circulation in the patient with a respiratory pathologic condition. Specific management of the somatic component, as well as the disease process, might have a beneficial impact on the clinical outcome.

Gastroenterology

It is not uncommon to find mechanical dysfunction in the midthoracic region of the spine when examining peptic ulcer patients. This dysfunction may inhibit the sympathetic motor innervation to the gastric tissues and result in an imbalance favoring the parasympathetic component. This pattern of dysfunction might contribute to hyperacidity and contractibility of the upper GI system. If the midthoracic dysfunction has a stimulatory effect on the sympathetic motor innervation from this area, one might observe a decrease in peristalsis and production of gastric secretions. The midthoracic dysfunction might also have an adverse impact on the sympathetic vasomotor supply and further render the gastric tissues more susceptible to a pathologic state and irritation from medications used for other conditions.

Some patients with duodenal symptomatology also have mechanical dysfunction in the rib cage and the middle and lower thoracic regions of the spine. These mechanical dysfunctions might impair diaphragmatic excursion and secondarily influence the associated fascias from the diaphragm to the contiguous structures, i.e, the ligament of Treitz, which inserts on the duodenum. A slight kinking of the duodenum, caused by cephalad traction by the ligament of Treitz, might occur and explain why the duodenal symptomatology may subside once the thoracic spine and rib cage dysfunctions are alleviated with manual therapy.

It is not uncommon for patients with thoracolumbar and low back pain to also have a history of irritable bowel syndrome, but the connection between the two problems has never been realized by either the patient or his or her physician. Frequently, as the low back pain subsides with manipulation, the patient also reports an improvement in the irritable bowel symptoms. This should not be surprising from an anatomic perspective. Patients with low back pain

frequently have somatic dysfunction in the thoracolumbar area of the spine, and this may have an inhibitory impact on the sympathetic motor innervation to the bowel, resulting in a predominance of parasympathetic motor input to the colon. Also, mechanical dysfunction of the bony pelvis might have a stimulatory impact on the sacral parasympathetic motor innervation to the colon, also contributing to colon irritability. The thoracolumbar dysfunction may have an adverse impact on the sympathetic ganglia in this region, altering the sympathetic vasomotor innervation to the colon.

Patients with hiatal hernias frequently report a decrease in their symptoms after manual therapy. Altered thoracic spine and rib cage mechanics might adversely affect diaphragmatic tone and excursion. Once the dysfunctions are alleviated with appropriate mechanical intervention, better diaphragmatic tone may result and less sliding of the hernia may occur, with a resulting decrease in symptoms. Mechanical dysfunctions in the midthoracic region might either stimulate or inhibit the sympathetic motor innervation to the esophagus and stomach, resulting in either hypo- or hyperperistaltic activity of the esophagus. Altered thoracic spine and rib cage mechanics could impair venous and lymphatic circulation from both the esophagus and stomach, further contributing to the symptoms of the hiatal hernia patient, especially if varices are present.

Neurology

Patients may have a symptom complex closely resembling a migraine headache. The main areas of somatic dysfunction are frequently the upper cervical and thoracic spine or rib cage regions. Secondary contraction of the suboccipital muscles can cause an entrapment of the greater occipital nerve, giving a unilateral pattern of head pain. Thoracic spine or rib cage dysfunction can also secondarily affect the function of the cervical area. Cervical spine dysfunction might secondarily affect the cervical fascial planes, which blend with the carotid sheath. Facilitation of the vagal innervation to the upper GI tract may occur as the vagus nerve passes through the cervical area within the carotid sheath. The patient may experience nausea and vomiting secondary to any cervical dysfunction. This pseudo-migraine complex is not associated with an aura.

In patients with true migraine, upper thoracic spine and rib cage mechanical dysfunction is frequently diagnosed. This might affect the vasomotor supply to the head and neck, contributing to vasomotor instability in some patients. Visualize an old clothes line, which consisted of two Ts with ropes strung in between them. Obviously, if one pole is twisted, it secondarily affects the position of the other pole. In the same way, mechanical dysfunction in the low back and pelvis may be completely asymptomatic but because of the long paravertebral muscles going up into the neck and the atlanto-occipital area, may produce compensatory soft tissue changes and pain in the suboccipital area. This could further contribute to both the migraine and pseudo-migraine symptom complex. Since lower extremity dysfunctions can alter the functional capabilities of the lumbar areas, sacrum, and pelvis, it can have an indirect impact on the cervical area. Upper extremity dysfunction may also impair cervical or thoracic spine or rib cage mechanical function and must also be evaluated and treated when somatic dysfunction is present. Thus, a comprehensive musculoskeletal evaluation ensures that each patient's overall specific somatic dysfunctional pattern has been managed rather than ineffectively treating only the symptomatic regions.

When a migraine patient responds poorly to ergotamine tartrate and caffeine (Cafergot) or propranolol hydrochloride (Inderal), one should become suspicious that somatic dysfunction might be significantly contributing to that patient's symptomatology. Thoracic somatic dysfunction, facilitating the sympathetic vasomotor system, is common with patients suffering from other vasomotor-type headaches. If the somatic dysfunction is contributing to the patient's symptomatology, alleviation of the somatic dysfunction will secondarily relieve the vascular headaches.

Primary Musculoskeletal Conditions

Several true mechanical conditions appear to benefit from manual therapy. The most obvious is the hypomobile joint. Once diagnosed by palpatory examination, the segment can be managed using the most appropriate technique selected according to the nature of the restrictive barrier. Secondary to hypomobility, there are usually areas of neurophysiologic hypermobility that develop either above or below the restricted segment. These areas become hypermobile in an effort to compensate for the hypomobile or restricted areas. This form of hypermobility subsides once the hypomobile somatic dysfunctions are effectively managed. Ligamentous strain can also result in hypermobility, but this form of hypermobility will not respond to manual therapy. Either form of hypermobility can be very painful but the clinical trap is to fail to understand the need for locating and properly managing the hypomobile areas. Interestingly, these hypomobile areas are frequently asymptomatic.

A common clinical example of this concept of hypomobility is a flexed somatic dysfunction at T12. This area when dysfunctional often displays a marked side-bending and rotational restrictive component. This early and dysfunctional flexion initiates a compensatory decrease of the normal lumbar lordotic curve. Additionally, the L5 segment frequently becomes compensatorily hypermobile and may result in either lumbosacral pain or sciatica. If this mechanical condition at T12 is not appropriately diagnosed and managed, manual therapy will frequently be directed ineffectively at the hypermobile and painful L5–S1 area. The patient is often incorrectly told "the L5 keeps going out" when in reality the hypomobile area at T12, the key area, has never been properly managed. Somatic dysfunction at T12 is frequently associated with pain arising at the thoracolumbar area, which then radiates along the T12 dermatome into the inguinal area, imitating the pain pattern of renal colic. The pain pattern resolves once the somatic dysfunction is effectively treated with manual therapy.

Three spinal deviation problems, scoliosis, kyphosis, and flat back, can often benefit from manual therapy. When these conditions are caused by structural anomalies, the goal of manual therapy would be to help the musculoskeletal system adapt to the structural variations and alleviate any pain. When structural anomalies are not a factor, the entire musculoskeletal system must be evaluated for contributing somatic dysfunction.

In a functional scoliotic patient, an anatomic short leg syndrome must be ruled out. If such a condition exists, appropriate heel lift therapy can be beneficial. When somatic dysfunction of the pelvis exists, an adaptive torquing of this structure can occur because of the movement potential within the sacroiliac joints. This can secondarily produce a functional short leg syndrome and result in a mild functional adaptive scoliosis. This condition responds favorably to specific manual therapy to the pelvis followed by treatment of the adaptive thoracic segments.

A functional kyphosis can develop when a pattern of flexed vertebral dysfunctions is present in the thoracic area. The same pattern can develop when a group of ribs are functionally maintained in a pattern of exhalation and unable to rise during inspiration.

Frequently a flat area or loss of kyphosis is noted in the normally kyphotic thoracic region. This can occur when a group of vertebrae are functionally maintained in a pattern of extension or the related ribs are maintained in a functional pattern of inspiration and unable to move through a complete expiratory excursion. With both the functional kyphotic and flat back syndromes, the rib cage and thoracic spinal regions must be evaluated, since the muscles from these areas can play a role in maintaining the deviational pattern.

The cervical region contributes both muscles and neurologic innervation to the thoracic spine, rib cage, and shoulder regions. Since the diaphragm takes its origin from the lower six ribs and is innervated by the phrenic nerve (C3–C5), improved diaphragmatic excursion is frequently observed once rib cage and cervical spine somatic dysfunction are alleviated with manual therapy. Thus a comprehensive musculoskeletal evaluation is required to effectively manage functional deviation conditions.

In a manual medicine practice, several other clinical problems are seen that could be classified as functional radicular syndromes. The patient may complain of neck and upper back pain, pain radiating down the arm, or numbness, tingling, or other paresthesias. The electromyographic and neurologic examination findings are usually unremarkable. The cervical x-ray films may or may not demonstrate disc narrowing with or without osteoarthritic changes. Muscle relaxants and nonsteroidal anti-inflammatory drugs frequently have been of little clinical value. It appears the symptoms complex can result from an entrapment of the neurovascular bundle coursing into the arm from the cervical region. Entrapment can occur with scalenus anticus and medius tightness secondary to somatic dysfunction of the upper thoracic spine and ribs 1 and 2. Entrapment can also occur when the upper thoracic spine and ribs 3–5 display somatic dysfunction. Since the pectoralis minor muscle takes its origin from the third, fourth, and fifth ribs, an increase in the tone of this muscle may develop once somatic dysfunction

is present. The outcome may result in a functional hyperabduction syndrome. Finally, it is also possible for entrapment to occur as the neurovascular bundle courses under a tight subclavius secondary to sternoclavicular or acromioclavicular somatic dysfunction. Specific manual management of any somatic dysfunction in the cervical or thoracic spine, rib cage, or upper extremity regions will frequently alleviate these clinical symptoms but only if the somatic dysfunction is the symptom-generating factor.

Gentle manual therapy techniques can be used to effectively treat somatic dysfunction even in the presence of imaged disc pathologic states. At times, the disc is asymptomatic but the mechanically generated pain is attributed to a herniated or bulging disc. Generally, high-velocity thrust techniques are contraindicated, but gentle muscle energy or functional techniques can be used as a differential diagnostic procedure to rule out the possibility of the pain being mechanically generated from tissue other than that affected by the disc.

Another mechanical condition is described as the T4 syndrome. The symptom complex consists of upper thoracic pain, which may be diffuse and widespread and constant or intermittent, associated with pain and paresthesias involving the upper extremities with or without a glovelike distribution. Usually there is no specific etiologic factor, but a history of trauma or strain may correlate with the onset of symptoms. Neurologic changes do not occur. Somatic dysfunction in the cervical and thoracic spine, rib cage, and upper extremities is frequently present and could produce an entrapment, by the related muscles, of the neurovascular bundle coursing into the arm. Also, the upper thoracic somatic dysfunction might stimulate both the sympathetic motor innervation to the spindles of the related arm muscles and the sympathetic vasomotor innervation to the vascular supply of the upper extremity musculature. Both of these mechanisms could contribute to increased muscle tone of the cervical and thoracic spine, rib cage, and upper extremity regions. Thus, several mechanical factors may by contributing to the development of the T4 syndrome. Specific manual management of any diagnosed somatic dysfunction will frequently benefit a patient experiencing the T4 syndrome.

Chronic fibromyositis is another condition frequently seen in a manual medicine practice. Some of these patients respond to manual therapy. The primary problems are musculoskeletal pain, insomnia, and painful localized trigger points. Some of these patients have widespread somatic dysfunction throughout the thoracic area. With these patients, it is postulated that the somatic dysfunction of the thoracic area facilitates the widely distributed sympathetic motor innervation to the related spindles. This could contribute to the diffuse increase of muscle tone throughout the body. Facilitation of the sympathetic vasomotor supply to the related muscles may also contribute to the clinical condition by generating a mild ischemic pain. The tender or trigger points frequently correlate with underlying somatic dysfunction. Occasionally, a chronic fibromyositis patient with marked and widespread somatic dysfunction in the thoracic area responds well to manual management. Other patients attain only temporary symptomatic relief of their chronic fibromyositic symptoms.

Summary

In conclusion, manual therapy is not a panacea. However, a wide spectrum of clinical symptomatology, both musculoskeletal and visceral, may develop secondary to somatic dysfunction. Because the musculoskeletal system makes up two-thirds of the total body mass, it may initiate a wide spectrum of neurophysiologic and mechanical alterations when somatic dysfunction is present. The clinician is challenged to incorporate a comprehensive functional evaluation of the musculoskeletal system as part of the management strategy for a broad spectrum of clinical conditions. Excellent clinical results will be realized only when skilled and specific manual therapy is used to manage the diagnosed somatic dysfunctional component of a patient's clinical condition. As in medicine, the manual therapy practitioner will cure some patients, help many, and should strive to comfort all.

Selected Readings

Basmajian JV, Nyberg R. Rational Manual Therapies. Baltimore: Williams & Wilkins, 1993.

Bone RC, Rosen RL. Quick Reference to Internal Medicine: Outline Format. New York: Igaku-shoin, 1994.

Bourdillon JF, Day EA, Bookhout MR. Spinal Manipulation (5th ed). London: Butterworth-Heinemann, 1992.

Bray JJ, Cragg PA, Macknight ADC et al. Lecture Notes on Human Physiology (3rd ed). Oxford, England: Blackwell, 1994.

Cailliet R. Pain: Mechanisms and Management. Philadelphia: FA Davis, 1993.

Cooper JR, Bloom FE, Roth RH. The Biochemical Basis of Neuropharmacology (6th ed). New York: Oxford University Press, 1991.

deGroot J, Chusid JG. Correlative Neuroanatomy (21st ed). Norwalk, CT: Appleton & Lange, 1991.

Despopoulos A, Silbernagl S. Color Atlas of Physiology (4th ed). New York: Thieme, 1991.

Frymoyer JW, Gordon SL. New Perspectives on Low Back Pain. Park Ridge, IL: American Academy of Orthopedic Surgeons, 1989.

Gilman S, Newman SW. Essentials of Clinical Neuroanatomy and Neurophysiology (8th ed). Philadelphia: FA Davis, 1992.

Goldstein M. The Research Status of Spinal Manipulative Therapy. Workshop Held at the National Institutes of Health. Bethesda, MD: U.S. Department of Health, Education, and Welfare, 1975.

Greenman PE. Concepts and Mechanisms of Neuromuscular Functions. Berlin: Springer, 1984.

Greenman PE. Principles of Manual Medicine. Baltimore: Williams & Wilkins, 1989.

Groer MW, Skekleton ME. Basic Pathophysiology—A Holistic Approach (3rd ed). St. Louis: Mosby, 1989.

Inman VT, Ralston HJ, Todd F. Human Walking. Baltimore: Williams & Wilkins, 1981.

Inman VT, Saunders JB, Eberhart HD. The major determinants in normal and pathological gait. J Bone Joint Surg [Am] 1953;356:543.

Korr IM. The Neurobiologic Mechanisms in Manipulative Therapy. New York: Plenum, 1977.

Lewit K. Manipulative Therapy in Rehabilitation of the Locomotor System (2nd ed). London: Butterworth-Heinemann, 1991.

Moore ML. Clinically Orientated Anatomy (2nd ed). Baltimore: Williams & Wilkins, 1985.

Mumenthaler M. Neurology (3rd ed). New York: Thieme, 1990.

Netter FH. The Ciba Collection of Medical Illustrations, Vol 1. Nervous System, Part I and II. West Caldwell, NJ: Ciba, 1986.

Netter FH. The Ciba Collection of Medical Illustrations, Vol. 8. Musculoskeletal System, Part I. West Caldwell, NJ: Ciba, 1987.

Patterson MM, Howell JN. The Central Connection: Somatovisceral/Viscerosomatic Interaction. The Proceedings of the 1989 American Academy of Osteopathy International Symposium. Athens, OH: University Classics, 1992.

Peterson B. The Collected Papers of Irvin M. Korr. Colorado Springs, CO: American Academy of Osteopathy, 1979.

Sinclair D. An Introduction to Functional Anatomy (5th ed). Oxford, England: Blackwell, 1975.

Slaby FJ, McCune SK, Summers RW. Gross Anatomy in the Practice of Medicine. Philadelphia: Lea & Febiger, 1994.

Snell RS. Clinical Anatomy for Medical Students (3rd ed). Boston: Little, Brown, 1986.

Soderberg GL. Kinesiology Application to Pathological Motion. Baltimore: Williams & Wilkins, 1986.

Vander AJ, Sherman JH, Luciano DS. Human Physiology, The Mechanisms of Body Function. New York: McGraw-Hill, 1985.

White AA, Panjabi MM. Clinical Biomechanics of the Spine (2nd ed). Philadelphia: Lippincott, 1990.

Chapter 14

Use and Abuse of Therapeutic Interventions

Mark A. Tomski

If you are not part of the solution, you are part of the problem.

—Eldridge Cleaver

The Problem

Therapeutics is the practical branch of medicine concerned with the treatment of disease. The therapist is one who is skilled in the practice of some type of therapy, and therapy is the treatment of a disease by various methods. Therein lies the problem. The problem is, as Maslow put it, "The whole world looks like a nail and your only tool is a hammer." As the title of this chapter implies, all therapies may be used appropriately or abused.

No therapeutic intervention is inherently wrong, but it may be wrongly used when applied to a condition it was not intended to treat. This can happen when a practitioner misdiagnoses a condition or when a practitioner overzealously continues to use an intervention in a futile cycle. The early chapters of this book laid a firm foundation in musculoskeletal diagnosis of the thoracic spine and rib cage region and provided the reader with the ability to make sound diagnostic assessments. The latter half of this book provided the reader with a variety of therapeutic interventions that can be used in the treatment of dysfunctions of the thoracic spine and ribs. However, the sound application of these therapies requires the practitioner to have a framework of knowledge on which to draw when selecting the type and duration of therapy. Intimately meshed

within this framework is the practitioner's ability to establish clear goals that must be set forth before applying the therapeutic intervention.

Therapeutic interventions may be categorized into curative, rehabilitative, or palliative (Table 14.1). Curative therapeutic interventions are aimed at treating the underlying mechanism of the dysfunction or disease state and restoring normal and usual bodily function. Rehabilitative therapeutic interventions are focused on restoring an ability to function again in a normal or near normal manner, while minimizing the residua of the initial dysfunctional or disease state. Palliative therapeutic interventions focus on reducing the severity of or alleviating the symptoms of the disease or dysfunction without curing the underlying disease state.

Many palliative therapeutic interventions have been wrongly labeled useless when in fact they may have properties that can be used to achieve curative or rehabilitative goals. An example is the use of heat as part of a therapeutic rehabilitation exercise regimen. On the other hand, many chemical agents are thought to be curative when they are only palliative and thus prevent rehabilitative interventions from being used. The bottom line is that practitioners must have the goal of the therapeutic regimen clear in their mind before embarking on any therapeutic intervention.

As a side note regarding the use of palliative therapeutic interventions, certain insurers may deny reimbursement for palliative therapeutic interventions because of the lack of a proper goal of either minimizing impairment or curing the underlying disease

Table 14.1. Categories of Therapeutic Intervention

	Curative	Rehabilitative	Palliative
Treatment aims	Cure underlying disease mechanism	May or may not cure underlying mechanism	Does not cure underlying mechanism
Functional goal	Restore normal bodily function	Restore normal or near-normal function	Reduce severity of symptoms

state. The need to be goal-oriented in the prescription of therapies has been emphasized by Tomski and Corsolini [1], while the functional aspects of these goals has been elaborated by Tomski and Mauldin [2]. A brief look at the application of select therapeutic interventions follows.

Nonsteroidal Anti-Inflammatory Analgesics

One of the most important developments in the management of acute pain with analgesic drugs has been the emergence of peripherally acting, nonsteroidal anti-inflammatory drugs (NSAIDs). The NSAIDs work most favorably in conjunction with narcotics and acetaminophen with respect to their ability to alleviate pain. The goal of treatment in their use must be considered. The NSAIDs with a short half-life and rapid onset to peak drug levels are ideal for treating brief, sudden painful events such as headache or acute injury. However, if the goal of therapy is to have long-term anti-inflammatory effects as well as analgesic activity, different NSAIDs with a longer half-life may be considered, especially in light of patient compliance rates of about 50% for any long-term use of medication.

The adverse effects of NSAIDs also must be considered, especially the potential for renal toxicity and the effects of GI intolerance and bleeding. The impairment of platelet function with long-term use of large doses of NSAIDs is a potentially serious side effect.

Physical Agents

The appropriate use of therapeutic physical agents must be planned with the goal of the therapy in mind. The palliative use of heat and cold gained the common pejorative term "fake and bake." However, the use of ice in the acute treatment of spinal pain is

appropriate. Later in treatment, the use of ice may still be appropriate in a palliative manner to assist with rehabilitation goals. The use of therapeutic heat is often appropriate. The reduction in pain that results when heat is applied is caused by the direct effects of temperature elevation on tissue and cellular functions. This warming effect may permit a patient to become more active in an exercise treatment regimen, thus providing palliative effects to achieve rehabilitation goals. However, heat and cold have no curative effects when applied at therapeutic doses in musculoskeletal conditions.

The use of modern medical electricity in the management of painful conditions has been recently reviewed by Shealy and Mauldin [3]. Here, too, the application of electricity either via transcutaneous electrical nerve stimulation or dorsal column stimulation is principally symptom relief. If that is the goal, it is appropriate; however, if one is attempting to provide a curative treatment modality, the use of electricity in this manner is not appropriate. Other forms of more palliative electrical therapy include inferential current therapy, cranial electrical stimulation, and pulsed electromagnetic therapy. These modalities differ significantly from functional electrical stimulation of denervated muscle where the goal is to prevent the atrophic, degenerative, and fibrotic effects of a nerve lesion.

Disability Prevention

It is essential that the goal of treatment focus on the patient's usual role before his or her painful dysfunction. While a person is under our care, he or she is only a patient. Patients have other roles such as husband, wife, wage earner, and so forth. With this in mind, the practitioner can focus on the issue of disability prevention. Whereas medicine and therapy have traditionally been quite good in evaluating issues related to impairment and pathology, they have been less than effective in evaluating issues dealing with disability. Practitioners do a grave disservice to their patients when they become overly involved in the promotion of disability. Urging patients to remain in the sick role by encouraging them to remain off work to "let things calm down" or urging them not to assume responsibility for their usual social roles by telling them to "take it easy" involves the practitioner in disability promotion rather than prevention. Disability prevention can best be practiced when we as clinicians set realistic expectations, outcomes, and goals for both ourselves and our patients. It is of the utmost importance to recognize as quickly as possible when a patient adopts the signs of the "sick role." Time must be spent educating the patient about the nature of the pain problem and the difference between hurt and harm. It is important for both the practitioner and the patient to forge a partnership to achieve functional goals. Poor selection of patients for any treatment intervention can lead to a poor outcome. That is why there are more than four textbooks devoted to the "failed back syndrome" in the literature. Is it truly a failed back syndrome, or is it a failed surgery syndrome? The focus of this textbook is on the manual medicine approach to treatment of spinal pain, but it is equally important to have a goal for a practitioner's manual therapeutic interventions besides joint mechanical function and the treatment of somatic dysfunction. Appropriate use of manual medicine will mobilize the patient to become more active in an overall exercise regimen, including aerobic conditioning, flexibility, and neuromuscular balance retraining. All too often, a practitioner will focus on the esoteric aspects of joint mobility and not look at the overall picture in a goal-oriented context. Manual therapy is important because if a joint does not move, a joint cannot appropriately exercise. However, if the practitioner focuses exclusively on the joint, the patient and person can be lost in the esoteria of the patient's lesion mechanics and the particular therapy du jour (i.e., muscle energy technique, high velocity thrust, or myofascial treatment, etc.).

Codependency

It is possible for the practitioner and patient to develop a symbiotic and codependent relationship. Treatment efficacy, however short-lived, can be in-toxicating and addictive. It is important for the practitioner to realize that getting the patient back to his or her usual role, rather than having the patient dependent on the practitioner for treatment, be it a modality or a hands-on approach, is essential. There are many nontraditional approaches that have a role in musculoskeletal medicine; prolotherapy [4, 5], neural therapy [6], and myofascial trigger point therapy [7] all have their place, but overzealous practitioners can use these treatments for the treatment approach itself rather than looking at the aim of the therapy.

Summary

To summarize, the appropriate use of therapeutic interventions in the management of pain and dysfunction can by summed up in one word—that word is "goals." Both the practitioner and the patient must have a goal, and this goal should be shared in a partnership between the patient and practitioner.

References

1. Tomski MA, Corsolini TB. Prescription of Rehabilitation Regimens in the Management of Pain. In MT Andary, MA Tomski (eds), Office Management of Pain. Philadelphia: Saunders, 1993;105–109.
2. Tomski MA, Mauldin CC. Functional medicine. Am J Phys Med 1990;69:108.
3. Shealy NC, Mauldin CC. Modern Medical Electricity in the Management of Pain. In MT Andary, MA Tomski (eds), Office Management of Pain. Philadelphia: Saunders, 1993;175–186.
4. Dorman TA, Ravin RH. Diagnosis and Injection Techniques in Orthopedic Medicine. Baltimore: Williams & Wilkins, 1991.
5. Hackett GS, Hemwall GA, Montgomery GA. Ligament and Tendon Relaxation Treated by Prolotherapy (5th ed). Oak Park, IL: Gustav A Hemwall, 1991.
6. Dosch P. Manual of Neural Therapy According to Huneke. Heidelberg, Germany: Haug, 1984.
7. Travell JG, Simons DG. Myofascial Pain and Dysfunction—The Trigger Point Manual. Baltimore: Williams & Wilkins, 1983.

Index